T0257631

Encyclopedia of Diabetes:
Clinical Issues of Type 1 Diabetes

Volume 08

Encyclopedia of Diabetes: Clinical Issues of Type 1 Diabetes
Volume 08

Edited by **Rex Slavin, Windy Wise and Roy Marcus Cohn**

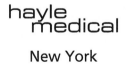

New York

Published by Hayle Medical,
30 West, 37th Street, Suite 612,
New York, NY 10018, USA
www.haylemedical.com

Encyclopedia of Diabetes: Clinical Issues of Type 1 Diabetes
Volume 08
Edited by Rex Slavin, Windy Wise and Roy Marcus Cohn

International Standard Book Number: 978-1-63241-150-1 (Hardback)

Contents

Preface

It is often said that books are a boon to mankind. They document every progress and pass on the knowledge from one generation to the other. They play a crucial role in our lives. Thus I was both excited and nervous while editing this book. I was pleased by the thought of being able to make a mark but I was also nervous to do it right because the future of students depends upon it. Hence, I took a few months to research further into the discipline, revise my knowledge and also explore some more aspects. Post this process, I begun with the editing of this book.

The book provides an overview of current developments in Type-1 Diabetes research across the world, focusing on distinct research fields significant to this disease. The areas covered are diabetes mellitus and complexities, psychological characteristics of diabetes and perspectives of diabetes pathogenesis. Top-notch investigators from across the world have contributed in this book. The book aims to elucidate understandable presentation of concepts on the basis of experiments and results from existing published reports as well as from research works of authors. The book will serve as a valuable source of reference for basic science and clinical investigators as well as for patients and their families.

I thank my publisher with all my heart for considering me worthy of this unparalleled opportunity and for showing unwavering faith in my skills. I would also like to thank the editorial team who worked closely with me at every step and contributed immensely towards the successful completion of this book. Last but not the least, I wish to thank my friends and colleagues for their support.

Editor

Part 1

Diabetes Mellitus and Complications

The Study of Glycative and Oxidative Stress in Type 1 Diabetes Patients in Relation to Circulating TGF-Beta1, VCAM-1 and Diabetic Vascular Complications

Vladimir Jakus[1], Jana Kostolanska[2],
Dagmar Michalkova[1] and Michal Sapak[3]
[1]*Institute of Medical Chemistry, Biochemistry and Clinical Biochemistry,
Faculty of Medicine, Comenius University, Bratislava*
[2]*Children Diabetological Center of the Slovak Republic,
1st Department of Pediatrics, Comenius University
and University Hospital for Children, Bratislava*
[3]*Institute of Medical Immunology, Faculty of Medicine,
Comenius University, Bratislava*
Slovakia

1. Introduction

Type 1 diabetes mellitus (T1DM) is one of most frequent autoimmune diseases and is characterized by absolute or nothing short of absolute endogenous insulin deficiency which results in hyperglycemia that is considered to be a primary cause of diabetic complications (DC) (Rambhade et al., 2010). T1DM leads to various chronic micro- and macrovascular complications. Diabetic nephropathy is a major cause of morbidity and mortality in patients with DM. Microvascular disease is the main determinant in the development of late complications in DM.

Persistent hyperglycemia is linked with glycation, glycoxidation, and oxidative stress (Aronson, 2008; Negre-Salvayre et al., 2009). During glycation and glycoxidation there are formed early, intermediate and advanced glycation products via Maillard reaction, glucose autoxidation and protein glycation. Accumulation of advanced glycation end products (AGEs) has several toxic effects and takes part in the development of DC, such as nephropathy (Kashihara et al, 2010), neuropathy, retinopathy and angiopathy (Peppa & Vlassara, 2005; Yamagishi et al., 2008; Goh & Cooper, 2008; Karasu, 2010). Higher plasma levels of AGEs are associated also with incident cardiovascular disease and all-cause mortality in T1DM (Nin et al., 2011). AGEs are believed to induce cellular oxidative stress through the interaction with specific cellular receptors (Ramasamy et al., 2005; Boulanger et al., 2006; Yamagishi, 2009; Mosquera, 2010). On the other side, carbonyl stress-induced tissue damage is caused by AGE precursors formed by hyperglycaemia, hyperlipidemia, nonenzymatic glycation, peroxidation of lipids and metabolic processes.

It has been suggested that the chronic hyperglycaemia in diabetes enhances the production of reactive oxygen species (ROS) from glucose autoxidation, protein glycation and glycoxidation, which leads to tissue damage (Son, 2007). Also, cumulative episodes of acute hyperglycaemia can be source of acute oxidative stress. A number of studies have summarized the relation between glycation and oxidation (Boyzel et al., 2010). The overproduction of ROS leads to oxidative modification of biologically important compounds and damage of them. Uncontrolled production of ROS often leads to damage of cellular macromolecules (DNA, lipids and proteins).

Some oxidation products or lipid peroxidation products may bind to proteins and amplify glycoxidation-generated lesions. Lipid peroxidation of polyunsaturated fatty acids, one of the radical reaction in vivo, can adequately reflect increased oxidative stress in diabetes. Advanced oxidation protein products (AOPP) are formed during oxidative stress by the action of chlorinated oxidants, mainly hypochlorous acid and chloramines. In diabetes the formation of AOPP is induced by intensified glycoxidation processes, oxidant-antioxidant imbalance, and coexisting inflammation (Piwowar, 2010a, 2010b). AOPP are supposed to be structurally similar to AGEs and to exert similar biological activities as AGEs, i.e. induction of proinflammatory cytokines in neutrophils, as well as in monocytes, and adhesive molecules (Yan et al., 2008). Accumulation of AOPP has been found in patients with chronic kidney disease (Bargnoux, et al., 2009). Further possible sources of oxidative stress are decreased antioxidant defenses, or alterations in enzymatic pathways.

Diabetes is associated also with inflammation (Navaro & Mora, 2006; Wautier et al., 2006; Devaraj et al., 2007; Hartge et al., 2007; Fawaz, et al., 2009 ; Van Sickle et al., 2009; Nobécourt et al., 2010). ROS are implicated also in the pathogenesis of the inflammatory response to ischemic-reperfusion which is exacerbated in diabetes. Oxidative stress during reperfusion is markedly balanced in diabetes and this appears to results from increased leukocyte recruitment and a higher capacity of diabetic leukocytes to generate ROS in response to stimulation. Several adhesion molecules are expressed on endothelial cells and participate in leukocyte adhesion to the endothelium. These molecules are important for monocyte–endothelium interaction in the initiation and progression of atherosclerosis. The monocyte–macrophage is a pivotal cell in atherogenesis. Cellular adhesion molecules mediate attachment and transmigration of leukocytes across the endothelial surface and are thought to play a crucial role in the early steps of atherogenesis (Seckin et al., 2006). Adhesion molecule VCAM-1 is not expressed under baseline conditions but is rapidly induced by proatherosclerotic conditions in rabbits, mice, and humans, including in early lesions. Initially, it is unclear whether VCAM-1 is simply a marker for atherogenesis or whether it acts in this disease pathway. AGEs promote VCAM-1 expression and atheroma formation in rabbits (Vlassara et al., 1995) and in cultured human endothelial cells (Schmidt et al., 1995). These results suggest the involvement of AGEs in the accelerated coronary atherosclerosis on diabetes (Zhang et al., 2003). Plasma concentrations of VCAM-1 are elevated also in T1DM patients with microalbuminuria and overt nephropathy (Schmidt et al., 1996; Clausen et al, 2000).

Diabetic nephropathy is characterized by specific morphological changes including glomerular basement membrane thickening, mesangial expansion and glomerular and tubulointersticial sclerosis. The first clinical manifestation of diabetic nephropathy is microalbuminuria, defined as a urinary albumin excretion rate of 20 to 200 microgram/min. Growth factor TGF-beta1 is one of profibrotic cytokines and is important mediator in the pathogenesis of diabetic nephropathy (Goldfarb & Ziyadeh, 2001; Schrijvers et al., 2004; Wang et al., 2005; Wolf & Ziyadeh, 2007). TGF-beta1 stimulates production of extracellular matrix components such as collagen-IV, fibronectin, proteoglycans (decorin, biglycan). TGF-beta1 may cause glomerulosclerosis and its one of the causal factor in myointimal hyperplasia after baloon injury of carotid artery. It mediates angiotensin-II modulator effect on smooth muscle cell growth. Besides profibrotic activity, TGF-beta1 has immunoregulatory function on adaptive immunity too. AGEs induce connective tissue growth factor-mediated renal fibrosis through TGF-beta1-independent Smad3 signalling (Zhou et al., 2004; Chung et al., 2010).

The present study investigates the relationship between diabetes complications presence, diabetes control (represented by actual levels of HbA1c (HbA1cA) and mean of HbA1c during the last 2 years (HbA1cP)), early glycation products (fructosamine (FAM)), serum advanced glycation end products (s-AGEs), lipid peroxidation products (LPO), advanced oxidation protein products (AOPP), profibrotic cytokines and adhesive molecules in patients with T1DM. We wanted to find a relationship of DC to glycative and oxidative stress parameters, circulating (serum) TGF-beta1 and soluble VCAM-1. Further, we aimed to compare measured parameters in groups –DC, one with DR, with DR combined with another DC and one with only DC another than DR and their combinations. The further aim of the present study was to evaluate if monitoring of circulating FAM, HbA1c, s-AGEs, AOPP, LPO in patients with T1DM could be useful to predict the diabetic complications development.

2. Study design and methods

2.1 Patients and design

The studied group consisted of 46 children and adolescents with T1DM regularly attending the 1st Department of Pediatrics, Children Diabetological Center of the Slovak Republic, University Hospital, Faculty of Medicine, Comenius University, Bratislava. They had T1DM with duration at least for 5 years. One of children was obese (BMIc 97 percentile) and three of them were of overweight (BMIc about 90 percentile). The file was divided into two subgroups: 20 persons without DC (-DC) and 46 those with them (+DC). Then the file of +DC patients was divided into several subgroups according to particular complications: the patients only with retinopathy, those with neuropathy combined with another kinds of DC and those with other than retinopathy to compare the parameters of glycative and oxidative stress and cytokines in each mentioned subgroups. The urine samples in our patients were collected 3 times overnight, microalbuminuria was considered to be positive when UAER was between 20 and 200 microgram/min in 2 samples. No changes (fundus diabetic retinopathy) were found by the ophtalmologist examining the eyes in subject without retinopathy. Diabetic neuropathy was confirmed by EMG exploration using the conductivity assessment of sensor and motor fibres of peripheral nerves. The controls file consists of 26 healthy children. The samples of EDTA capillary blood were used to determine of HbA1c and serum samples were used to determine of FAM, s-AGEs, AOPP and VCAM-1. The samples of serum were stored in -18°C/-80°C.

2.2 Parameter analysis
2.2.1 Determination of UAER

UAER was determined by means of immunoturbidimetric assay (Cobas Integra 400 Plus, Roche, Switzerland), using the commercial kit 400/400Plus. The assay was performed as a part of patients routine monitoring in Department of Laboratory Medicine, University Hospital, Bratislava.

2.2.2 Determination of fructosamine

For the determination of fructosamine we used a kinetic, colorimetric assay and subsequently spectrophotometrical determination at wavelength 530 nm. We used 1-deoxy-1-morpholino-fructose (DMF) as the standard. Serum samples were stored at -79°C and were defrost only once. This test is based on the ability of ketoamines to reduce nitroblue tetrazolium (NBT) to a formazan dye under alkaline conditions. The rate of formazan formation, measured at 530 nm, is directly proportional to the fructosamine concentration. Measurements were carried out in one block up to 5 samples. To 3 ml of 0.5 mmol/l NBT were added 150 microliters of serum and the mixture was incubated at 37°C for 10 minutes. The absorbance was measured after 10 min and 15 min of incubation at Novaspec analyzer II, Biotech (Germany).

2.2.3 Determination of glycated hemoglobin HbA1c

HbA1c was determined from EDTA capillary blood immediately after obtained by the low-pressure liquid chromatography (LPLC) (DiaSTAT, USA) in conjunction with gradient elution. Before testing hemolysate is heated at 62-68°C to eliminate unstable fractions and after 5 minutes is introduced into the column. Hemoglobin species elute from the cation-exchange column at different times, depending on their charge, with the application of buffers of increasing ionic strength. The concentration of hemoglobins is measured after elution from the column, which is then used to quantify HbA1c by calculating the area under each peak. Instrument calibration is always carried out when introducing a new column set procedure (Bio-RAD, Inc., 2003).

2.2.4 Determination of serum AGEs

Serum AGEs were determined as AGE-linked specific fluorescence, serum was diluted 20-fold with deionized water, the fluorescence intensity was measured after excitation at 346 nm, at emission 418 nm using a spectrophotometer Perkin Elmer LS-3, USA. Chinine sulphate (1 microgram/ml) was used to calibrate the instrument. Fluorescence was expressed as the relative fluorescence intensity in arbitrary units (A.U.).

2.2.5 Determination of serum lipoperoxides

Serum lipid peroxides were determined by iodine liberation spectrophotometrically at 365 nm (Novaspec II, Pharmacia LKB, Biotech, SRN). The principle of this assay is based on the oxidative activity of lipid peroxides that will convert iodide to iodine. Iodine can then simply be measured by means of a photometer at 365 nm. Calibration curves were obtained using cumene hydroperoxide. A stoichiometric relationship was observed between the amount of organic peroxides assayed and the concentration of I_3 produced (El-Saadani et al., 1989).

2.2.6 Determination of serum AOPP

AOPP were determined in the plasma using the method previously devised by Witko-Sarsat et al. (1996), modified by Kalousova et al. (2002). Briefly, AOPP were measured by spectrophotometry on a reader (FP-901, Chemistry Analyser, Labsystems, Finland) and were calibrated with chloramine-T solutions that in the presence of potassium iodide absorb at 340 nm. In standard wells, 10 microliters of 1.16 M potassium iodide was added to 200 microliters of chloramine-T solution (0–100 micromol/l) followed by 20 microliters of acetic acid. In test wells, 200 microliters of plasma diluted 1:5 in PBS was placed to cell of 9 channels, and 20 microliters of acetic acid was added. The absorbance of the reaction mixture is immediately read at 340 nm on the reader against a blank containing 200 microliters of PBS, 10 microliters of potassium iodide, and 20 microliters of acetic acid. The chloramine-T absorbance at 340 nm being linear within the range of 0 to 100 micromol/l, AOPP concentrations were expressed as micromoles per liter of chloramine-T equivalents.

2.2.7 Determination of TGF- beta1

Quantitative detection of TGF- beta1 in serum was done by enzyme linked immunosorbent assay, using human TGF-beta1 ELISA-kit (BMS249/2, Bender MedSystem).
Brief description of the method: into washed, with anti-TGF-beta1 precoated microplate were added prediluted (1:10) sera (100 microliters) and "HRP-Conjugate" (50 microliters) as a antihuman-TGF-beta1 monoclonal antibody and incubated for 4 hour on a rotator (100rpm). After microplate washing (3 times) "TMB Substrate Solution" (100 microliters) was added and was incubated for 10 minutes. Enzyme reaction was stopped by adding "Stop Solution" (100 microliters). The absorbance of each microwell was readed by HumaReader spectrophotometer (Human) using 450 nm wavelength. The TGF-beta1 concentration was determined from standard curve prepared from seven TGF-beta1 standard dilutions. Each sample and TGF-beta1 standard dilution were done in duplicate.

2.2.8 Determination of serum soluble form of adhesion molecule VCAM-1

For serum soluble form of VCAM-1 (sVCAM-1) estimating we used bead-based multiplex technology and Athena Multi-LyteTM Luminex 100 xMAP (multi-analyte profiling) analyser. We used RnD systems manufacturer kits: „Human Adhesion Molecule MultiAnalyte Profiling Base Kit" and „Fluorokine® MAP Human sVCAM-1/CD106 Kit".
Analyte-specific antibodies are pre-coated onto color-coded microparticles. Microparticles, standards and samples are pipetted into wells and the immobilized antibodies bind the analytes of interest. After washing away any unbound substances, a biotinylated antibody cocktail specific to the analytes of interest are added to each well. Following a wash to remove any unbound biotinylated antibody, streptavidin-phycoerythrin conjugate (Streptavidin-PE), which binds to the captured biotinylated antibody, is added to each well. A final wash removes unbound Streptavidin-PE and the microparticles are resuspended in buffer and read using the Luminex analyzer. One laser is microparticle-specific and determines which analyte is being detected. The other laser determines the magnitude of the phycoerythrin-derived signal, which is in direct proportion to the amount of analyte bound (R&D Systems, Inc. 2010).

2.2.9 Statistical analysis

Shapiro-Wilk test was performed to the test the distribution of all continuous variables. The variables with normal distribution were compared by one way ANOVA test followed by Bonferroni´s post-test and the results was expressed as mean ± SD. Since the evaluated variables did not have normal distribution, we compared them with Kruskal–Wallis non-parametric analysis of variance (ANOVA) followed by Bonferroni´s post-test and the results was expressed as median (1st quartile, 3rd quartile). The Fisher´s test was used to compare the subgroups in regard to diabetic retinopathy and other complications presence/absence. Pearson´s test with correlation coefficient r or Spearman´s one with Spearman's rank correlation coefficient R in case of small count of variables were then used to evaluate the association between parameters described within the text, in all studied patients and in diabetic and non-diabetic subgroups. P values less than 0.05 were accepted as being statistically significant. All statistical analyses were carried out using Excel 2003, Origin 8 and BioSTAT 2009.

3. Results

Clinical and biochemical characteristics of the patients with T1DM without and with diabetic complications and controls (CTRL) are reported in Table 1.

	CTRL	n	T1DM -DC	n	T1DM +DC	N
Age (yrs.)	9.0(6.1,14.0)	26	14.4(12.4, 17.9)[ab]	20	16.4(15.1, 17.6)[a]	26
DD (yrs.)	-	0	6(5.5, 8.1)[b]	20	10.0(7.9, 12.9)	26
HbA1cA (%)	5.0 ± 0.3	18	8.3 ± 1.4 [ab]	20	10.4 ± 1.4[a]	26
FAM (mmol/l)	1.67 ± 0.31	24	2.64 ± 0.38 [ab]	20	3.06 ± 0.48[a]	26
s-AGEs (A.U.)	54.9 ± 9.9	22	64.4 ± 10.1 [ab]	20	71.8 ± 11.6	24
AOPP (micromol/l)	58.8(52.0, 71.8)	11	43.3(42.6, 60.4)	17	78.2(49.5, 114.6)	20
LPO (nmol/ml)	100(88, 110)	10	106(105, 161)	19	127(109, 152)[a]	17
TGF-beta1 (ng/ml)	3.30 ± 3.41	8	5.9 ± 4.14[b]	10	10.49 ± 4.55[a]	16
VCAM-1 (ng/ml)	12.6 ± 3.7	15	17.1 ± 3.1	19	17.4 ± 3.3[a]	26

[a] significant difference in comparison with CTRL
[b] significant difference in comparison with +DC group T1DM

Table 1. Clinical and biochemical characteristics of the patients with T1DM and controls

As seen, HbA1c and FAM were significantly elevated in both diabetic groups in comparison with controls and also in +DC vs. –DC those. Serum AGEs were significantly elevated in +DC compared to –DC and also to controls, but the difference between –DC and controls was not significant. The levels of AOPP were evidently higher in +DC compared to controls, but the difference was not significant. The levels of LPO were significantly elevated in +DC vs. controls, the differences between both diabetic groups and between –DC vs. controls were not significant. The levels of TGF-beta1 similarly to s-AGEs were significantly elevated in +DC compared to –DC and also to controls, but the difference between –DC and controls was not significant (Fig. 1). In terms of the VCAM-1 values, only between +DC and controls there were found significant difference there (Fig. 2).
The levels of TGF-beta1 are significantly elevated in +DC compared to –DC (10.49 ± 4.55 vs. 5.9 ± 4.14 ng/ml, p<0.05) and also to controls (10.49 ± 4.55 vs. 3.30 ± 3.41ng/ml, p<0.05), but the difference between –DC and controls (5.9 ± 4.14 vs. 3.30 ± 3.41ng/ml, p>0.05) was not statistically significant.

3.1 The relationships between clinical and biochemical parameters
3.1.1 The subgroup of patients with T1DM without diabetic complications
The relationships characterized by Pearson´s correlation coefficient r or Spearman´s coefficient R between the parameters described within the text are reported in Table 2. As seen, we found significant linear correlations of FAM with HbA1cA (r=0.676), LPO with HbA1cP (r=-0.507) and AOPP (R=0.671). The relationship between LPO (y) and HbA1cP(x) is possible to describe by non-linear equation $y=19x^2-354x+1752$ (R=0.632, R^2=0.400, p<0.05). VCAM-1 significantly correlated with age (r=-0.478), HbA1cA (r=0.653, Fig. 3), HbA1cP (r=0.501) and with FAM (r=0.630, Fig. 4).

The Study of Glycative and Oxidative Stress in Type 1 Diabetes Patients in Relation to Circulating TGF-Beta1,
VCAM-1 and Diabetic Vascular Complications

9

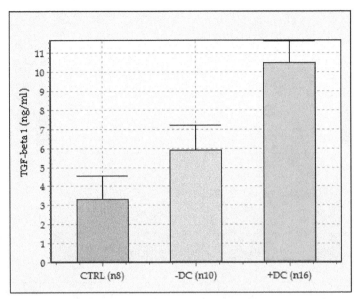

Fig. 1. Comparison of TGF-beta1 levels of patients with T1DM and controls

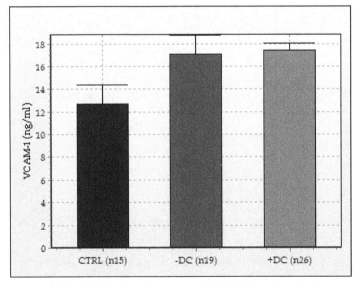

Fig. 2. Comparison of VCAM-1 levels of patients with T1DM and controls

The levels of VCAM-1 are significantly elevated in +DC compared to controls (17.4 ± 3.3 vs.
12.6 ± 3.7 ng/ml, p<0.05). The values of VCAM-1 in –DC subgroup differ obviously from
those in controls, but the difference is non statistically significant (17.1 ± 3.1 vs. 12.6 ± 3.7
ng/ml, p>0.05). There are similar levels in both diabetic subgroups ((17.4 ± 3.3 vs. 17.1 ± 3.1
ng/ml, p>>0.05).

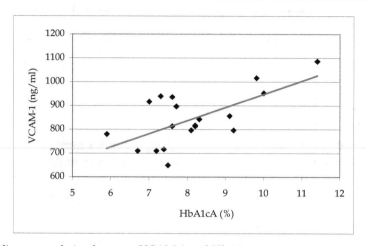

Fig. 3. The linear correlation between VCAM-1 and HbA1cA

	DD (yrs.)	HbA1cA	HbA1cP	FAM	s-AGEs	AOPP	LPO	TGF-beta1	VCAM-1
Age (yrs.)	0.205	-0.267	-0.232	-0.328	-0.030	0.130†	0.334	0.406†	-0.478△
DD (yrs.)	N	0.152	-0.008	0.326	-0.256	-0.193†	-0.001	0.036†	0.089
HbA1cA (%)		N	0.748△	0.676△	0.217	-0.298†	-0.398	-0.588†	0.653△
HbA1cP (%)			N	0.433	0.302	-0.400†	-0.507△	-0.042†	0.501△
FAM (mmol/l)				N	0.134	0.081†	-0.260	-0.224†	0.630△
s-AGEs (A.U.)					N	0.197†	0.270	0.006	0.068
AOPP (micromol/l)						N	0.671†△	0.477†	-0.447†
LPO (nmol/ml)							N	0.200†	-0.404
TGF-beta1 (ng/ml)								N	-0.578†

Table 2. The relationships between the parameters in patients with T1DM without diabetic complications († R, △ p<0.05)

In this subgroup LPO and VCAM-1 were in association also with other parameters, but those were not statistically significant. Non linear statistically significant relationship with regression line equation $y=0.33x^2 - 4.10x + 28.26$ was found between VCAM-1(y) and HbA1cA(x) (R=0.694, R^2=0.481, p<<0.05).

3.1.2 The subgroup of patients with T1DM with diabetic complications
The relationships characterized by Pearson´s correlation coefficient r or Spearman´s coefficient R between the parameters described within the text are reported in Table 3.

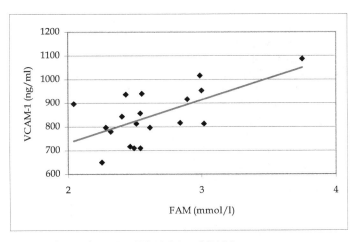

Fig. 4. The linear correlation between VCAM-1 and FAM

	DD (yrs.)	HbA1cA	HbA1cP	FAM	s-AGEs	AOPP	LPO	TGF-beta1	VCAM-1
Age (yrs.)	0.448△	-0.295	-0.422△	-0.023	-0.068	-0.165	-0.044†	0.541†△	0.067
DD (yrs.)	N	-0.070	-0.110	-0.170	-0.069	-0.034	-0.297†	0.247†	0.009
HbA1cA (%)		N	0.539△	0.581△	0.221	0.278	0.123†	-0.429†	0.006
HbA1cP (%)			N	0.3405	0.247	0.116	0.127†	-0.679†△	0.291
FAM (mmol/l)				N	0.479△	0.538△	0.471†	-0.708†△	0.183
s-AGEs (A.U.)					N	0.119†	0.125†	-0.356†	0.432△
AOPP (micromol/l)						N	0.355†	-0.545†	-0.026
LPO (nmol/ml)							N	-0.612†	-0.174†
TGF-beta1 (ng/ml)								N	-0.069†

(† R, △ p<0.05)

Table 3. The relationships between parameters described within the text in patients with T1DM with diabetic complications

As seen, in +DC subgroup we found significant correlations of FAM with HbA1cA (r=0.581), s-AGEs with FAM (r=0.479) and AOPP with FAM (r=0.538). LPO correlated with FAM (r=0.471), but this relation is not statistically significant (p=0.056). TGF-beta1 correlated with age (R=0.541), HbA1cP (R=-0.679) and FAM (R=-0.708). Statistically significant moderate linear correlation was found between VCAM-1 and s-AGEs (r=0.432). Moderate relationships were found also between TGF-beta1 and oxidative stress parameters, but those were not statistically significant.

3.1.3 Controls

As seen in Table 4, there were found moderate negative relation on the border of significance between AOPP and FAM (R=-0.627, p=0.05) and strong relation between AOPP and s-AGEs (R=0.855) in controls. TGF-beta1 was in statistically significant relation with age (R=-0.838) and s-AGEs (R=-0.757) and moderate, but not significant relationship was found with LPO (R=0.478). Slight relationship were found between VCAM-1 and FAM (R=0.366) and also between VCAM-1 and s-AGEs (R=0.267).

	HbA1cA	FAM	s-AGEs	AOPP	LPO	TGF-beta1	VCAM-1
Age (yrs.)	0.354†	-0.249	-0.008	0.193†	0.026†	-0.838†∆	-0.052†
HbA1cA (%)	N	0.109†	-0.133†	-0.022†	0.189†	-0.024†	-0.068†
FAM (mmol/l)		N	-0.143	-0.627†■	-0.162†	0.276†	0.366†
s-AGEs (A.U.)			N	0.855†∆	-0.382†	-0.757†∆	0.267†
AOPP (micromol/l)				N	-0.286†	N	0.069†
LPO (nmol/ml)					N	0.478†	0.037†
TGF-beta1 (ng/ml)						N	0.152†

(† R, p<0.05, ■ p=0.05)

Table 4. The relationships between the parameters in controls

3.2 The parameters of glycative and oxidative stress, TGF-beta1 and VCAM-1 with regard to presence/absence of retinopathy and/or other complications

We compared described parameters between subgroups with/without diabetic retinopathy. The results of Fisher´s post-test (p values) are reported in table 5.

Subgroups	FAM	HbA1cA	s-AGEs	AOPP	LPO	TGF-beta1	VCAM-1
DR vs. DR+O	NS	NS	NS	NS	NS	NA	NS
DR vs. ODC	0.055	NS	0.055	NS	<0.05	<0.05	NS
DR vs. -DC	NS	0,01	NS	NS	NS	<0.05	NS
DR+O vs. ODC	0.052	NS	0,05	NS	NS	NA	NS
DR+O vs. -DC	NS	<0.05	NS	NS	NS	NA	NS
ODC vs. -DC	<0.05	<0.05	<0.05	NS	NS	NS	NS

(DR – having diabetic retinopathy only, DR+ODC – having diabetic retinopathy and another complications, ODC – having only other diabetic complications except diabetic retinopathy-DC – having no complications, NS – non-significant difference, NA – not available)

Table 5. The differences in measured parameters between subgroups of patients with T1DM with regard to presence/absence of diabetic retinopathy and/or other (O) complications

The Study of Glycative and Oxidative Stress in Type 1 Diabetes Patients in Relation to Circulating TGF-Beta1,
VCAM-1 and Diabetic Vascular Complications

13

FAM were significantly elevated in patients having diabetic complications only other than diabetic retinopathy compared to –DC (3.10(2.93, 3.54) vs. 2.54(2.42, 2.91) mmol/l, p<0.05, Fig. 5). HbA1c levels are elevated in patients having diabetic retinopathy against to –DC (9.8(9.6, 10.2) vs. (7.9(7.4, 9.1)%, p<0.05), in subgroup of patients having diabetic retinopathy with other complication/s compared to -DC (10.4(8.6, 11.2) vs. (7.9(7.4, 9.1) %, p<0.05, Fig.6) and also the subgroup of patients having diabetic complications only other than diabetic retinopathy compared to –DC (10.5(10.0, 11.1 vs. (7.9(7.4, 9.1) %, p<0.05, Fig. 6). Serum AGEs were significantly higher in subgroup with only other diabetic complications than diabetic retinopathy compared to –DC one (74.8(71.2, 76.5) vs. 61.9(58.9, 71.0) A.U., Fig. 7), and non-significantly higher in patients with retinopathy only than in those with others DC and also in patients with DR and another DC compared to ODC group, however, p-values were only slightly higher than 0.05 (Fig. 7). The values of LPO were significantly elevated in patients with complications other than retinopathy compared to those with retinopathy only (138(129, 165) vs. 101(93, 109) nmol/ml, Fig. 8). No significant differences were found between others in LPO. There were the significant differences between patients having only diabetic retinopathy vs. –DC in TGF-beta1 levels (14.17(13.32, 15.52) vs. 5.7(2.23, 8.71) ng/ml, p<0.05, Fig. 9) and also between subgroup of patients having only diabetic retinopathy and those having diabetic complications other than diabetic retinopathy (14.17(13.32, 15.52) vs. 9.05(5.29, 10.39) ng/ml, p=0.05, Fig. 9). Neither AOPP parameters nor VCAM-1 showed any significant differences between subgroups with regard to presence/absence diabetic retinopathy or other diabetic complications.

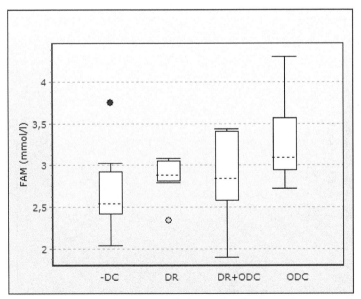

Fig. 5. The values of FAM in subgroups of patients with T1DM with regard to diabetic retinopathy presence/absence (DR – having diabetic retinopathy only, DR+ODC – having diabetic retinopathy and another complications, ODC – having only other diabetic complications except diabetic retinopathy, -DC – having no complications)

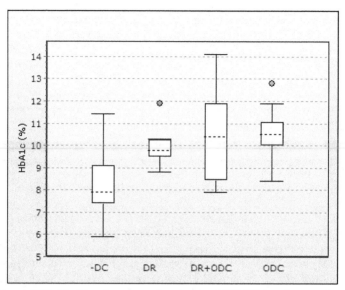

Fig. 6. The values of HbA1c in subgroups of patients with T1DM with regard to diabetic retinopathy presence/absence (DR – having diabetic retinopathy only, DR+ODC – having diabetic retinopathy and another complications, ODC – having only other diabetic complications except diabetic retinopathy, -DC – having no complications)

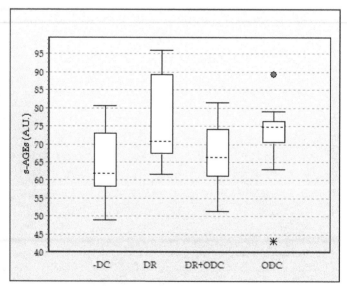

Fig. 7. The values of s-AGEs in subgroups of patients with T1DM with regard to diabetic retinopathy presence/absence (DR – having diabetic retinopathy only, DR+ODC – having diabetic retinopathy and another complications, ODC – having only other diabetic complications except diabetic retinopathy, -DC – having no complications)

The Study of Glycative and Oxidative Stress in Type 1 Diabetes Patients in Relation to Circulating TGF-Beta1,
VCAM-1 and Diabetic Vascular Complications

15

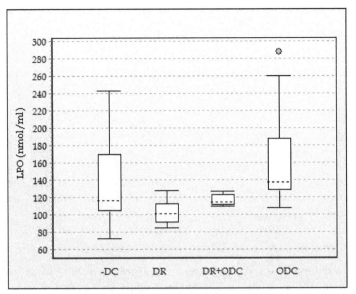

Fig. 8. The values of LPO in subgroups of patients with T1DM with regard to diabetic
retinopathy presence/absence (DR – having diabetic retinopathy only, DR+ODC – having
diabetic retinopathy and another complications, ODC – having only other diabetic
complications except diabetic retinopathy, -DC – having no complications)

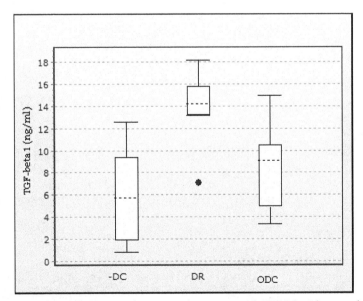

Fig. 9. The values of TGF-beta1 in subgroups of patients with T1DM with regard to diabetic
retinopathy presence/absence (DR – having diabetic retinopathy only, ODC – having only
other diabetic complications except diabetic retinopathy, -DC – having no complications)

4. Conclusion

Our results suggest the relation of glycation and oxidation to profibrotic cytokines, vascular molecules and diabetic complications. Serum AGEs were connected with complications other than retinopathy more than just with retinopathy, nevertheless, some relation of retinopathy and s-AGEs was found (p-values were only slightly higher than 0.05). Lipoperoxides showed some relation to DR since higher in patients with retinopathy than in those with other DC, whereas AOPP did not show any relation to any DC. It seems that in our patients TGF-beta1 and VCAM-1 are linked with the development of DC, but only TGF-beta1 showed some linkage to diabetic retinopathy.

We ought to keep in mind the fact our investigation concerns the children and adolescents. Maybe the study of older patients with T1DM would show more, especially about VCAM-1 and its relation to glycative and oxidative stress and consequently to development of retinopathy/other complications.

5. Acknowledgment

This work is supported by the Vega Grant 1-0375-09 from the Ministry of Education, Sciences, Research and Sport of Slovak Republic. Authors thank Mr. Ľ. Barak, M.D., Mrs. E. Jancova, M.D., Mrs. A. Stanikova, M.D., Mrs. D. Tomcikova, M.D. for assistance with subject recruitment and assessment and Mrs. J. Kalninova, RN.D. and Mrs. E. Tomeckova for technical assistance.

6. References

Bio-Rad, a.s. (2003). *DiaSTAT Hemoglobin A1c Program*. Bio-Rad laboratories Inc., Hercules CA, USA retrieved from http://www.embeediagnostics.com/equip/glycol/diastat.htm April 28th 2009.

R&D Systems, a.s. (2010). Fluorokine MAP. Human Adhesion Molecule MultiAnalyte Profiling Base K. retrieved from http://www.rndsystems.com/product_results.aspx?m=2246&c=87 March 1th 2011.

Aronson, D. (2008). Hyperglycemia and pathobiology of diabetic complications. *Advances in Cardiology*, Vol. 45, pp. 1-16, ISSN 0065-2326

Bargnoux, A.S., Morena, M., Badiou, S., Dupuy, A.M., Canaud, B., Cristol, J.P. & Groupe de travail de la SFBC: Biologie des fonctions renales et de ľ insuffisance renale (2009). Carbonyl stress and oxidatively modified proteins in chronic renal failure. *Annales de Biologie Clinique (Paris)*, Vol.67, No.2, (March 2009), pp. 153-158, ISSN 0003-3898

Boulanger, E., Wautier, J.L., Dequiedt, P. & Schmidt, A.M. (2006). Glycation, glycoxidation and diabetes mellitus. *Nephrologie et Therapeutique*, Vol.2, Suppl.1, (January 2006), pp. S8-S16, ISSN 1769-7255

Boyzel, R., Bruttmann, G, Benhamou, P.Y., Halimi, S. & Stanke-Labesque, F. (2010). Regulation of oxidative stress and inflammation by glycaemic control: evidence for reversible activation of the 5-lipoxygenase pathway in type 1 diabetes, but not in diabetes 2. *Diabetologia*, Vol.53, No.9, pp. 2068-2070, ISSN 0012-186X

Clausen, P., Jacobsen, P., Rossing, K., Jensen, J.S., Parving, H.H. & Feldt-Rasmussen, B. (2000). Plasma concentration of VCAM-1 and ICAM-1 are elevated in patients with Type 1 diabetes mellitus with microalbuminuria and overt nephropathy. *Diabetic Medicine*, Vol.17, No.9, pp. 644-649, ISSN 0742-3071

Devaraj, S., Cheung, A.T., Jialal, I., Griffen, S.C., Nguyen, D., Glaser, N., & Aoki, T. (2007). Evidence of increased inflammation and microcirculatory abnormalities in patients with type 1 diabetes and their role in microvascular complications. *Diabetes*, Vol.56, No.11, (November 2007), pp. 2790-2796, ISSN 0012-1797

El-Saadani, M., Esterbauer, H., el-Sayed, M., Goher, M., Nassar, A.Y. & Jürgens, G. (1989). A spectrophotometric assay for lipid peroxides in serum lipoproteins using a commercially available reagent. *Journal of Lipid Research*, Vol.30, No.4, (April 1989), pp. 627-630, ISSN 0022-2275

Fawaz, L., Elwan, A.E., Kamel, Y.H., Farid, T.M., Kamel, A. & Mohamed, W.A. (2009). Value of C-reactive protein and IL-6 measurements in type 1 diabetes mellitus. *Archives of Medical Science*, Vol.5, No.3, pp. 383-390, ISSN 1734-1922

Goh, S.Y. & Cooper M.E. (2008). Clinical review: The role of advanced glycation end products in progression and complications of diabetes. *Journal of Clinical Endocrinology and Metabolism*, Vol.93, No.4, (January 2008), pp.1143-1152, ISSN 0021-972X

Goldfarb, S. & Ziyadeh, F.N. (2001). TGF-beta: a crucial component of the pathogenesis of diabetic nephropathy. *Transactions of the American Clinical and Climatological Association*, Vol.112, pp.27-33 , ISSN 0065-7778

Hartge, M.M., Unger, T. & Kintscher, U. (2007). The endothelium and vascular inflammation in diabetes. *Diabetes and Vascular Disease Research*, Vol.4, No.2, (June 2007), pp. 84-88, ISSN 1479-1641

Chung, A.C.K., Zhang, H., Kong, Y.Z., Tan, J.J., Huang, X.R., Kopp, J.B. & Lan, H.Y. (2010). Advanced glycation end-products induce tubular CTGF via TGF-beta-independent Smad3 signalling. *Journal of the American Society of Nephrology*, Vol.21, No.2, (February 2010), pp. 249-260, ISSN 1046-6673

Kalousova, M., Škrha, J. & Zima, T. (2002). Advanced glycation end-products and advanced oxidation protein products in patients with diabetes mellitus. *Physiological Research*, Vol.51, No.6, pp. 597–604, ISSN 0862-8408

Karasu, C. (2010). Glycoxidative stress and cardiovascular complications in experimentally-induced diabetes: effects of antioxidant treatment. *The Open Cardiovascular Medicine Journal*, Vol.4, (Nov 2010), pp. 240-256, ISSN 1874-1924

Kashihara, N., Haruna, Y., Kondeti, V.K. & Kanvar, Y.S. (2010). Oxidative stress in diabetic nephropathy. *Current Medicinal Chemistry*, Vol.17, No.34, (December 2010), pp. 4256-4269, ISSN 0929-8673

Mosquera, J.A. (2010). Role of the receptor for advanced glycation end products (RAGE) in inflammation. *Investigación Clínica*, Vol.51, No.2, (June 2010), pp. 257-268, ISSN 0535-5133

Navarro, J.F., & Mora, C. (2006). Diabetes, inflammation, proinflammatory cytokines, and diabetic nephropathy. *The Scientific World Journal*, pp. 6908-6917, ISSN 1537-744X

Negre-Salvayre, A., Salvayre, R., Auge, N., Pamplona, R. & Portero-Otin, M. (2009). Hyperglycemia and glycation in diabetic complications. *Antioxidants & Redox Signaling,* Vol. 11, No.12, (December 2009), pp. 3071-3109, ISSN 1523-0864

Nin, J.W., Jorsai, A., Ferreira, J., Schalwijk, C.G., Prins, M.H., Parving, H.H., Tarnow, L., Rossing, P. & Stehouwer, C.D. (2011). Higher plasma levels of advanced glycation end products are associated with incident cardiovascular disease and all-cause mortality in type 1 diabetes: A 12-year follow-up study. *Diabetes Care,* Vol.34, No.2, (February 2011), pp. 442-447, ISSN 0149-5992

Nobécourt, E., Tabet, F., Lambert, G., Puranik, R., Bao, S., Yan, L., Davies, M.J., Brown, B.E., Jenkins, A.J., Dusting, G.J., Bonnet, D.J., Curtiss, L.K., Barter, P.J. & Rye, K.A. (2010). *Arteriosclerosis, Thrombosis, and Vascular Biology,* Vol.30, No.4, (April 2010), pp. 766-772, ISSN 1079-5642

Peppa, M. & Vlassara, H. (2005). Advanced glycation end products and diabetic complications: A General overview. *Hormones,* Vol.4, No.1, pp. 28-37, ISSN 1109-3099

Piwovar, A. (2010a). Advanced oxidation products. Part I. Mechanism of the formation, characteristics and property. *Polski Merkuriusz Lekarski,* Vol.28, No.164, (February, 2010), pp. 166-169, ISSN 1426-9686

Piwovar, A. (2010b). Advanced oxidation products. Part II. The significance of oxidation protein products in the pathomechanism of diabetes and its complications. *Polski Merkuriusz Lekarski,* Vol.28, No.165, (March, 2010), pp. 227-230, ISSN 1426-9686

Ramasamy, R., Vannucci, S. J., Yan, S. S., Herold, K., Yan, S. F. & Schmidt A. M. (2005). Advanced glycation end products and RAGE: a common thread in aging, diabetes, neurodegeneration, and inflammation. *Glycobiology,* Vol.15, No.7, pp. 16R–28R, ISSN 0959-6658

Rambhade, S., Chakraborty, A.K., Patil, U.K., & Rambhade, A. (2010). Diabetes mellitus- Its complications, factors influencing complications and prevention - An Overview. *Journal of Chemical and Pharmaceutical Research,* Vol.2, No.6, pp. 7-25, ISSN 0975-7384

Seckin, D, Ilhan, N., Ilhan, N. & Ertugrul, S. (2006). Glycaemic control, markers of endothelial cell activation and oxidative stress in children with type 1 diabetes mellitus. *Diabetes Research and Clinical Practice,* Vol.73., (August 2006), pp. 191-197, ISSN 0168-8227

Schmidt, A.M., Hori, A., Jing, X.C., Jian, F.L., Crandall, J. Zhang, J., Cao, R., Shi, D.Y., Brett, J. & Stern, D. (1995). Advanced glycation endproducts interacting with their endothelial receptor induce expression of vascular cell adhesion molecule-1 (VCAM-1) in cultured human endothelial cells and in mice: A potential mechanism for the accelerated vasculopathy of diabetes. *Journal of Clinical Investigation,* Vol.96, No.3, pp.1395-1403, ISSN 0021-9738

Schmidt, A.M., Crandall, J., Hori, O., Cao, R. & Lakatta, E. (1996). Elevated plasma levels of vascular adhesion molecule (VCAM-1) in diabetic patients with microalbuminuria: A marker of vascular dysfunction and progressive vascular

The Study of Glycative and Oxidative Stress in Type 1 Diabetes Patients in Relation to Circulating TGF-Beta1,
VCAM-1 and Diabetic Vascular Complications

19

disease. *British Journal of Haematology*, Vol.92, No.3, pp. 747-750, ISSN 0007-1048

Schrijvers, B.F., De Vriese, A.S. & Flyvbjerg, A. (2004). From hyperglycemia to diabetic kidney disease: The role of metabolic, hemodynamic, intracellular factors and growth factors/cytokines. *Endocrine Reviews*, Vol.25, No.6, (December 2004), pp. 971-1010, ISSN 0163-769X

Son, S.M. (2007). Role of vascular reactive oxygen species in development of vascular abnormalities in diabetes. *Diabetes Research and Clinical Practice*, Vol. 77, Suppl. 1, pp. S65–S70, ISSN 0168-8227

Van Sickle, B.J., Simmons, J., Hall, R., Raines, M., Ness, K. & Spagnoli, A. (2009). Increased circulating IL-8 is associated with reduced IGF-1 and related to poor metabolic control in adolescents with type 1 diabetes mellitus. *Cytokine*, Vol.48, No.3, pp. 290-294, ISSN 1043-4666

Vlassara, H., Fuh, H., Donnelly, T. & Cybulsky, M. (1995). Advanced glycation endproducts promote adhesion molecule (VCAM-1, ICAM-1) expression and atheroma formation in normal rabbits. *Molecular Medicine (Cambridge, Mass.)*, Vol.1, No.4, (May 1995), pp. 447-456, ISSN 1076-1551

Wang, W., Koka, V. & Lan, H.Y. (2005). Transforming growth factor-β and Smad signalling in kidney diseases. *Nephrology*, Vol.10, No.1, (February 2005), pp. 48-56, ISSN 1320-5358

Wautier, J.L., Boulanger, E. & Wautier, M.P. (2006). Postprandial hyperglycemia alters inflammatory and hemostatic parameters. *Diabetes and Metabolism*, Vol.32, No.HS2, (September 2006), pp. 2S34-2S36, ISSN 1262-3636

Witko-Sarsat, V., Friedlander, M., Capeillère-Blandin, C., Nguyen-Khoa, T., Nguyen, A. T., Zingraff, J., Jungers, P. & Descamps-Latscha, B. (1996). Advanced oxidation protein products as a novel marker of oxidative stress in uremia. *Kidney Internatinal*, Vol. 49, No.5, (May 1996), pp. 1304-1313, ISSN 0085-2538

Wolf, G. & Ziyadeh, F.N. (2007). Cellular and molecular mechanisms of proteinuria in diabetic nephropathy. *Nephron-Physiology*, Vol.106, No.2, (June 2007), pp. 26-31, ISSN 1660-2137

Yamagishi, S. Ueda, S. Matsui, T., Nakamura, K. & Okuda, S. (2008). Role of advanced glycation end products (AGEs) and oxidative stress in diabetic retinopathy. *Current Pharmaceutial Design*, Vol.14, No.10, pp. 962-968, ISSN 1381-6128

Yamagishi, S. (2009). Advanced glycation end products and receptor-oxidative stress system in diabetic vascular complications. *Therapeutic Apheresis and Dialysis*, Vol.13, No.6, (December 2009), pp. 534-539, ISSN 1744-9979

Yan S.F., Ramasamy, R. & Schmidt, A.M. (2008). Mechanisms of disease: advanced glycation end products and their receptors in inflammation and diabetes complications. *Nature Clinical Practice Endocrinology Metabolism*, Vol.4, No.5, (May 2008), pp. 285-293, ISSN 1745-8366

Zhang, L., Zalewski, A., Liu, Y., Mazurek, T., Cowan, S., Martin, J.L., Hofmann, S.M., Vlassara, H. & Shi, Y. (2003). Diabetes induced oxidative stress and low-grade inflammation in porcine coronary arteries. *Circulation*, Vol.108, No.4, (July 2003), pp. 472-478, ISSN 0009-7322

Zhou, G., Li C. & Cai, L. (2004). Advanced glycation end-products induce connective tissue
    growth factor-mediated renal fibrosis predominantly through transforming growth
    factor β-independent pathway. *American Journal of Pathology*, Vol.165, No.6,
    (December 2004), pp. 2033-2043, ISSN 0002-9440

2

Lipid Disorders in Type 1 Diabetes

Bruno Vergès
Service Endocrinologie, Diabétologie et Maladies Métaboliques
Dijon University Hospital
France

1. Introduction

Cardiovascular disease is the major cause of death in persons with type 1 diabetes (Libby et al., 2005). Dyslipidemia has been shown to be a significant coronary heart disease risk factor in type 1 diabetes (Soedamah-Muthu et al., 2004; Grauslund et al., 2010). Thus, it seems important to pay attention to lipid abnormalities, in patients with type 1 diabetes, in order to reduce cardiovascular disease in this population.

Patients with type 1 diabetes show lipid disorders, mostly qualitative abnormalities of lipoproteins, which may promote atherogenesis. The pathophysiology of these lipid abnormalities is not totally explained, but hyperglycemia and peripheral hyperinsulinemia, due to the subcutaneous route of insulin administration, are likely to play a role. After a brief review of lipoprotein metabolism and some information on the role of insulin on lipid metabolism, quantitative abnormalities then qualitative abnormalities of lipoproteins, in type 1 diabetes, will be discussed.

2. Brief review of lipoprotein metabolism

Lipoproteins, which transport non-water soluble cholesterol and triglycerides in plasma, are spherical particles composed of a central core of non-polar lipids (cholesterol esters, triglycerides) and a surface monolayer of phospholipids, free cholesterol and apolipoproteins. Lipoproteins are generally classified according to their density as chylomicron, Very Low Density Lipoprotein (VLDL), Intermediate Density Lipoprotein (IDL), Low Density Lipoprotein (LDL) and High Density Lipoprotein (HDL). An overview of lipoprotein metabolism is shown in Figure 1.

2.1 Chylomicrons

Chylomicrons, the largest lipoprotein particles, are responsible for the transport of dietary triglycerides and cholesterol. Chylomicrons are composed of triglycerides (85-90%), cholesterol esters, phospholipids and apolipoproteins (mainly apoB48 but also apoA-I and apoA-IV). The formation of chylomicrons takes place in the enterocytes, and the process associating the lipid components (triglycerides, cholesterol esters, phospholipids) and the apoB48 is performed by the MTP (Microsomal Tranfer Protein). Chylomicrons are secreted into the lymphatic circulation before entering the bloodstream. In plasma, triglycerides of chylomicrons are hydrolyzed by the lipoprotein lipase leading to the formation of smaller, triglyceride-poorer particles known as chylomicron-remnants. Chylomicron-remnants are cleared by the liver through LDL B/E receptor or LRP receptor (LDL-receptor related protein).

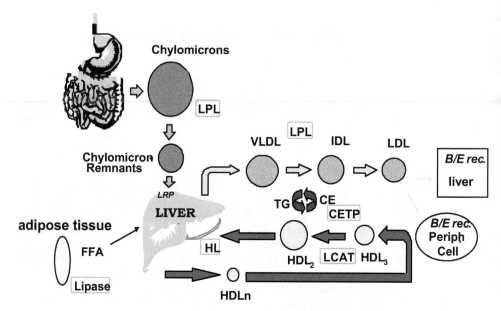

VLDL: Very Low Density Lipoprotein; *IDL*: Intermediate Density Lipoprotein, *LDL*: Low Density Lipoprotein; *HDL*: High Density Lipoprotein; *LPL*: LipoProtein Lipase; *HL*: Hepatic Lipase; *CETP*: Cholesteryl Ester Transfer Protein; *LCAT*: Lecithin-Cholesterol Acyl Transferase; *FFA*: Free Fatty Acids ; *B/E rec.*: B/E receptor (LDL receptor); *TG*: Triglycerides; *CE*: Cholesterol Esters; *ABCA1*: ATP Binding Cassette A1 transporter.

Fig. 1. Human lipoprotein metabolism.

2.2 VLDLs and IDLs

VLDL particles, which are secreted by the liver, consist of endogenous triglycerides (55% to 65%), cholesterol, phospholipids and apolipoproteins (apoB100 as well as apoCs and apoE). In the hepatocyte, the formation of VLDL occurs in two major steps. In the first step, which takes place in the rough endoplasmic reticulum, apoB is co-translationally and post-translationally lipidated by the MTP (Microsomal Tranfer Protein). MTP transfers lipids (mainly triglycerides but also cholesterol esters and phospholipids) to apoB. This first step leads to the formation of pre-VLDL (Olofsson et al., 2000). In the second step, pre-VLDL is converted to VLDL in the smooth membrane compartment. This step is driven by ADP ribosylation factor-1 (ARF-1) and its activation of phospholipase D, needed for the formation of VLDL from pre-VLDL (Olofsson , 2000).

In plasma, triglycerides of VLDLs are hydrolyzed by the lipoprotein lipase. As VLDLs become progressively depleted in triglycerides, a portion of the surface including phospholipids and apolipoproteins C and E is transferred to HDLs. This metabolic cascade leads to the formation of IDL particles, which are either cleared by the liver through LDL B/E receptor or further metabolized to form LDLs. The enzyme, hepatic lipase, which has both triglyceride lipase and phospholipase activities, is involved in this metabolic process generating LDL particles from IDLs.

2.3 LDLs
LDL is the final product of the VLDL-IDL-LDL cascade. LDL is the main cholesterol-bearing lipoprotein in plasma. Each LDL particle contains one molecule of apoB100, which plays an important role in LDL metabolism, particularly recognition of its dedicated LDL B/E receptor. Clearance of LDL is mediated by the LDL B/E receptor. Seventy percent of LDL B/E receptors are located on hepatic cells and 30% on the other cells of the body.

2.4 HDLs
HDL particles are secreted by the hepatocytes as small lipid-poor lipoproteins, containing mostly apoA-I, which receive, in the circulation, phospholipids, apoCs and apoE from chylomicrons and VLDLs. Nascent or lipid-poor HDLs get from peripheral cells free cholesterol and phospholipids through ABCA1 transporter (ATP Binding Cassette A1 transporter), allowing the transport of free cholesterol and phospholipids from the cell cytoplasm into the HDL particles (Oram & Lawn, 2001). Within HDL particles, free cholesterol is esterified by LCAT (Lecithin Cholesterol AcylTransferase) leading to the formation of HDL_3 particles. The fusion of 2 HDL_3 particles, which is promoted by PLTP (PhosphoLipid Transfer Protein), leads to the formation of one larger size HDL_2 particle. HDL_2 lipoproteins, rich in cholesterol ester, are degraded by the hepatic lipase and the endothelial lipase, leading to the formation of HDL remnant particles that are cleared by the liver after recognition by SR-B1 receptor (Scavenger Receptor class B type 1) (Jian et al., 1998).

2.5 Lipid transfer proteins
Lipoprotein metabolism is largely influenced by lipid transfer proteins. Among these, two play an important role: CETP (Cholesteryl Ester Transfer Protein) and PLTP (PhosphoLipid Transfer Protein). CETP facilitates the transfer of triglycerides from triglyceride-rich lipoproteins (mainly VLDLs) toward HDLs and LDLs and the reciprocal transfer of cholesteryl esters from HDLs and LDLs toward VLDLs (Lagrost, 1994). PLTP facilitates the transfer of phospholipids and α-tocopherol between lipoproteins. PLTP is also involved in the formation of HDL_2 lipoproteins from HDL_3 particles (Lagrost et al., 1998). Any modification of CETP or PLTP activities is likely to promote significant qualitative abnormalities of lipoproteins.

3. Insulin and lipoprotein metabolism

Insulin plays a central role in the regulation of lipid metabolism (Vergès, 2001). The main sites of action of insulin on lipoprotein metabolism are shown in Figure 2.

In adipose tissue, insulin inhibits the hormone-sensitive lipase. Thus, insulin has an anti-lipolytic action, promoting storage of triglycerides in the adipocytes and reducing release of free fatty acids from adipose tissue in the circulation.

Insulin inhibits VLDL production from the liver. In normal subjects, it has been shown that insulin induces a 67% decrease of VLDL-triglyceride production and a 52% decrease of VLDL-apoB production (Lewis et al., 1993; Malmström et al., 1998). Insulin reduces VLDL production by diminishing circulating free fatty acids (due to its antilipolytic effect), which are substrates for VLDL, but also by a direct inhibitory effect in the hepatocyte (Malmström et al., 1998). Insulin is a potent activator of lipoprotein lipase (LPL), promoting the catabolism of triglyceride-rich lipoproteins and reducing, as a consequence, plasma triglyceride level. Insulin not only enhances LPL activity (Brunzell et al., 1998), but has also a direct positive effect on LPL gene, promoting LPL synthesis (Fried etal., 1993). Insulin promotes the clearance of LDL, by increasing LDL B/E receptor expression and activity (Chait et al., 1979, Mazzone et al., 1984).

Insulin acts also on HDL metabolism by activating LCAT and hepatic lipase activities (Ruotolo et al., 1994).

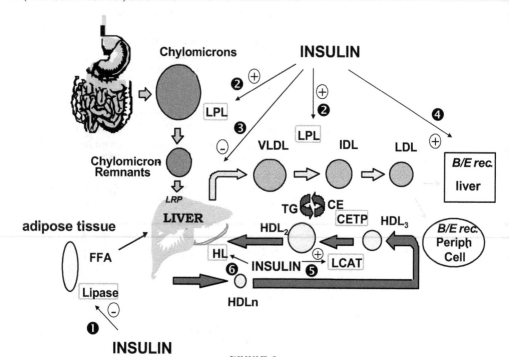

VLDL: Very Low Density Lipoprotein; IDL: Intermediate Density Lipoprotein, LDL: Low Density Lipoprotein; HDL: High Density Lipoprotein; LPL: LipoProtein Lipase; HL: Hepatic Lipase; CETP: Cholesteryl Ester Transfer Protein; LCAT: Lecithin-Cholesterol Acyl Transferase; FFA: Free Fatty Acids ; B/E rec.: receptor B/E (LDL receptor); TG: Triglycerides; CE: Cholesterol Esters. 1: insulin inhibits hormone-sensitive lipase. 2 : insulin activates LipoProtein Lipase (LPL). 3: insulin inhibits hepatic VLDL production. 4: insulin increases LDL B/E receptor expression. 5: insulin activates LCAT. 6: insulin activates Hepatic Lipase (HL).

Fig. 2. Main effects of insulin on lipoprotein metabolism.

4. Quantitative lipid abnormalities in type 1 diabetes

4.1 Untreated (diabetic ketoacidosis) type 1 diabetes

In type 1 diabetic patients with diabetic ketoacidosis, quantitative lipid abnormalities are observed, due to insulin deficiency.

Triglyceride-rich lipoproteins (chylomicrons, VLDLs) are increased leading to hypertriglyceridemia. This is mainly due to decreased lipoprotein lipase activity (Vergès, 2001; Dullaart, 1995). Diabetic ketoacidosis is a situation of severe insulin deficiency with reduced lipoprotein lipase activity as a consequence, because insulin usually stimulates its activity. Decreased lipoprotein lipase activity leads to profound reduction of triglyceride-rich lipoprotein catabolism (Taskinen, 1987). In this condition of severe insulin deficiency, reduced catabolism of triglyceride-rich lipoproteins is, by far, the main factor involved in hypertriglyceridemia. This hypertriglyceridemia resolves rapidly after well titrated insulin therapy (Weidman et al., 1982).

LDL-cholesterol is decreased during diabetic ketoacidosis (Weidman et al., 1982). This fall in plasma LDL-cholesterol level is the direct consequence of the reduction of triglyceride-rich lipoprotein catabolism, due to decreased lipoprotein lipase activity (see above).

In diabetic ketoacidosis, HDL-cholesterol level is significantly decreased (Weidman et al., 1982). This is a consequence of hypertrigliceridemia observed in this condition. Indeed, the augmented level of plasma triglyceride-rich lipoproteins drives, through CETP, the transfer of triglycerides from triglyceride-rich lipoproteins to HDLs leading to the formation of triglyceride-rich HDL particles. HDLs enriched in triglycerides become very good substrate for hepatic lipase, leading to increase their catabolism and, thus, to decrease plasma HDL-cholesterol level. This low HDL-cholesterol condition resolves rapidly after well titrated insulin therapy (Weidman et al., 1982).

4.2 Treated type 1 diabetes

Patients with treated type 1 diabetes may show quantitative lipid disorders. In a prospective study performed in 895 young subjects with type 1 diabetes, 20.1% had plasma triglycerides above 1.7 mmol/l, 9.6% had LDL-cholesterol above 3.4 mmol/l and 25.9% had non-HDL cholesterol above 3.4 mmol/l (Marcovecchio et al., 2009). It has been shown that abnormal lipid levels, in type 1 diabetes, predict worse cardiovascular outcomes (Soedamah-Muthu et al., 2004). HbA1c has been shown to be independently correlated with LDL-cholesterol, non-HDL cholesterol and triglyceride levels, indicating that these disorders were mostly observed in patients with poor glycemic control (Marcovecchio et al., 2009). In a British follow-up study of 229 children with type 1 diabetes, LDL cholesterol and non-HDL cholesterol values increased with duration of diabetes (Edge et al., 2008). In that study, total cholesterol, triglycerides and non-HDL cholesterol were positively correlated with HbA1c and around 10% of the patients had lipid values outside recommendations (Edge et al., 2008). In a large study performed in 29 979 patients with type 1 diabetes, multivariate analyses showed a significant positive association between HbA1c and total cholesterol (p<0.0001), LDL cholesterol (p<0.0001) and a significant negative association between HbA1c and HDL cholesterol (p<0.0001) (Schwab et al., 2009). In the Diabetes Control and Complications Trial (DCCT), HbA1c correlated positively with total cholesterol, LDL-cholesterol and triglycerides at baseline (The DCCT Research Group, 1992). Data from the Coronary Artery Calcification in type 1 diabetes (CACTI) study, which examined 652 patients with type 1 diabetes, have shown, in patients not using hypolipidemic agents, that a higher HbA1c was associated with significantly higher levels of total cholesterol, triglycerides, LDL cholesterol and non-HDL cholesterol (Maahs et al., 2010). In that study, 1% change in HbA1c was associated with an increase of 0.101 mmol/l (4 mg/dl) for total cholesterol, of 0.052 mmol/l (4.5 mg/dl) for triglycerides, of 0.103 mmol/l (4 mg/dl) for LDL cholesterol and of 0.129 mmol/l (5 mg/dl) for non-HDL cholesterol (Maahs et al.,

2010). In a recent study, performed in 512 young patients with type 1 diabetes and in 188 healthy age-matched controls, patients with suboptimal control (HbA1c ≥ 7.5%) had much more lipid quantitative disorders than patients with optimal control (HbA1c<7.5%) (Guy et al., 2009). All these data suggest that quantitative lipid abnormalities are more frequent, when type 1 diabetes is not well controlled.

In addition, some patients with type 1 diabetes may have insulin resistance, in situation of abdominal obesity and/or family history of type 2 diabetes. Such patients have been shown to have greater dyslipidemia (Purnell et al., 2003). In a recent study performed in 60 young type 1 diabetic patients and 40 adults with type 1 diabetes, it has been shown, using hyperinsulinemic clamp studies, that lower glucose infusion (more insulin resistance) was associated with lower levels of HDL cholesterol in youths with type 1 diabetes and with higher levels of triglycerides and higher triglyceride/HDL ratio in both youths and adults (Maahs et al., 2011). These data indicate that insulin resistance may be an additional factor that could induce quantitative lipid abnormities in some type 1 diabetic patients with a background of insulin resistance (abdominal obesity, family history of type 2 diabetes). In this chapter we will consider only the typical situation of type 1 diabetes without insulin resistance.

4.2.1 Treated type 1 diabetes with poor or suboptimal glycemic control

In case of poor or suboptimal control, patients with type 1 diabetes may show increased plasma triglyceride levels (Dullaart,1995). This hypertriglyceridemia is due to increased production of VLDL, promoted by elevated circulating free fatty acids secondary to the relative insulin deficiency (Nikkilä & Kekki, 1973).

Type 1 diabetic patients with poor or suboptimal glycemic control show increased LDL-cholesterol levels as compared to non–diabetic individuals and type 1 diabetic patients with optimal glycemic control (Dullaart, 1995; Guy et al., 2009). Indeed, in this condition, VLDL production is increased (see above), when catabolism of triglyceride-rich lipoproteins is not importantly decreased, which leads to increase LDL production (Dullaart, 1995).

4.2.2 Treated type 1 diabetes with optimal glycemic control

In well controlled type 1 diabetes, the lipid profile is totally different than in poorly controlled type 1 diabetes (Dullaart, 1995; Nikkilä & Kekki, 1973).

Plasma triglycerides are normal or slightly decreased (Dullaart, 1995; Nikkilä & Kekki, 1973). This slight decrease in plasma triglycerides may be observed with intense insulin therapy because of increased down control of VLDL production by augmented plasma insulin levels as a consequence of the subcutaneous route of insulin delivery (Dashti & Wolfbauer, 1987; Taskinen, 1992). Furthermore, in patients with well controlled type 1 diabetes, peripheral hyperinsulinemia has been shown to be associated with increased lipoprotein lipase activity that could be an additional factor responsible for decreased plasma triglycerides (Nikkilä et al., 1977).

Plasma LDL-cholesterol level is normal or slightly decreased (Winocour et al., 1986). This slight decrease in plasma LDL-cholesterol may be observed with intense insulin therapy as a consequence of decreased VLDL production by peripheral hyperinsulinemia (see above).

Plasma HDL-cholesterol level is normal or slightly increased in well controlled type 1 diabetic patients (Dullaart, 1995). Some studies have shown an increase in HDL subfraction 2 (Eckel et al., 1981; Kahri et al., 1993), when others have found an increase in HDL subfraction 3 (Winocour et al., 1986). It has also been reported that elevation of HDL in type 1 diabetic patients with good glycemic control was caused by an increase of HDL particles containing only apoA-I (LpA-I) (Kahri et al., 1993). This increase in plasma HDL-cholesterol could be the consequence of the elevated Lipoprotein Lipase/Hepatic Lipase ratio that is observed in patients with well controlled type 1 diabetes (increased Lipoprotein Lipase activity and normal Hepatic Lipase activity) (Kahri et al., 1993). The increased Lipoprotein Lipase activity observed in these patients is likely to be due to peripheral hyperinsulinemia as a consequence of the subcutaneous route of insulin administration (Kahri et al., 1993).

4.2.3 Subcutaneous insulin therapy versus intraperitoneal insulin therapy

Intensive subcutaneous insulin therapy results in normalization of plasma glucose, but at the expense of peripheral hyperinsulinemia, which is likely to modify lipoprotein metabolism (as discussed above). Implantable insulin pumps with intraperitoneal insulin administration mimic the physiologic route of insulin delivery and are likely to restore the normal portal-peripheral insulin gradient. For this reason, several studies have been performed to analyze the modification of lipoprotein metabolism after replacement of subcutaneous insulin therapy by intraperitoneal insulin therapy. Plasma triglycerides have been found increased in one study (Selam et al., 1989) and unchanged in three other studies (Bagdade & Dunn, 1996; Ruotolo et al., 1994; Duvillard et al., 2005). Total cholesterol and apoB were found unchanged (Bagdade & Dunn, 1996; Ruotolo et al., 1994; Duvillard et al., 2005). HDL-cholesterol has been found decreased (Selam et al., 1989) or not modified (Bagdade & Dunn, 1996; Ruotolo et al., 1994; Duvillard et al., 2007). The discrepancies of these studies that may be due to confounding factors such as degree of glycemic control and peripheral insulin levels during subcutaneous insulin therapy. Further studies are needed to clearly evaluate the effect of intraperitoneal insulin administration on lipoprotein metabolism.

4.2.4 Type 1 diabetes with nephropathy

In type 1 diabetic patients with nephropathy and overt albuminuria, elevated plasma levels of total cholesterol, triglycerides and LDL-cholesterol are observed whereas HDL-cholesterol is decreased due to a fall in HDL_2 (Dullaart ,1995; Taskinen, 1992; Jensen et al., 1987). In the EURODIAB IDDM Complications study, macroalbuminuria was associated with significantly increased plasma triglycerides, cholesterol, LDL-cholesterol and LDL/HDL ratio in both sexes and decreased HDL-cholesterol in women (Mattock et al., 2001).

Some quantitative lipid modifications are also observed in type 1 diabetic patients with microalbuminuria. Microalbuminuric patients compared with normoalbuminuric patients show increased plasma apoB (Jones et al., 1989, Dullaart et al, 1989a; Jay et al., 1991), LDL cholesterol (Jones et al., 1989, Dullaart et al, 1989a) and apoB/apoA1 ratio (Dullaart et al, 1989a; Jay et al., 1991). A positive correlation has been found between urinary albumin excretion rate and plasma apoB and apoB/apoA1 ratio (Dullaart et al, 1989a). In the EURODIAB IDDM Complications study, microalbuminuria was associated with increased plasma triglycerides (Mattock et al., 2001). In a prospective study performed in 895 young subjects with type 1 diabetes, total cholesterol and non-HDL cholesterol were independently related to longitudinal changes in albumin-to-creatinine ratio (Marcovecchio et al., 2009). The mechanisms responsible for these lipoprotein abnormalities in type 1 diabetic patients with microalbuminuria remain unclear.

Moreover, serum lipids have been shown to be associated with the progression of nephropathy in type 1 diabetes. In a prospective study performed in 152 patients with type 1 diabetes followed for 8-9 years, LDL-cholesterol was an independent factor associated with progression of nephropathy (Thomas et al., 2006).

5. Qualitative lipid abnormalities in type 1 diabetes

Several qualitative abnormalities of lipoproteins are observed in patients with type 1 diabetes, even in those with good metabolic control, who do not have significant quantitative lipid changes. These qualitative lipid abnormalities are not totally reversed by optimal glycemic control and are likely to be atherogenic.

5.1 VLDLs

VLDLs from patients with type 1 diabetes are frequently enriched in esterified cholesterol at the expense of triglycerides leading to an increased VLDL cholesterol/triglyceride ratio (Rivellese et al., 1988; Bagdade et al., 1991a). It has been suggested that this compositional changes may be due to increased cholesteryl ester transfer between lipoproteins (Bagdade et al., 1991a). It has been shown that the VLDL cholesterol/triglyceride ratio was significantly reduced with intraperitoneal insulin therapy (Dunn, 1992). Furthermore, the free cholesterol /lecithin ratio within the peripheral layer of VLDL particles is increased (Dullaart, 1995; Bagdade et al., 1991a). Such increase in the free cholesterol /lecithin ratio within the peripheral layer of lipoproteins has been shown to raise the risk for cardiovascular events possibly by reducing fluidity and stability of lipoproteins (Kuksis, 1982). Moreover, VLDLs from patients with type 1 diabetes have been shown, in vitro, to induce abnormal response of cellular cholesterol metabolism in human macrophages (Klein et al., 1989).

5.2 LDLs

In patients with type 1 diabetes, LDLs are often enriched in triglycerides and increased number of small dense LDL particles is observed (Guy et al., 2009; Lahdenperä et al., 1994; James & Pometta, 1990; Skyrme-Jones et al., 2000). In a study performed in 2657 patients with type 1 diabetes, it has been shown that dense LDL increased with HbA1c with buoyant LDL shifting toward dense LDL for HbA1c values above 8% (Albers et al., 2008). It has been shown that the presence of small dense LDL particles is associated with increased cardiovascular risk (Austin et al., 1990). Many data indicate that small dense LDL particles have atherogenic properties. Indeed, small dense LDL particles have reduced affinity for the LDL B/E receptor and are preferentially taken up by macrophages, through the scavenger receptor, leading to the formation of foam cells. Small dense LDL particles have higher affinity for intimal proteoglycans than large LDL particles which may favor the penetration of LDL particles into the arterial wall (Chapman et al., 1998). It has been shown that subjects with small dense LDL particles show an impaired response to endothelium dependent vasodilator acetylcholine (Vakkilainen et al., 2000). Moreover, small dense LDL particles show an increased susceptibility to oxidation (Tribble et al., 1992). A reduction of the proportion of small dense LDL particles has been reported after optimization of glycemic control in patients with type 1 diabetes (Caixàs et al., 1997).

The free cholesterol /lecithin ratio within the peripheral layer of LDL particles is increased (Dullaart, 1995; Bagdade et al., 1991a). In patients with type 1 diabetes, glycation of ApoB occurs within LDL in parallel with plasma hyperglycemia. It has been shown that apoB glycation reduces significantly LDL binding to the B/E receptor even when apoB glycation is moderate (Witztum et al., 1982; Steinbrecher et al, 1984). Furthermore, glycated LDLs are preferentialy taken up by macrophages through the scavenger receptor, leading to the formation of foam cells in the arterial wall. In patients with type 1 diabetes, advanced glycation end products-modified LDL have been shown to be positively associated with increased intima media thickness (IMT) (Lopes-Virella et al., 2011).

Moreover, patients with type 1 diabetes may show an increased oxidation of LDL which is promoted by glycemic excursions (de Castro et al., 2005). Increased urinary excretion of malondialdehyde, reflecting enhanced lipid peroxidation, has been reported in patients with type 1 diabetes (Hoeldtke et al., 2009). Oxidative modification of LDL results in rapid uptake by macrophages, leading to foam cell formation. Oxidized LDLs produce chemotactic effects on monocytes by increasing the synthesis of adhesion molecules, such as ICAM-1 (intercellular adhesion Molecule 1) by endothelial cells. Oxidized LDLs stimulate the formation by macrophages of cytokines, such as TNFα or IL1, which amplify the inflammatory atherosclerotic process. It has recently been shown that oxidized LDL particles were significantly associated with progression and increased levels of IMT in type 1 diabetes (de Castro et al., 2005).

5.3 HDLs

HDL particles from patients with type 1 diabetes are often enriched in triglycerides (Dullaart, 1995; Bagdade et al., 1991a). This modification has been attributed to increased cholesteryl ester transfer between lipoproteins (Bagdade et al., 1991a). In HDL particles from patients with type 1 diabetes, sphingomyelin/lecithin ratio within the peripheral layer is augmented, which may increase HDL rigidity (Bagdade & Subbaiah, 1989). These alterations are not totally reversed after achievement of optimal glycemic control (Bagdade et al., 1991b). ApoA-I within HDL is glycated in patients with type 1 diabetes, which may impair the HDL-mediated reverse cholesterol pathway. Indeed, it has been shown that HDL particles containing glycated apoA-I were less effective to promote cholesterol efflux from the cells (Fievet et al., 1992).

In addition to their role in the reverse cholesterol pathway, HDLs have anti-oxidative, anti-inflammatory, anti-thrombotic and vasorelaxant properties, potentially anti-atherogenic (Link et al., 2007). Some of these properties have been shown to be reduced in patients with type 1 diabetes. Indeed, a significant reduction of the activity of paraoxonase, an anti-oxidative enzyme associated with HDLs, is observed in patients with type 1 diabetes (Boemi et al., 2001; Ferretti et al., 2004). As a consequence, HDLs from patients with type 1 diabetes protect less efficiently erythrocyte membranes and LDL particles against oxidative damage than HDLs from normal individuals (Boemi et al., 2001; Ferretti et al., 2004). Furthermore, using rabbit aorta rings, it has been shown that HDL from patients with type 1 diabetes are no more able to prevent the endothelium dependent vasoconstriction induced by oxidized LDL, whereas HDL from normal individuals can prevent it (Perségol et al., 2007).

5.4 Lipid transfer proteins

In some studies, an increased cholesteryl ester transfer between lipoproteins (Bagdade et al., 1991a; Bagdade et al., 1994) or an augmented activity of CETP (Colhoun et al., 2001) have been found in normolipidemic patients with type 1 diabetes. In some other studies, increased CETP activity has been reported only in type 1 diabetic patients that smoke or those having microalbuminuria (Dullaart et al., 1989b; Dullaart et al., 1991). This augmented CETP activity may explain the increase in free cholesterol/ triglycerides ratio within VLDL and its decrease within HDL. Some studies have shown a positive correlation between CETP activity and hyperglycemia (Ritter & Bagdade, 1994; Chang et al., 2001). However, the main factor which is likely to be responsible for increased CETP activity, in type 1 diabetes, could be peripheral hyperinsulinemia secondary to the subcutaneous route of insulin administration. Indeed, peripheral hyperinsulinemia has been shown to be responsible for increased lipoprotein lipase activity in patients with type 1 diabetes (Nikkilä et al., 1977) and it has been reported that lipoprotein lipase, in presence of VLDL, enhances CETP activity (Sammett & Tall,1985; Pruneta et al., 1999). Moreover, it has been shown, in patients with type 1 diabetes, that the increase in both lipoprotein lipase and CETP activities was abolished when insulin was administrated intraperitoneously with implantable insulin pumps, mimicking the physiologic portal route or after pancreatic graft (Bagdade et al., 1994; Bagdade et al., 1996).

Increased PLTP activity has been reported in patients with type 1 diabetes (Colhoun et al., 2001). In this study, PLTP activity was positively correlated with CETP activity, LDL-cholesterol and HDL-cholesterol (Colhoun et al., 2001). The reasons and consequences of this increased PLTP activity are not clear.

6. Conclusion

In conclusion, quantitative lipid abnormalities are observed in patients with poorly controlled type 1 diabetes (increased triglyceride and LDL-cholesterol levels) or with micro- or macroalbuminuria (increased triglycerides and LDL-cholesterol, decreased HDL-cholesterol). Patient with optimally controlled type 1 diabetes show normal or slightly decreased triglycerides and LDL-cholesterol levels and sometimes increased HDL-cholesterol levels. Qualitative abnormalities of lipoproteins are observed in patients with type 1 diabetes, even in good glycemic control. These abnormalities are not fully explained by hyperglycemia and may partly be due to peripheral hyperinsulinemia associated with the subcutaneous route of insulin administration. The exact consequences of these qualitative lipid changes on the development of cardiovascular disease in type 1 diabetes are still unknown.

7. References

Albers JJ, Marcovina SM, Imperatore G, Snively BM, Stafford J, Fujimoto WY, Mayer-Davis EJ, Petitti DB, Pihoker C, Dolan L & Dabelea DM. (2008). Prevalence and determinants of elevated apolipoprotein B and dense low-density lipoprotein in youths with type 1 and type 2 diabetes. *J Clin Endocrinol Metab.*; 93: 735-42

Austin MA, King MC, Vranizan KM & Krauss RM. (1990). Atherogenic lipoprotein phenotype : a proposed genetic marker for coronary heart disease risk. *Circulation*; 82, 495-506.

Bagdade JD & Subbaiah PV. (1989). Whole-plasma and high-density lipoprotein subfraction surface lipid composition in IDDM men. *Diabetes*; 38: 1226-30.

Bagdade JD, Ritter MC & Subbaiah PV. (1991a). Accelerated cholesteryl ester transfer in plasma of patients with insulin dependent diabetes mellitus. *Eur J Clin Invest*, 21, 161-167.

Bagdade JD, Helve E & Taskinen MR. (1991b). Effects of continuous insulin infusion therapy on lipoprotein surface and core lipid composition in insulin-dependent diabetes mellitus. *Metabolism*; 40: 445-9.

Bagdade JD, Dunn FL, Eckel RH & Ritter MC. (1994). Intraperitoneal insulin therapy corrects abnormalities in cholesteryl ester transfer and lipoprotein lipase activities in insulin-dependent diabetes mellitus. *Arterioscler Thromb*; 14: 1933-9.

Bagdade JD & Dunn FL. (1996). Improved lipoprotein surface and core lipid composition following intraperitoneal insulin delivery in insulin-dependent diabetes mellitus. *Diabetes Metab*; 22: 420-6.

Bagdade JD, Ritter MC, Kitabchi AE, Huss E, Thistlethwaite R, Gabfr O et al. (1996). Differing effects of pancreas-kidney transplantation with systemic versus portal venous drainage on cholesteryl ester transfer in IDDM subjects. *Diabetes Care*; 19:1108-12.

Boemi M, Leviev I, Sirolla C, Pieri C, Marra M & James RW. (2001). Serum paraoxonase is reduced in type 1 diabetic patients compared to non-diabetic, first degree relatives; influence on the ability of HDL to protect LDL from oxidation. *Atherosclerosis*; 155: 229-35.

Brunzell JD, Schwartz RS, Eckel RH & Goldberg AP. (1981). Insulin and adipose tissue lipoprotein lipase activity in humans. *Int J Obes*; 5: 685-94.

Caixàs A, Ordóñez-Llanos J, de Leiva A, Payés A, Homs R & Pérez A. (1997). Optimization of glycemic control by insulin therapy decreases the proportion of small dense LDL particles in diabetic patients. *Diabetes*; 46: 1207-13.

Chait A, Bierman EL & Albers JJ. (1979). Low-density lipoprotein receptor activity in cultured human skin fibroblasts. Mechanism of insulin-induced stimulation. *J Clin Invest*; 64:1309-19.

Chang CK, Tso TK, Snook JT, Huang YS, Lozano RA & Zipf WB. (2001). Cholesteryl ester transfer and cholesterol esterification in type 1 diabetes: relationships with plasma glucose. *Acta Diabetol*, 38: 37-42.

Chapman MJ, Guerin M & Bruckert E. (1998). Atherogenic, dense low-density lipoproteins. Pathophysiology and new therapeutic approaches. *Eur Heart J*; 19 (Suppl A): A24-30.

Colhoun HM, Scheek LM, Rubens MB, Van Gent T, Underwood SR, Fuller JH et al. (2001). Lipid transfer protein activities in type 1 diabetic patients without renal failure and nondiabetic control subjects and their association with coronary artery calcification. *Diabetes*; 50: 652-9.

Dashti N, Wolfbauer G. (1987). Secretion of lipids, apolipoproteins, and lipoproteins by human hepatoma cell line, HepG2: effects of oleic acid and insulin. *J Lipid Res*; 28: 423-36.

de Castro SH, Castro-Faria-Neto HC & Gomes MB. (2005). Association of postprandial hyperglycemia with in vitro LDL oxidation in non-smoking patients with type 1 diabetes--a cross-sectional study. *Rev Diabet Stud*; 2: 157-64.

Dullaart RP, Dikkeschei LD & Doorenbos H. (1989a). Alterations in serum lipids and apolipoproteins in male type 1 (insulin-dependent) diabetic patients with microalbuminuria. *Diabetologia*; 32: 685-9.

Dullaart RP, Groener JE, Dikkeschei LD, Erkelens DW & Doorenbos H. (1989b). Increased cholesteryl ester transfer activity in complicated type 1 (insulin-dependent) diabetes mellitus--its relationship with serum lipids. *Diabetologia*; 32:14-9.

Dullaart RP, Groener JE, Dikkeschei BD, Erkelens DW & Doorenbos H. (1991). Elevated cholesteryl ester transfer protein activity in IDDM men who smoke. Possible factor for unfavorable lipoprotein profile. *Diabetes Care*; 14: 338-41.

Dullaart RP. (1995). Plasma lipoprotein abnormalities in type 1 (insulin-dependent) diabetes mellitus. *Neth J Med*; 46: 44-54.

Dunn FL. (1992). Plasma lipid and lipoprotein disorders in IDDM. *Diabetes*, 41 (Suppl 2): 102-6.

Duvillard L, Florentin E, Baillot-Rudoni S, Lalanne-Mistrich ML, Brun-Pacaud A, Petit JM, Brun JM, Gambert P & Vergès B (2005). Comparison of apolipoprotein B100 metabolism between continuous subcutaneous and intraperitoneal insulin therapy in type 1 diabetes. *J Clin Endocrinol Metab*; 90: 5761-4.

Duvillard L, Florentin E, Baillot-Rudoni S, Lalanne-Mistrich ML, Brun-Pacaud A, Petit JM, Brun JM, Gambert P & Vergès B. (2007). No change in apolipoprotein AI metabolism when subcutaneous insulin infusion is replaced by intraperitoneal insulin infusion in type 1 diabetic patients. *Atherosclerosis*; 194: 342-7.

Eckel RH, Albers JJ, Cheung MC, Wahl PW, Lindgren FT & Bierman EL. (1981). High density lipoprotein composition in insulin-dependent diabetes mellitus. *Diabetes*; 30: 132-8.

Edge JA, James T & Shine B. (2008). Longitudinal screening of serum lipids in children and adolescents with Type 1 diabetes in a UK clinic population. *Diabet Med.*; 25: 942-8.

Ferretti G, Bacchetti T, Busni D, Rabini RA & Curatola G. (2004). Protective effect of paraoxonase activity in high-density lipoproteins against erythrocyte membranes peroxidation: a comparison between healthy subjects and type 1 diabetic patients. *J Clin Endocrinol Metab*; 89: 2957-62.

Fievet C, Theret N, Shojaee N, Duchateau P, Castro G, Ailhaud G et al. (1992). Apolipoprotein A-I-containing particles and reverse cholesterol transport in IDDM. *Diabetes*; 41 (Suppl 2): 81-5.

Fried SK, Russell CD, Grauso NL & Brolin RE. (1993). Lipoprotein lipase regulation by insulin and glucocorticoid in subcutaneous and omental adipose tissues of obese women and men. *J Clin Invest*; 92: 2191-8.

Grauslund J, Jørgensen TM, Nybo M, Green A, Rasmussen LM & Sjølie AK. (2010). Risk factors for mortality and ischemic heart disease in patients with long-term type 1 diabetes. *J Diabetes Complications*; 24: 223-8.

Guy J, Ogden L, Wadwa RP, Hamman RF, Mayer-Davis EJ, Liese AD et al. (2009). Lipid and lipoprotein profiles in youth with and without type 1 diabetes: the SEARCH for Diabetes in Youth case-control study. *Diabetes Care*; 32: 416-20.

Hoeldtke RD, Bryner KD, Corum LL, Hobbs GR & Van Dyke K. (2009). Lipid peroxidation in early type 1 diabetes mellitus is unassociated with oxidative damage to DNA. *Metabolism*; 58: 731-4.

James RW & Pometta D. (1990). Differences in lipoprotein subfraction composition and distribution between type I diabetic men and control subjects. Diabetes; 39: 1158-64.

Jay RH, Jones SL, Hill CE, Richmond W, Viberti GC, Rampling MW et al. (1991). Blood rheology and cardiovascular risk factors in type 1 diabetes: relationship with microalbuminuria. *Diabet Med*; 8: 662-7.

Jensen T, Borch-Johnsen K, Kofoed-Enevoldsen A & Deckert T. (1987). Coronary heart disease in young type 1 (insulin-dependent) diabetic patients with and without diabetic nephropathy: incidence and risk factors. *Diabetologia*; 30:144-8.

Jian B, de la Llera-Moya M, Ji Y, Wang N, Phillips MC, Swaney JB et al. (1998). Scavenger receptor class B type I as a mediator of cellular cholesterol efflux to lipoproteins and phospholipid acceptors. *J Biol Chem*; 273:5599-606.

Jones SL, Close CF, Mattock MB, Jarrett RJ, Keen H & Viberti GC. (1989). Plasma lipid and coagulation factor concentrations in insulin dependent diabetics with microalbuminuria. *BMJ*; 298: 487-90.

Kahri J, Groop PH, Viberti G, Elliott T & Taskinen MR. (1993). Regulation of apolipoprotein A-I-containing lipoproteins in IDDM. *Diabetes*; 42:1281-8.

Klein RL, Lyons TJ & Lopes-Virella MF. (1989). Interaction of very-low-density lipoprotein isolated from type I (insulin-dependent) diabetic subjects with human monocyte-derived macrophages. *Metabolism*; 38:1108-14.

Kuksis A, Myher JJ, Geher K, Jones GJ, Breckenridge WC, Feather T et al. (1982). Decreased plasma phosphatidylcholine/free cholesterol ratio as an indicator of risk for ischemic vascular disease. *Arteriosclerosis*; 2: 296-302.

Lagrost L, Desrumaux C, Masson D, Deckert V & Gambert P. (1998). Structure and function of the plasma phospholipid transfer protein. *Curr Opin Lipidol*; 9: 203-9.

Lagrost L. (1994). Regulation of cholesteryl ester transfer protein (CETP) activity: review of in vitro and in vivo studies. *Biochim Biophys Acta*; 1215: 209-36.

Lahdenperä S, Groop PH, Tilly-Kiesi M, Kuusi T, Elliott TG, Viberti GC et al. (1994). LDL subclasses in IDDM patients: relation to diabetic nephropathy. *Diabetologia*; 37: 681-8.

Lewis GF, Uffelman KD, Szeto LW, Weller B & Steiner G. (1993). Effects of acute hyperinsulinemia on VLDL triglyceride and VLDL apo B production in normal weight and obese individuals. *Diabetes*; 42: 833-42.

Libby P, Nathan DM, Abraham K, Brunzell JD, Fradkin JE, Haffner SM, Hsueh W, Rewers M, Roberts BT, Savage PJ, Skarlatos S, Wassef M, Rabadan-Diehl C & National Heart, Lung, and Blood Institute; National Institute of Diabetes and Digestive and Kidney Diseases Working Group on Cardiovascular Complications of Type 1 Diabetes Mellitus. (2005). Report of the National Heart, Lung, and Blood Institute-National Institute of Diabetes and Digestive and Kidney Diseases Working Group on Cardiovascular Complications of Type 1 Diabetes Mellitus. *Circulation*; 111: 3489-93.

Link JJ, Rohatgi &, de Lemos JA. (2007). HDL cholesterol: physiology, pathophysiology, and management. *Curr Probl Cardiol*; 32: 268-314.

Lopes-Virella MF, Hunt KJ, Baker NL, Lachin J, Nathan DM, Virella G & Diabetes Control and Complications Trial/Epidemiology of Diabetes Interventions and Complications Research Group. (2011). Levels of oxidized LDL and advanced glycation end products-modified LDL in circulating immune complexes are strongly associated with increased levels of carotid intima-media thickness and its progression in type 1 diabetes. *Diabetes*; 60: 582-9

Maahs DM, Ogden LG, Dabelea D, Snell-Bergeon JK, Daniels SR, Hamman RF & Rewers M. (2010). Association of glycaemia with lipids in adults with type 1 diabetes: modification by dyslipidaemia medication. *Diabetologia*; 53: 2518-25.

Maahs DM, Nadeau K, Snell-Bergeon JK, Schauer I, Bergman B, West NA, Rewers M, Daniels SR, Ogden LG, Hamman RF & Dabelea D. (2011). Association of insulin sensitivity to lipids across the lifespan in people with Type 1 diabetes. *Diabet Med.*; 28:148-55.

Malmström R, Packard CJ, Caslake M, Bedford D, Stewart P, Yki-Jarvinen H et al. (1998). Effects of insulin and acipimox on VLDL1 and VLDL2 apolipoprotein B production in normal subjects. *Diabetes*; 47: 779-87.

Marcovecchio ML, Dalton RN, Prevost AT, Acerini CL, Barrett TG, Cooper JD et al. (2009). Prevalence of Abnormal Lipid Profiles and the Relationship with the Development of Microalbuminuria in Adolescents with Type 1 Diabetes. *Diabetes Care*; 32: 658-663.

Mattock MB, Cronin N, Cavallo-Perin P, Idzior-Walus B, Penno G, Bandinelli S et al. (2001). EURODIAB IDDM Complications Study. Plasma lipids and urinary albumin excretion rate in Type 1 diabetes mellitus: the EURODIAB IDDM Complications Study. *Diabet Med*; 18: 59-67.

Mazzone T, Foster D & Chait A. (1984). In vivo stimulation of low-density lipoprotein degradation by insulin. *Diabetes*; 33: 333-8.

Nikkilä EA & Kekki M. (1973). Plasma triglyceride transport kinetics in diabetes mellitus. *Metabolism*; 22:1-22.

Nikkilä EA, Huttunen JK & Ehnholm C. (1977). Postheparin plasma lipoprotein lipase and hepatic lipase in diabetes mellitus. Relationship to plasma triglyceride metabolism. *Diabetes*; 26:11-21.

Olofsson SO, Stillemark-Billton P & Asp L. (2000). Intracellular assembly of VLDL: two major steps in separate cell compartments. *Trends Cardiovasc Med*; 10: 338-45.

Oram JF & Lawn RM. ABCA1. (2001). The gatekeeper for eliminating excess tissue cholesterol. *J Lipid Res*; 42:1173-9.

Perségol L, Foissac M, Lagrost L, Athias A, Gambert P, Vergès B & Duvillard L. (2007). HDL particles from type 1 diabetic patients are unable to reverse the inhibitory effect of oxidised LDL on endothelium-dependent vasorelaxation. *Diabetologia*; 50: 2384-7.

Pruneta V, Pulcini T, Lalanne F, Marçais C, Berthezène F, Ponsin G et al. (1999). VLDL-bound lipoprotein lipase facilitates the cholesteryl ester transfer protein-mediated transfer of cholesteryl esters from HDL to VLDL. *J Lipid Res*; 40:2333-9.

Purnell JQ, Dev RK, Steffes MW, Cleary PA, Palmer JP, Hirsch IB, Hokanson JE & Brunzell JD. (2003). Relationship of family history of type 2 diabetes, hypoglycemia, and autoantibodies to weight gain and lipids with intensive and conventional therapy in the Diabetes Control and Complications Trial. *Diabetes*; 52: 2623-9.

Ritter MC & Bagdade JD. (1994). Contribution of glycaemic control, endogenous lipoproteins and cholesteryl ester transfer protein to accelerated cholesteryl ester transfer in IDDM. *Eur J Clin Invest*; 24: 607-14.

Rivellese A, Riccardi G, Romano G, Giacco R, Patti L, Marotta G et al. (1988). Presence of very low density lipoprotein compositional abnormalities in type 1 (insulin-dependent) diabetic patients; effects of blood glucose optimisation. *Diabetologia*; 31: 884-8.

Ruotolo G, Parlavecchia M, Taskinen MR, Galimberti G, Zoppo A, Le NA et al. (1994). Normalization of lipoprotein composition by intraperitoneal insulin in IDDM. Role of increased hepatic lipase activity. *Diabetes Care*; 17: 6-12.

Sammett D & Tall AR. (1985). Mechanisms of enhancement of cholesteryl ester transfer protein activity by lipolysis. *J Biol Chem*; 260: 6687-97.

Schwab KO, Doerfer J, Naeke A, Rohrer T, Wiemann D, Marg W, Hofer SE, Holl RW & German/Austrian Pediatric DPV Initiative. (2009). Influence of food intake, age, gender, HbA1c, and BMI levels on plasma cholesterol in 29,979 children and adolescents with type 1 diabetes--reference data from the German diabetes documentation and quality management system (DPV). *Pediatr Diabetes.*; 10: 184-92.

Selam JL, Kashyap M, Alberti KG, Lozano J, Hanna M, Turner D et al. (1989). Comparison of intraperitoneal and subcutaneous insulin administration on lipids, apolipoproteins, fuel metabolites, and hormones in type I diabetes mellitus. *Metabolism*; 38: 908-12.

Skyrme-Jones RA, O'Brien RC, Luo M & Meredith IT. (2000). Endothelial vasodilator function is related to low-density lipoprotein particle size and low-density lipoprotein vitamin E content in type 1 diabetes. *J Am Coll Cardiol*; 35: 292-9.

Soedamah-Muthu SS, Chaturvedi N, Toeller M, Ferriss B, Reboldi P, Michel G, Manes C, Fuller JH & EURODIAB Prospective Complications Study Group. (2004). Risk factors for coronary heart disease in type 1 diabetic patients in Europe: the EURODIAB Prospective Complications Study. *Diabetes Care*; 27: 530-7.

Steinbrecher UP & Witztum JL. (1984). Glucosylation of low-density lipoproteins to an extent comparable to that seen in diabetes slows their catabolism. Diabetes; 33:130-4.

Taskinen MR. (1987). Lipoprotein lipase in diabetes. *Diabetes Metab Rev*; 3:551-70.

Taskinen MR. (1992). Quantitative and qualitative lipoprotein abnormalities in diabetes mellitus. *Diabetes*; 41 (Suppl 2):12-7.

The DCCT Research Group. (1992). Lipid and lipoprotein levels in patients with IDDM diabetes control and complication. Trial experience. *Diabetes Care*; 15: 886-94.

Thomas MC, Rosengård-Bärlund M, Mills V, Rönnback M, Thomas S, Forsblom C et al. (2006). Serum lipids and the progression of nephropathy in type 1 diabetes. *Diabetes Care*; 29: 317-22.

Tribble DL, Holl LG, Wood PD & Krauss RM. (1992). Variations in oxidative susceptibility among six low density lipoprotein subfractions of differing density and particle size. *Atherosclerosis*; 93: 189-99.

Vakkilainen J, Makimattila S, Seppala-Lindroos A, Vehkavaara S, Lahdenpera S, Groop PH et al. (2000). Endothelial dysfunction in men with small LDL particles. *Circulation*; 102: 716-21.

Vergès B. (2001). Insulin sensitiviy and lipids. *Diabetes Metab*; 27: 223-7.

Weidman SW, Ragland JB, Fisher JN Jr, Kitabchi AE & Sabesin SM.J. (1982). Effects of insulin on plasma lipoproteins in diabetic ketoacidosis: evidence for a change in high density lipoprotein composition during treatment. *J Lipid Res*; 23: 171-82.

Winocour PH, Durrington PN, Ishola M & Anderson DC. (1986). Lipoprotein abnormalities in insulin-dependent diabetes mellitus. *Lancet*; 1: 1176-8.

Witztum JL, Mahoney EM, Branks MJ, Fisher M, Elam R & Steinberg D. (1982). Nonenzymatic glucosylation of low-density lipoprotein alters its biologic activity. *Diabetes*; 31: 283-91.

3

Diet, Lifestyle and Chronic Complications in Type 1 Diabetic Patients

S. S. Soedamah-Muthu[1], S. Abbring[1] and M. Toeller[2]
[1]Division of Human Nutrition, Wageningen University, Wageningen
[2]Department of Endocrinology, Diabetology and Rheumatology
Heinrich-Heine-University Duesseldorf
[1]Netherlands
[2]Germany

1. Introduction

Diabetes mellitus is with 220.000 deaths per year the eighth leading cause of death in high income countries (World Health Organization (WHO) 2008). In 2007, over 740.000 people in the Netherlands were suffering from diabetes and this number is expected to grow to 1.3 million people in 2025 (National Institute for Public Health and the Environment (RIVM) 2010). Worldwide approximately 285 million people had the disease in 2010 and this number will increase till 438 million in 2030 (World Diabetes Foundation (WDF) 2010). In 2000, diabetes was most prevalent in India with 31.7 million cases. China (20.8 million cases) and the United States (17.7 million cases) were on the second and third place. Diabetes also has a great economic impact on the individual, nation healthcare system and economy (International Diabetes Federation (IDF) 2010).

Type 1 diabetes accounts for 5% of all cases of diabetes worldwide. Of this 5% the vast majority are children. In type 1 diabetes the body does not produce insulin (American Diabetes Association (ADA) 2010).The disease has a strong genetic component, inherited mainly through the HLA complex but the exact cause is unknown. Most likely there is an environmental trigger in genetically susceptible people that causes an immune reaction. The body's white blood cells mistakenly attack the insulin-producing pancreatic β-cells (U.S. National Library of Medicine 2011). Putative environmental triggers include viruses (e.g. enteroviruses), environmental toxins (e.g. nitrosamines) or foods (e.g. early exposure to cow's milk proteins, cereals or gluten) (Daneman D 2006). This 'food' trigger explains why type 1 diabetes is less common in people who were breastfed and in those who first ate solid foods at later ages (Sadauskaitė-Kuehne V et al. 2004; American Diabetes Association (ADA) 2010).

People with type 1 diabetes also have an increased risk of developing some serious and life threatening complications. This involves acute complications, like hyperglycaemia and hypoglycaemia which can lead to a coma, but also chronic complications (National Institute for Public Health and the Environment (RIVM) 2007). Chronic complications can be subdivided into macrovascular and microvascular complications. Cardiovascular disease is the major macrovascular complication and includes mainly myocardial infarction and stroke (American Diabetes Association (ADA) 2010). The risk for cardiovascular disease, is 4-8 times higher for people with type 1 diabetes (Soedamah-Muthu SS et al. 2006). The major microvascular complications are diabetic nephropathy, diabetic neuropathy and diabetic retinopathy (American Diabetes Association (ADA) 2010). Of the patients with type 1 diabetes approximately 29% develop persistent microalbuminuria (urinary albumin excretion rate between 30 and 300 mg/24 h) after 20 years. Of these 29%, 34% progressed further to persistent macroalbuminuria (urinary albumin excretion rate > 300 mg/24 h). Persistent microalbuminuria is a risk factor for the development of diabetic nephropathy. Microalbuminuria can be seen as an early marker of diabetic kidney disease (Hovind P 2004). Also retinopathy is a common microvascular complication. The 25-year cumulative incidences of any visual impairment and severe visual impairment are 13% and 3%, respectively. Diabetic retinopathy is an important cause of visual impairment (Klein R et al. 2010). Finally the high incidence of lower extremity amputations also stresses how serious the complications of type 1 diabetes are. The overall 25-year incidence of lower extremity amputations is 10.1% in 943 American type 1 diabetic patients (Sahakyan K et al. 2011). These complications account for the major morbidity and mortality associated with type 1 diabetes, so it is very important to treat them (Daneman D 2006).

In type 1 diabetes, special attention is paid to balancing the insulin dose with episodes of activity and the quantity and timing of food intake to prevent acute episodes of hypoglycaemia and hyperglycaemia (Franz MJ et al. 2003). This is important because these acute complications can lead to a coma, but also because a high blood glucose concentration (glycosylated hemoglobin (HbA1c) ≥ 7%) in people with diabetes increases the risk for macrovascular as well as microvascular complications. Other risk factors for these chronic complications are smoking, obesity, physical inactivity, high blood pressure and high cholesterol levels. Also people with a longer history of diabetes have a higher risk (National Institute for Public Health and the Environment (RIVM) 2007). Furthermore it is important to realise that the microvascular complications lie on the pathway between diabetes and cardiovascular disease. Nephropathy for example is an important risk factor for cardiovascular disease in people with type 1 diabetes (Jensen T et al. 1987).

Recent studies have shown that people with type 1 diabetes eat a more atherosclerosis-prone diet. This includes a high intake of energy from saturated fat and a low intake of fiber, fruits and vegetables, which could increase the risk of the development of atherosclerosis. An atherogenic diet may contribute to the risk of cardiovascular disease (Øverby NC et al. 2006; Snell-Bergeon JK et al. 2009). It has been demonstrated that 80%-90% of type 2 diabetes and coronary heart disease cases can be prevented by healthy lifestyle behavior with a focus on healthy diet and exercise.(Stampfer et al. 2000; Hu et al. 2001; Yusuf et al. 2004) These studies suggest that there could be a potential role for diet in type 1 diabetes to reduce the risk of cardiovascular disease.

There are more studies suggesting that diet (including alcohol) can play an important role in treating the complications of diabetes (Franz MJ et al. 2003; Franz et al. 2010). Several studies have reviewed nutritional recommendations for people with diabetes (Franz MJ et al. 2003; Toeller M July 2010). But most of these recommendations combine both type 1 as well as type 2 diabetes. Furthermore they are general and not always specific for the different type of complications. An overview of the relationship between diet (including alcohol) and complications in type 1 diabetic patients is lacking. Also the effect of lifestyle (including physical activity and dietary patterns) on complications is still not elucidated for type 1 diabetic patients. Lack of physical activity together with an atherogenic diet could enhance development of complications especially in high risk type 1 diabetic patients.

In the following paragraphs of this bookchapter the literature on associations between diet (including alcohol) and lifestyle and chronic complications in type 1 diabetic patients will be summarized. Since 'diet' and 'lifestyle' are broad terms the focus will be on macronutrients (carbohydrates (including fiber), proteins and fats (including cholesterol), alcohol, physical activity and dietary patterns. The paragraphs are divided by nephropathy, retinopathy and CVD. In the final paragraphs all recommendations on diet and lifestyle in patients with type 1 diabetes will be put in perspective with the current literature.

2. Diet, lifestyle and nephropathy

Eighteen studies reported an association between macronutrients and type 1 diabetic nephropathy. Of these, thirteen reported results for the association between protein and nephropathy. The other five focussed on other dietary macronutrients such as fat, cholesterol or carbohydrate in relation with nephropathy. There were also three studies that reported results for protein as well as carbohydrate or fats and nephropathy. Furthermore one study reported an association between alcohol consumption and nephropathy in type 1 diabetic patients and one study reported an association between physical activity and nephropathy in type 1 diabetic patients. No studies were found examining the effect of glycaemic index/glycaemic load on nephropathy in type 1 diabetic patients.

2.1 Macronutrients
2.1.1 Protein
Of the thirteen studies that reported an association between protein and nephropathy there were three cross-sectional studies (Toeller M et al. 1997; Riley MD& Dwyer T 1998; O'Hayon BE et al. 2000), one case control study (Möllsten AV et al. 2001), two cohort studies (Jibani MM et al. 1991; Barsotti G et al. 1998), six randomized controlled trials (Brouhard BH& LaGrone L 1990; Zeller K et al. 1991; Dullaart RP et al. 1993; Raal FJ et al. 1994; Hansen HP et al. 1999; Hansen HP et al. 2002) and a pilot study (Percheron C et al. 1995). These will be discussed in the following paragraphs by study design.
The three cross-sectional studies were not consistent in their conclusions on the effect of protein on diabetic nephropathy. O'Hayon et al. (O'Hayon BE et al. 2000) failed to show a significant relationship between dietary protein intake and markers of early nephropathy, other than creatinine clearance. Toeller et al. (Toeller M et al. 1997) found a significant relationship between dietary protein intake and urinary albumin excretion rate (AER). A higher AER was particularly found in people consuming more than 20% of their dietary food energy as protein. Riley et al. (Riley MD& Dwyer T 1998) even found the opposite, a decreased prevalence of microalbuminuria at high relative intakes of protein.
In the case-control study (Möllsten AV et al. 2001) total protein intake was not associated with the presence of microalbuminuria, but a diet including a high amount of fish protein seemed to decrease the risk. Furthermore they could not confirm an association between a high total animal protein intake and having microalbuminuria. In contrast to this finding , Jibani et al. (Jibani MM et al. 1991) found in their cohort study that a predominantly vegetarian diet (low in animal protein) may have an important beneficial effect on diabetic nephropathy without the need for a heavily restricted total protein intake. But they were not able to determine if the reduction in total protein intake rather than the reduction in the fraction of animal origin was primarily responsible for the fall in the fractional albumin clearance. Another (Barsotti G et al. 1998) cohort study showed that a low protein diet has a protective effect on the residual renal function in type 1 diabetic patients.

In conclusion, these studies were not consistent in their conclusions on the effect of protein restriction on type 1 diabetic nephropathy. Furthermore there is not enough evidence for recommendations about the preferred type of dietary protein.

Of the six randomized controlled trials reporting an association between protein and nephropathy (**Table 1**), four have reported a decline in glomerular filtration rate (GFR) during the low protein diet (protein intake of approximately 0.8 g/kg/day) (Brouhard BH& LaGrone L 1990; Dullaart RP et al. 1993; Hansen HP et al. 1999; Hansen HP et al. 2002). In one of these four this decline was greater in the low protein diet group than in the usual protein diet group, but this difference was not significant (Hansen HP et al. 1999). In two studies this decline was greater in the usual protein diet group than in the low protein group (Brouhard BH& LaGrone L 1990; Hansen HP et al. 2002). Among these 2 studies, one (Brouhard BH& LaGrone L 1990) found a decline that was significantly greater in the usual protein group. Another study showed a decline in GFR in the low protein diet group, but did not directly compare this with the usual protein group (Dullaart RP et al. 1993). Only one study(Raal FJ et al. 1994) reported an increase in GFR during the low protein diet, but this increase was not significant. Zeller et al. (Zeller K et al. 1991) used iothalamate clearance and creatinine clearance to assess renal function. The rates of decline in both iothalamate and creatinine clearence were significantly slower in the patients in the study-diet group than in those in the control-diet group.

Five trials reported an effect of protein on albuminuria (Brouhard BH& LaGrone L 1990; Dullaart RP et al. 1993; Raal FJ et al. 1994; Hansen HP et al. 1999; Hansen HP et al. 2002). In three of these five trials there was a decline in albuminuria in the low protein diet group as well as in the usual protein diet group (Dullaart RP et al. 1993; Hansen HP et al. 1999; Hansen HP et al. 2002). Two of these three showed a significant greater decline in albuminuria in the low protein diet group than in the usual protein diet group (Dullaart RP et al. 1993; Hansen HP et al. 1999). The other two trials showed a decline in albuminuria in the low protein diet group and an increase in the usual diet protein group (Brouhard BH& LaGrone L 1990; Raal FJ et al. 1994). One of these (Brouhard BH& LaGrone L 1990) found a significant difference between the diet groups. Furthermore, another (pilot) study (Percheron C et al. 1995) also found a decline in albuminuria and in creatinine clearance. They conclude that moderately (protein intake of approximately 1.2 g/kg/day) rather than severely protein restricted diets (protein intake of approximately 0.8 g/kg/day) should be recommended, because of the lack of compliance with severely protein restricted diets. The only trial (Hansen HP et al. 2002) that determined the effect of dietary protein restriction on survival and progression to end stage renal disease (ESRD) in diabetic nephropathy reported a relative risk of 0.23 (95% CI: 0.07-0.72) for ESRD in patients assigned to a low-protein diet compared with patients assigned to a usual protein diet.

In conclusion, protein restriction (protein intake of approximately 0.8 g/kg/day, **Table 1**) had a positive significant effect on albuminuria, but no effect on GFR was found.

2.1.2 Carbohydrate

Two cross-sectional studies (Watts GF et al. 1988; Riley MD& Dwyer T 1998) examined the association between carbohydrates and nephropathy. In one study (Watts GF et al. 1988) type 1 diabetic patients with microalbuminuria consumed a significantly smaller percentage of total energy as carbohydrate compared with patients with normal albumin excretion. In the other study (Riley MD& Dwyer T 1998) no significant association between energy adjusted carbohydrate intake and microalbuminuria was found. This could be due to their

Ref.	Study pop.	Age (mean or range)	Study duration	Exposure	Results Mean protein intake (g/kg/day)	GFR	Albuminuria
Hansen (2002) (Hansen HP et al., 2002)	n=82	18-60	4 years	LPD (0.6 g/kg/day) vs. UPD	LPD: 0.89 UPD: 1.02	LPD: mean decline 3.8 ml/min/yr UPD: mean decline 3.9 ml/min/yr	LPD: mean decline 148 mg/24 h UPD: mean decline 107 mg/24 h
Hansen (1999) (Hansen HP et al., 1999)	n=29	18-60	8 weeks	LPD (0.6 g/kg/day) vs. UPD	LPD: 0.8 UPD: 1.1	LPD: mean decline 8.6 ml/min/1,73m² UPD: mean decline 2.5 ml/min/1,73m²	LPD: mean decline 28.7% UPD: mean decline 0.0%
Raal (1994) (Raal FJ et al., 1994)	n=22	20-41	6 months	Unrestricted protein diet (>1.6 g/kg/day) vs. moderately protein-restricted diet (0.8 g/kg/day)	LPD: 0.87 UPD: 2.00	LPD: mean increase 3 ml/min/1,73m² UPD: mean decline 8 ml/min/1,73m²	LPD: mean decline 1.02 g/day UPD: mean increase 0.34 g/day
Dullaart (1993) (Dullaart RP et al., 1993)	n=30	40,8	2 years	LPD (0.6 g/kg/day) vs. UPD	LPD: 0.79		LPD: mean decline 26%* UPD: mean decline 5%*
Zeller (1991) (Zeller K et al., 1991)	n=35	18-60	mean: 34.7 months	LPLP (0.6g/kg/day protein; 500-1000 mg phosphorus) vs. Control diet (1.0 g/kg/day protein; 1000 mg phosphorus)	LPLP: 0.72 Control: 1.08	LPLP: IC: decline of 0.0043 ml/s/mo CC: 0.0055 ml/s/mo Control: IC: decline of 0.0168 ml/s/mo CC: 0.0135 ml/s/mo	
Brouchard (1990) (Brouchard BH& LaGrone L 1990)	n=15	18-49	12 months	LPD (0.6 g/kg/day) vs. UPD	LPD: 1.3 UPD: 1.5	LPD: decline 0.28 ml/min/1,73m²/mo UPD: decline 0.68 ml/min/1,73m²/mo	LPD: mean decline 407 µg/min UPD: mean increase 1055 µg/min

* after adjustment for MAP (mean arterial pressure) and diabetes duration
GFR: glomerular filtration rate; LPD: low protein diet; UPD: usual protein diet; LPLP: low protein, low phosphorus; IC: iothalamate clearance; CC: creatinine clearance

Table 1. Randomized controlled trials; protein and diabetic nephropathy

study design (cross-sectional), due to a substantial measurement error in the food frequency questionnaires (FFQs) and due to the low response rate (61.2%) for participation.

2.1.3 Fat/cholesterol

Four cross-sectional studies reported an association between fat and/or cholesterol and nephropathy (Watts GF et al. 1988; Bouhanick B 1995; Riley MD& Dwyer T 1998; Toeller M et al. 1999 [1]). One study (Riley MD& Dwyer T 1998) found no significant association between energy adjusted monounsaturated fat intake or energy adjusted polyunsaturated fat intake and microalbuminuria, but reported a positive association between usual dietary saturated fat intake and microalbuminuria. Another study (Watts GF et al. 1988) found a significant positive association between total fat intake and microalbuminuria. Another study (Bouhanick B 1995) examined the relationship between fat intake and glomerular hyperfiltration (GFR > 173 ml/min/1.73m²), a marker for diabetic nephropathy, in type 1 diabetic patients. They found that excess fat intake may contribute to hyperfiltration in type 1 diabetic patients. Finally the fourth study(Toeller M et al. 1999 [1]) found a higher intake of cholesterol, total fat and saturated fat in Eastern Europe compared to Southern or North-Western Europe. They also found more frequent acute and chronic complications (including nephropathy) in Eastern Europe people. Since it was a cross-sectional study they could not conclude if this was due to the high intake of cholesterol, total fat and/or saturated fat.

These cross-sectional studies show that there seems to be a detrimental effect of total dietary fat intake as well as saturated fat intake on type 1 diabetic nephropathy. No association between energy adjusted MUFA and energy adjusted PUFA and microalbuminuria was found.

In a case-control study (Möllsten AV et al. 2001), no association between total fat intake and microalbuminuria was found. In a prospective study (Cárdenas C et al. 2004) a progression of nephropathy with greater saturated fatty acid (SFA) consumption and lesser polyunsaturated fatty acid consumption (PUFA) was demonstrated. Specifically with higher SFA-to-PUFA and SFA-to-MUFA ratios. Another prospective cohort study (Lee CC et al. 2010) found an association between PUFA and microalbuminuria. They found that dietary n-3 PUFAs (eicosapentaenoic acid and docosahexaenoic acid) are inversely associated with the degree but not with the incidence of albuminuria in type 1 diabetes (Lee CC et al. 2010).

In conclusion these prospective studies are consistent with the cross-sectional studies about the detrimental effect of saturated fat on type 1 diabetic nephropathy. The effect of total fat intake on nephropathy is still not elucidated. The cross-sectional study of Watts et al. (Watts GF et al. 1988) and the case control study of Möllsten et al. (Möllsten AV et al. 2001) were in contrast with each other. Also the effect of PUFAs on nephropathy is still doubtful, but there seems to be an inverse association between n-3 PUFAs and the degree of albuminuria.

2.1.4 Alcohol

In the EURODIAB Prospective Complications Study (Beulens et al. 2008) the association between alcohol and nephropathy was analysed cross-sectionally. They found that moderate alcohol consumers (30-70 g alcohol per week) had a lower risk of diabetic nephropathy, with an odds ratio of 0.36 (95% CI: 0.18-0.71). This association was most pronounced for the consumption of wine.

2.1.5 Physical activity

There were no prospective studies on physical activity and type 1 diabetic nephropathy. One cross-sectional study (Kriska AM et al. 1991) found the lowest occurrence of diabetic nephropathy in people being 7+ hours a week physically active (sports and leisure physical activity).

3. Diet, lifestyle and retinopathy

Only two studies reported results for the association between macronutrients and type 1 diabetic retinopathy. Furthermore two studies reported an association between alcohol consumption and diabetic retinopathy and one study reported an association between physical activity and diabetic retinopathy. No studies were found examining the effect of glycaemic index/glycaemic load on retinopathy in type 1 diabetic patients.

3.1 Macronutrients

In post-hoc analyses (Cundiff DK& Nigg CR 2005) a positive association between total dietary fat, saturated fat and MUFA with retinopathy progression and retinopathy risk factors (mean arterial pressure, LDL/HDL cholesterol ratio, serum triglycerides, HbA1c, body mass index, and insulin utilization) was found. Furthermore, a negative association between carbohydrates and dietary fiber with retinopathy progression and risk factors was found. In addition to this, another cross-sectional study(Toeller M et al. 1999 [1]) reported a higher intake of cholesterol, total fat and saturated fat in Eastern Europe compared to Southern or North-Western Europe. They also found more frequent acute and chronic complications (including retinopathy) in Eastern European people. As with nephropathy, they could not conclude if this was due to the high intake of cholesterol, total fat and/or saturated fat.

In conclusion there is limited research on the effect of diet on diabetic retinopathy. The results of the post hoc analyses should be interpreted carefully, since it is a retrospective analysis which can generate hypotheses but not prove them.

3.1.2 Alcohol

In cross-sectional analyses of the EURODIAB Prospective Complications Study (Beulens et al. 2008) moderate alcohol consumers (30-70 g alcohol per week) had a lower risk of diabetic proliferative retinopathy, with an odds ratio of 0.60 (95% CI: 0.37-0.99). This association was most pronounced for the consumption of wine. Another cross-sectional study (Moss SE et al. 1992) examined whether alcohol consumption was associated with type 1 diabetic retinopathy. They found that moderate alcohol consumption was inversely associated with the prevalence of retinopathy (OR=0.49, 95% CI: 0.27-0.92) in patients with type 1 diabetes.

3.1.3 Physical activity

One cross-sectional study (Kriska AM et al. 1991) examined the relationship between physical activity and the occurrence of retinopathy in type 1 diabetic patients. They found no association between physical activity (sports and leisure physical activity) and occurrence of retinopathy.

4. Diet, lifestyle and cardiovascular disease

Eight studies reported an association between macronutrients and CVD in type 1 diabetic patients. Of these eight, six are cross-sectional studies (Toeller M et al. 1999 [1,2,3]; Helgeson 2006; Øverby NC et al. 2006; Snell-Bergeon JK et al. 2009). Only Strychar et al. (Strychar I et al. 2009) and Georgopoulos et al. (Georgopoulos A et al. 2000) performed a randomized controlled trial. One study reported an association between lifestyle risk factors (including alcohol) and atherosclerosis, which is often the underlying cause of CVD (Bishop et al. 2009). Eight studies reported an association between physical activity and CVD risk factors (Kriska AM et al. 1991; Lehmann R et al. 1997; Fuchsjäger-Mayrl G et al. 2002; Herbst A et al. 2007; Valerio G et al. 2007; Bishop et al. 2009; Trigona B et al. 2010; Seeger JPH et al. 2011), and two studies reported an association with dietary patterns (Gunther ALB et al. 2008; Liese AD et al. 2011). Furthermore no studies were found examining the effect of glycaemic index/glycaemic load on CVD in type 1 diabetic patients.

4.1 Macronutrients
Data on the relationship between macronutrients and incident CVD is lacking in patients with type 1 diabetes. Limited information on macronutrients is available from cross-sectional studies. Main focus was on fat, in particularly saturated fat, and fiber and CVD risk factors were used as a proxy for CVD events.

4.2 Cross-sectional studies on fat and fiber in relation to CVD
In more detail, one cross-sectional study (Øverby NC et al. 2006) found a higher than recommended percentage of energy intake from fat and saturated fat among type 1 diabetic patients compared with healthy same-age control subjects and a lower than recommended intake of fiber. They conclude that this higher intake of energy from saturated fat and this lower intake of energy from dietary fiber, vegetables and fruits could increase the risk of atherosclerosis, which is often the underlying cause of CVD. Another study (Helgeson 2006) reported a higher than recommended percentage of energy intake from fat and saturated fat among type 1 diabetic patients, but they did not study associations with CVD or CVD risk factors. Another cross-sectional study (Toeller M et al. 1999 [2]) found similar associations between dietary fiber and CVD. Higher fiber intake had a protective significant effect against CVD in type 1 diabetic women but not in men. In type 1 diabetic men it leads to positive changes of the serum cholesterol pattern (higher HDL, lower LDL, lower ratio total cholesterol:HDL cholesterol). In another study (Toeller M et al. 1999 [3]) a significant increase in energy adjusted total and LDL-cholesterol levels was associated with higher intakes of total fat, saturated fat and cholesterol. This was associated with a higher prevalence of CVD, although after adjusting for dietary fiber intake, these associations were attenuated. A third study by Toeller et al. (Toeller M et al. 1999 [1]) found a higher intake of cholesterol, total fat and saturated fat in Eastern Europe compared to Southern or North-Western Europe. They also found more frequent acute and chronic complications (including CVD) in Eastern European people. However, since it was a cross-sectional study they could not conclude if this was due to the high intake of cholesterol, total fat and/or saturated fat. In the CACTI study (Snell-Bergeon JK et al. 2009) found an increased risk of CVD in type 1 diabetic patients eating high amounts of fat and saturated fat. Carbohydrates were negatively correlated with CHD risk factors (higher total cholesterol, LDL cholesterol, obesity, poorer glycaemic control). Furthermore higher intakes of fat and protein were associated with greater odds of coronary artery calcium (CAC), which is a strong predictor for coronary

events approximating CVD risk. The opposite was true for carbohydrate intake, higher intake was associated with a reduced odds of CAC.

In conclusion a higher intake of total fat as well as saturated fat is positively correlated with CVD or CVD risk factors (atherosclerosis and CAC in these studies) and a higher intake of carbohydrate is negatively correlated with CVD or CVD risk factors. Furthermore dietary fiber is independently related to a lower risk for CVD in type 1 diabetic women. Since all these studies were cross-sectional, they could only look at the intake of certain nutrients and the prevalence of CVD or CVD risk factors at a certain time point. They could not conclude if these are related to each other and if the nutrients are responsible for the lower or higher prevalence of CVD.

4.3 Randomized controlled trials

Two randomized controlled trials reported an association between macronutrients and CVD (**Table 2**), but demonstrated conflicting conclusions. In one trial (Strychar I et al. 2009), the authors concluded that a diet lower in carbohydrate and higher in MUFA might be preferable to a diet higher in carbohydrate and lower in MUFA for type 1 diabetic patients. This was solely based on the positive effect on triglyceride (TG) levels and plasminogen activator inhibitor 1 levels (PAI-1) in the first diet. A significant decrease in PAI-1 was found after 6 months in the lower carbohydrate and higher MUFA diet. In the other diet there was a significant increase after 6 months of follow up. PAI-1 is an inhibitor of fibrinolysis, a process that degrades blood clots. A lower level of PAI-1 means less inhibition and more degradation of blood clots, which means a lower chance of developing atherosclerosis. Also a decrease in TG levels was found after 6 months following the low carbohydrate/high MUFA diet, although this decrease was not significant. In the other diet group there was an increase in TG levels, also this increase was not significant. Furthermore they conclude that the lower carbohydrate/higher MUFA diet was only a proper choice for nonobese individuals with weight control since this diet had induced a weight gain of 2% (1.6 kg) after 6 months. The other trial (Georgopoulos A et al. 2000) found exactly the opposite using a crossover design. They found that a diet high in carbohydrates might be preferable to a diet high in MUFA. Mainly because of the higher atherosclerotic risk due to more and bigger very low-density lipoprotein (VLDL) particles in the last diet. Furthermore the TG levels did not significantly differ between the two diets in this study.

In conclusion, these trials show that the effect of carbohydrate or MUFA on cardiovascular disease risk factors in type 1 diabetic patients is still not elucidated. Although they recommend exactly the opposite (higher intake of MUFA preferable vs. higher intake of carbohydrate preferable) they both found that a high MUFA or a high carbohydrate diet did not affect the TG levels. Their conclusions are based on PAI-1 and VLDL levels, which are not such a good predictors for atherosclerosis (and by extension CVD) as TG levels are. Furthermore none of these randomized controlled trials examined the potential positive effect of dietary fiber on CVD or the potential negative effect of saturated fat found in cross-sectional studies.

4.4 Alcohol

One cross-sectional study (Bishop et al. 2009) reported findings on the association between alcohol and cardiovascular disease. No significant association was found between alcohol consumption (±13.8 drinks/month) and CAC, a marker of coronary artery atherosclerosis (adjusted OR=0.9, 95% CI: 0.8-1.1, p=0.15). The positive effect of moderate alcohol

Ref.	Study pop.	Age (mean or range)	Study duration	Exposure	Results		
					PAI-1 (ng/ml) (mean ± SD)	TG (mmol/l) (mean ± SD)	VLDL (mg/l) (mean ± SEM)
Strychar (2009) (Strychar I et al., 2009)	n=30	37.9	6 months	diet high in CH/low in fat* vs. diet low in CH/high in fat**	HCLF: change after 6 mo: -12.8 ± 27.0 LCHF: change after 6 mo: + 14.2 ± 24.5	HCLF: change after 6 mo: -0.03 ± 0.22 LCHF: change after 6 mo: +0.14 ± 0.46	
Georgopoulos (2000) (Georgopoulos A et al., 2000)	n=19	22-47	4 weeks	diet high in MUFA*** vs. diet high in CH****		High MUFA: 0.89 ± 0.39 High CH: 0.90 ± 0.36	High MUFA: 31.4 ± 7.4 High CH: 20.0 ± 3.8

* 54-57% CH, 27-30% total fat (10% MUFA)
** 43-46% CH, 37-40% total fat (20% MUFA)
*** 40% total fatty acids (25% MUFA, 6% PUFA, 9% saturated), 45% CH and 15% protein
**** 24% total fatty acids (9% MUFA, 6% PUFA, 9% saturated), 61% CH and 15% protein
PAI-1: plasminogen activator inhibitor 1; TG: triglycerides; VLDL: very low-density lipoprotein; SD: standard deviation; SEM: standard error of mean; CH: carbohydrate; MUFA: monounsaturated fatty acid; HCLF: high carbohydrate, low fat; LCHF: low carbohydrate, high fat

Table 2. Randomized controlled trials; diet and cardiovascular disease

consumption on CVD as in the general population is not confirmed for type 1 diabetic patients in this study. However, this could also be due to the kind of study (cross-sectional) and the fact that markers for CVD were used instead of CVD as endpoint. There are no prospective studies which have addressed the relation between alcohol and CVD in type 1 diabetic patients.

4.5 Physical activity

Of the eight studies that reported an association between physical activity and CVD there were five cross-sectional studies (Kriska AM et al. 1991; Herbst A et al. 2007; Valerio G et al. 2007; Bishop et al. 2009; Trigona B et al. 2010) and three trials (Lehmann R et al. 1997; Fuchsjäger-Mayrl G et al. 2002; Seeger JPH et al. 2011). No prospective cohort studies were found. The studies will be discussed in the following paragraphs by study design.

One study (Kriska AM et al. 1991) examined the relationship between physical activity and the occurrence of CVD in type 1 diabetic patients. They found the lowest occurrence of CVD in people being 4-7 hours a week physical active (sports and leisure physical activity). The other four cross-sectional studies examined an association between physical activity and CVD risk factors. They all found a positive association. Another two studies (Herbst A et al. 2007; Valerio G et al. 2007) found that increased frequency of regular physical activity was associated with lower TG levels. One of these (Herbst A et al. 2007) found besides the positive association with TG levels also a positive significant association between regular physical activity and HDL cholesterol levels. Another study (Trigona B et al. 2010) found that 60 min/day of moderate-to-vigorous physical activity was associated with an enhanced endothelial function in type 1 diabetic patients. Impaired endothelial function is considered as an early sign of atherosclerosis, which is often the underlying cause of CVD. And finally, (Bishop et al. 2009) a significant inverse association between physical activity and CAC, a marker of coronary artery atherosclerosis, was demonstrated.

In conclusion all these studies found a beneficial effect of physical activity on cardiovascular risk factors. However, since all these studies were cross-sectional, they could only look at physical activity and the prevalence of CVD or CVD risk factors at a certain time point. They could not conclude if these are related to each other and if physical activity was responsible for the lower prevalence of CVD.

The three trials reporting an association between physical activity and cardiovascular disease risk factors (**Table 3**) were consistent in their conclusions. They all emphasize an important role for physical activity in type 1 diabetic patients. Two studies (Fuchsjäger-Mayrl G et al. 2002; Seeger JPH et al. 2011) examined the association between physical activity and brachial artery flow-mediated dilation (FMD). Endothelial dysfunction is reflected by an impaired FMD response and is an early sign of atherosclerosis. An increase in FMD was found in type 1 diabetic patients following an exercise training program (endurance sports; on average 2 times a week 60 minutes, **Table 3**). In both trials this increase was significant (p=0.038 and p=0.040 respectively). Two studies (Lehmann R et al. 1997; Fuchsjäger-Mayrl G et al. 2002) examined the impact of physical activity on lipid related cardiovascular risk factors (LDL cholesterol, HDL cholesterol and TG). They both found a decrease in LDL cholesterol levels in the training group, but only in one of these (Lehmann R et al. 1997) this decrease was significant (p=0.02). An additional effect was reported in one of these studies (Lehmann R et al. 1997) with a significant increase in HDL cholesterol levels (p=0.03) in the training group. No effect of physical activity on TG levels

Ref.	Study pop.	Age (mean)	Study duration	Exposure	Results VO$_{2max}$	FMD (%)	Triglycerides (mmol/L)	LDL cholesterol (mmol/L)	HDL cholesterol (mmol/L)
Seeger (2011) (Seeger JPH et al., 2011)	n=7	10.9	18 weeks	18 week exercise training program*	Mean increase: 2.0 ml/kg/min	Mean increase: 4.9			
Fuchsjäger-Mayrl (2002) (Fuchsjäger-Mayrl G et al., 2002)	n=23	37.5	4 months	TrGr: 4 mo exercise training program** C: type 1 diabetic patients following usual lifestyle	TrGr: mean increase: 7.6 ml/kg/min C: mean increase: 0.1 ml/kg/min	TrGr: mean increase: 3.3 C: mean increase: 0.7	TrGr: mean decline: 0.2 C: mean increase: 0.2	TrGr: mean decline: 0.3 C: mean decline: 0.2	TrGr: mean decrease: 0.2 C: mean decrease: 0.2
Lehmann (1997) (Lehmann R et al., 1997)	n=20	33.0	3 months	3 month exercise training program***	Mean increase: 178 ml/min		Mean increase: 0.09	Mean decline: 0.4	Mean increase: 0.16

* two times a week: first day: 30 min running exercise (intervals) and 30 min group-based activities such as ball games, short relay races, running techniques and stretching; second day: individual exercise session at home involved 30 min of interval running and a 10-min warm-up and cooling down (including stretching)

** first 2 weeks: two times a week 1 hour stationary cycling, during the remaining study period three times a week 1 hour stationary cycling

*** 135 min per week endurance sports (biking, long-distance running, or hiking)

VO$_{2max}$: peak oxygen uptake; FMD: flow mediated dilation; LDL: low-density lipoprotein; HDL: high-density lipoprotein; TrGR: training group; C: control group

Table 3. Randomized controlled trials; physical activity and cardiovascular disease risk factors

was found in both studies. Furthermore all three studies (Lehmann R et al. 1997; Fuchsjäger-Mayrl G et al. 2002; Seeger JPH et al. 2011) assessed physical fitness by VO_{2max} (peak oxygen uptake). They all found a positive significant association between physical activity and VO_{2max}. The relation between physical fitness and CVD was not examined.

In conclusion the three trials show that physical activity improves physical fitness as well as endothelial function in type 1 diabetic patients. A positive effect on lipid related cardiovascular risk factors was only found in one study (Lehmann R et al. 1997).

4.6 Dietary patterns

Two cross-sectional studies reported an association between dietary patterns, in this case the 'Dietary Approaches to Stop Hypertension' (DASH) diet, and CVD risk factors (Gunther ALB et al. 2008; Liese AD et al. 2011). No cross-sectional or prospective studies were found examining the effect of a Mediterranean diet or a Western diet on CVD in type 1 diabetic patients.

One study (Gunther ALB et al. 2008) reported an association between adherence to the DASH diet and hypertension in type 1 diabetic patients. They found that a higher adherence to this diet amongst type 1 diabetic patients was inversely related to hypertension (OR=0.6, 95% CI: 0.4-0.9, p=0.007). They did not investigate a possible association between the DASH diet and CVD, but used hypertension as the main risk factor for CVD. Another study (Liese AD et al. 2011) reported a possible association between the DASH diet and other CVD risk factors (total cholesterol, LDL cholesterol, HDL cholesterol, TG, LDL particle density, apolipoprotein B, body mass index (BMI), waist circumference, and adipocytokines) than blood pressure. A significant and inverse association between the DASH diet and LDL/HDL ratio was found. An estimated 0.07 lower LDL/HDL ratio was found in the highest adherence group compared with the lowest adherence group. No significant association was found between LDL particle density, BMI, waist circumference, adipocytokines, or TG and the DASH diet.

In conclusion a positive effect of adherence to the DASH diet on hypertension and LDL/HDL ratio, which are important risk factors for CVD, was found. Unfortunately there were no studies found examining the effect of dietary patterns on CVD events.

5. Current recommendations on diet and lifestyle in patients with type 1 diabetes put in perspective

Overall, fiber and saturated fat intake play an important role in type 1 diabetic patients, with a beneficial and detrimental effect on the chronic complications respectively. Many researchers have shown the inappropriate intake of these nutrients in patients with type 1 diabetes. A protein restriction diet helped reduce micro/macro albuminuria in known type 1 diabetic patients with nephropathy, however, the compliance was low. Also moderate alcohol intake and physical activity may have beneficial effects in type 1 diabetic patients. Most of the findings are consistent with the guidelines for type 1 diabetic patients (**Table 4**). The main limitations are the lack of prospective studies on diet and lifestyle in type 1 diabetics, lack of randomized controlled trials and the limited number of studies on dietary cholesterol, protein, carbohydrates, fat, fiber and no cardiovascular morbidity data. The available studies, with their limitations, all indicate that diet and lifestyle play an important role in preventing chronic complications of type 1 diabetes. To put the findings in the literature in perspective, current nutritional recommendations are evaluated in the

	Evidence grade A*	Evidence grade B**	Evidence grade C-E***
Carbohydrate[1]	Metabolic characteristics suggest the most appropriate intake: vegetables, legumes, fruits, wholegrain foods, naturally occurring foods rich in fiber; Fiber intake should be ideally ≈ 20 g/1000 kcal/day; Low glycaemic index foods provided other attributes of these foods are appropriate; Moderate amounts of free sugars (up to 50 g/day)	There is no justification for the recommendation of very low carbohydrate diets in persons with diabetes; Cereal-based foods should, whenever possible, be wholegrain and high in fiber	Consider quantity, sources and distribution of CHO to facilitate near-normal long-term glycaemic control; Timing and dosage of insulin or hypoglycaemic agents should match quantity and nature of CHO; Daily consumption of 5 servings of fiber-rich vegetables or fruits and 4 servings of legumes per week help to achieve recommended fiber intake; Total free sugars should not exceed 10% total energy
Dietary fat[1]	Saturated and trans-unsaturated fatty acids <10% total energy (<8% if LDL cholesterol is elevated); Dietary cholesterol <300 mg/day (further reduction of LDL is elevated)	Oils rich in mono-unsaturated fatty acids are encouraged (10-20% total energy), total fat <35% total energy; 2-3 servings of oily fish/week and plant sources of n-3 fatty acids (e.g. rapeseed oil, soybean oil, nuts) are recommended	Polyunsaturated fatty acids should not exceed 10% total daily energy; Total fat intake should not exceed 35% total energy
Protein[1]	0.8 g/kg normal body weight in patients with type 1 diabetes and established nephropathy	10-20% total energy in patients with no evidence of nephropathy	Insufficient evidence for recommendations about the preferred type of dietary protein; For type 1 diabetes with incipient nephropathy and type 2 diabetes with incipient or established nephropathy no firm recommendations regarding protein restriction
Alcohol[1]		Moderate use up to 10 g/day for women and up to 20 g/day for men is possible; In patients treated with insulin or insulin secretagogues alcohol should be taken with carbohydrate to avoid hypoglycaemia	Intake should be limited in overweight, hypertensive, hypertriglyceridemic individuals as well as during pregnancy and in advanced neuropathy
Physical[2] Activity	90 to 150 minutes of accumulated moderate-intensity aerobic physical activity per week as well as resistance/ strength training three times per week is recommended		

[1] obtained from DNSG EASD: Diabetes and Nutrition Study Group of the European Association for the Study of Diabetes(Toeller M July 2010);
[2] obtained from ADA: American Diabetic Association(American Diabetes Association (ADA) 2011)
* Evidence grade A: evidence obtained from meta-analyses of randomized controlled trials or at least one randomized controlled trial
** Evidence grade B: evidence obtained from at least one well designed and controlled study without randomization, well-designed quasi-experimental or non-experimental descriptive study
*** Evidence grade C-E: evidence obtained from expert committee reports or opinions and/or clinical experiences of respected authorities

Table 4. Nutritional recommendations for persons with type 1 and type 2 diabetes

following paragraphs at a macronutrient level. **Table 4** summarizes the nutritional recommendations as well as the lifestyle recommendations for type 1 and type 2 diabetic patients. These recommendations are for all diabetic patients in general, based in the majority of cases on evidence from type 2 diabetic patients.

5.1 Carbohydrates

The 'Diabetes and Nutrition Study Group of the European Association for the Study of Diabetes' (DNSG EASD) guidelines for persons with type 1 and type 2 diabetes (**Table 4**) recommend that the most appropriate intake of carbohydrates consists of vegetables, legumes, fruits, wholegrain foods and naturally occurring foods rich in fiber. The fiber intake should be ideally ≈ 20 g/1000 kcal/day. Cross-sectional data of the EURODIAB Complications Study showed an inverse association between fiber and LDL cholesterol and a positive association between fiber and HDL cholesterol. In addition dietary fiber was inversely and significantly related to CVD (Toeller M et al. 1999 [2]). This effect was already found with a fiber intake of approximately 8.1 g/1000 kcal, which is below the recommended intake. The average fiber intake in type 1 diabetic patients is 8.1 g/1000 kcal, but the recommended intake is 20 g/1000 kcal. Recommendation was only achieved in 0.4% of the type 1 diabetic population (Toeller M et al. 1996). Data from the EURODIAB Prospective Complication Study on fiber intake measured at baseline by 3-day food diaries and presented by each center is given in **Figure 1**. As seen in this figure, even the 10 g/1000 kcal recommended fiber intake by the 'American Diabetes Association' (ADA) was hardly achieved by type 1 diabetic patients. Only Finnish type 1 diabetic patients achieved the ADA fiber recommendation of 10 g/1000 kcal **Figure 1**). Keeping in mind that these samples are clinic based and not population based and that these figures may not exactly reflect the current nutritional intake, however it gives an indication of the status on fiber intake. Although positive effects were already found on CVD with a fiber intake of 8.1 g/1000 kcal, we assume that effects could be probably even higher when recommended levels of fiber intake are reached. Unfortunately, this positive effect of fiber on CVD and CVD risk factors was only found in cross-sectional studies. This makes it very difficult to distinguish cause and effect. Further research in prospective studies or randomized controlled trials is needed to ascertain the role of fiber in CVD.

DNSG EASD do not recommend a low carbohydrate diet for type 1 and type 2 diabetic patients (**Table 4**). A low carbohydrate diet does not produce beneficial health effect. It is more acceptable to avoid too much foods high in fast available carbohydrates, foods high in fat and cholesterol. An earlier quote (Helgeson 2006) expressed this precisely: 'families of adolescents with diabetes may be more concerned that the sugar in candy is going to translate into high blood glucose levels today than that the fat in potato chips will translate into cardiovascular disease in 10 years'.

5.2 Fat

The DNSG EASD guidelines for dietary fat for persons with type 1 and type 2 diabetes recommend a saturated and trans-unsaturated fatty acid consumption of <10% of the total energy intake (<8% if LDL cholesterol is elevated). Total fat intake should not exceed 35% of total energy and dietary cholesterol should be <300 mg/day (**Table 4**). Saturated fat is an important risk factor for diabetic nephropathy, diabetic retinopathy as well as CVD (Riley

MD& Dwyer T 1998; Toeller M et al. 1999 [3]; Cárdenas C et al. 2004; Cundiff DK& Nigg CR 2005). The recommended intake is <10% of the total energy intake which was only achieved by a small minority (14%) (Toeller M et al. 1996). Data from the EURODIAB Prospective Complication Study on saturated fatty acid intake measured at baseline by 3-day food diaries and presented by each center is given in **Figure 2**. The even lower saturated fatty acid recommendation of <7% total energy of the ADA was not achieved by any of the centers (**Figure 2**). All centers indicated in **Figure 2** exceed the recommendation of <7% saturated fat of the total energy intake. Type 1 diabetic patients from Italy had the lowest intake of saturated fatty acids, but this intake was still too high (**Figure 2**). Again, keeping in mind that these samples are clinic based and not population based and that these figures may not exactly reflect the current nutritional intake.

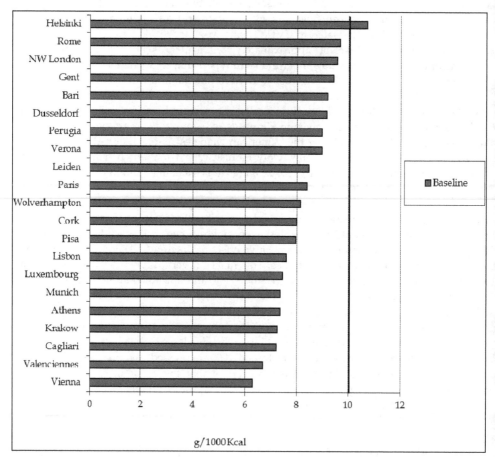

Fig. 1. Mean fiber intake in 1102 individuals with type 1 diabetes across Europa (Toeller M, Soedamah-Muthu 2011)

Furthermore the DNSG EASD guidelines recommend oils rich in MUFA (10-20% total energy) and that PUFA should not exceed 10% of total energy intake (**Table 4**). There were only a few studies examining the effect of MUFA or PUFA on chronic complications in type 1 diabetic patients. A positive association was found between MUFA and retinopathy (Cundiff DK& Nigg CR 2005) but no association was found between MUFA and PUFA and microalbuminuria (Riley MD& Dwyer T 1998). These conclusions are based on post-hoc analyses and a cross-sectional study respectively and should therefore be interpreted carefully. Also the conclusion of Strychar et al. (Strychar I et al. 2009) to recommend a diet higher in MUFA and lower in carbohydrate for nonobese type 1 diabetic individuals to reduce CVD risk factors is doubtful. Their conclusion is based on PAI-1 and VLDL levels, which are not such a good predictors for atherosclerosis (and by extension CVD) as TG levels are. And a high MUFA diet did not alter TG levels. Furthermore, the small study population of 30 subjects limits the power of their conclusions. In order to make accurate recommendations concerning MUFA and PUFA intake for type 1 diabetic patients more research with more participants (preferably in a prospective study) is needed.

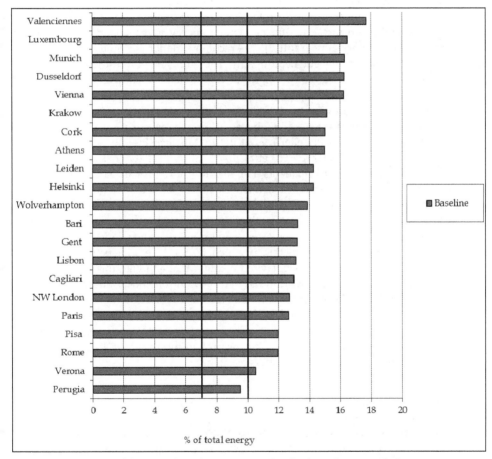

Fig. 2. Mean saturated fatty acid intake in 1102 individuals with type 1 diabetes across Europe (Toeller M, Soedamah-Muthu 2011)

The recommendation of the DNSG EASD to consume 2-3 servings of oily fish/week and plant sources of n-3 fatty acids (**Table 4**) is consistent with the findings in studies specific for type 1 diabetes. The prospective cohort study of Lee et al. (Lee CC et al. 2010) found that dietary n-3 PUFAs (eicosapentaenoic acid and docosahexaenoic acid) are inversely associated with the degree but not with the incidence of albuminuria in type 1 diabetes. A hypothesis is that n-3 PUFAs decrease urinary AER via anti-inflammatory mechanisms. It decreases lipopolysaccharide-induced nuclear factor-kB (NF-kB) activation and monocyte chemoattractant protein (MCP)-1 expression in human renal tubular cells (Lee CC et al. 2010). Further prospective studies and randomized controlled trials are needed to confirm this hypothesis.

5.3 Protein

With regards to protein, the DNSG EASD guidelines recommend an intake of 0.8 g/kg normal body weight in patients with type 1 diabetes and established nephropathy. There are no firm recommendations regarding protein intake for type 1 diabetic patients with incipient nephropathy. An intake of 10-20% of total energy is recommended for patients with no evidence of nephropathy (**Table 4**). The recommendation for protein intake is most important for patients with diabetic nephropathy. The guideline of a restricted protein diet which contains 0.8 g/kg normal body weight for type 1 diabetic patients with established nephropathy was demonstrated by previous research. Several randomized controlled trials showed that protein normalization (protein intake of approximately 0.8 g/kg/day, **Table 1**) had a positive significant effect on albuminuria, although no effect on GFR was found (Brouhard BH& LaGrone L 1990; Zeller K et al. 1991; Dullaart RP et al. 1993; Raal FJ et al. 1994; Hansen HP et al. 1999; Hansen HP et al. 2002). Even a relative risk of 0.23 (95% CI: 0.07-0.72) was found for ESRD in patients assigned to a low protein diet compared with patients assigned to a usual protein diet (Hansen HP et al. 2002). A hypothesis is that excessive protein intake causes renal vasodilatation and glomerular excessive perfusion leading to a raised glomerular transcapillary hydraulic pressure gradient ending in proteinuria and glomerular damage, conversely, will prevent kidney damage (Percheron C et al. 1995). So, indeed protein restriction is beneficial for type 1 diabetic patients with established nephropathy. However, we have to mention that although this beneficial effect of a restricted protein intake was found in randomized controlled trials, the sample size of these trials were really small (maximum of 82 people). Furthermore, we have to consider the feasibility of a protein intake of 0.8 g/kg/day. Percheron et al. (Percheron C et al. 1995) showed that even with this intake the compliance is poor. Further studies with a larger sample size are needed to find a cutoff point for protein intake which would still have a positive effect on diabetic nephropathy and its feasibility.

Alcohol

The DNSG EASD guidelines for alcohol for persons with type 1 and type 2 diabetes recommend a moderate use up to 10 g/day for women and up to 20 g/day for men (**Table 4**). In prior studies, moderate alcohol consumers (30-70 g alcohol per week) had a lower risk of diabetic nephropathy (OR=0.36, 95% CI: 0.18-0.71) and diabetic retinopathy (OR=0.60, 95% CI: 0.37-0.99) in patients with type 1 diabetes (Beulens et al. 2008). Alcohol has favourable effects on HDL-cholesterol, inflammation and inhibition of platelet aggregation

(Beulens et al. 2008). Because of this favourable effects we expect a beneficial effect on CVD, however to date no association was found between alcohol and CVD in type 1 diabetes patients (Bishop et al. 2009). In this cross-sectional study, markers for CVD were used instead of CVD as endpoint. Also the association between alcohol and diabetic nephropathy and diabetic retinopathy was only observed in cross-sectional studies. So the current recommendations for alcohol are confirmed by research in type 1 diabetes, but only based on cross-sectional studies, and especially for the association between alcohol and CVD in type 1 diabetic patients more research is needed.

5.4 Physical activity
There are no specific guidelines concerning physical activity for type 1 diabetic patients. The guidelines mentioned in **Table 4** are only for type 2 diabetic patients. However, it was shown that the guidelines for type 2 diabetic patients are also applicable for type 1 diabetic patients. Several randomized controlled trials (**Table 3**) showed that physical activity (endurance sports; on average 2 times a week 60 minutes) improves physical fitness as well as endothelial function in type 1 diabetic patients (Lehmann R et al. 1997; Fuchsjäger-Mayrl G et al. 2002; Seeger JPH et al. 2011). Especially the improvement in endothelial function is important since endothelial dysfunction is an early sign of atherosclerosis, which is often the underlying cause of CVD. Also a positive effect on lipid related cardiovascular risk factors was found in one study (Lehmann R et al. 1997). However, also this conclusion should be interpreted carefully. Although the evidence is gained from randomized controlled trials, the conditions of these trials are really disappointing. They had a maximum sample size of 23 people, and a minimum sample size of only 9 people. The follow-up period was relatively short, up to four months. The studies of Lehman et al. (Lehmann R et al. 1997) and Seeger et al. (Seeger JPH et al. 2011) not even used a control group. Furthermore CVD risk factors were used instead of CVD as endpoint. So the studies are in agreement with the guidelines but more research in better performed randomized controlled trials is needed to confirm this positive effect of physical activity on CVD in type 1 diabetic patients.

6. Conclusion

A diet high in fiber, low in saturated fat, moderate in protein intake with moderate alcohol consumption as well as physical activity can be recommended for type 1 diabetic patients to prevent complications. Inspite of the lack of large robust prospective studies, using the available evidence, we can conclude that diet as well as lifestyle could play an important role in preventing longterm complications of type 1 diabetes.

7. References

American Diabetes Association (ADA). (2010). "Diabetes Basics." Retrieved 24 March, 2011, from http://www.diabetes.org/diabetes-basics/.

American Diabetes Association (ADA). (2011). "Recommendations Summary Diabetes Mellitus (DM): Physical Activity." Retrieved 19 April, 2011, from http://www.adaevidencelibrary.com/template.cfm?template=guide_summary&key=2062.

Barsotti G, Cupisti A, et al. (1998). "Dietary treatment of diabetic nephropathy with chronic renal failure." Nephrology, dialysis, transplantation 13(8): 49-52.

Beulens, J. W. J., J. S. Kruidhof, et al. (2008). "Alcohol consumption and risk of microvascular complications in type 1 diabetes patients: the EURODIAB Prospective Complications Study." Diabetologia 51(9): 1631-1638.

Bishop, F. K., D. M. Maahs, et al. (2009). "Lifestyle risk factors for atherosclerosis in adults with type 1 diabetes." Diabetes and Vascular Disease Research 6(4): 269-275.

Bouhanick B, S. S., Berrut G, Bled F, Simard G, Lejeune JJ, Fressinaud P, Marre M. (1995). "Relationship between fat intake and glomerular filtration rate in normotensive insulin-dependent diabetic patients." Diabète and Métabolisme 21(3): 168-172.

Brindisi MC, Bouillet B, et al. (2010). "Cardiovascular complications in type 1 diabetes mellitus: review." Diabetes & Metabolism.

Brouhard BH and LaGrone L (1990). "Effect of dietary protein restriction on functional renal reserve in diabetic nephropathy." The American Journal of Medicine 89(4): 427-431.

Cárdenas C, Bordiu E, et al. (2004). "Polyunsaturated fatty acid consumption may play a role in the onset and regression of microalbuminuria in well-controlled type 1 and type 2 diabetic people: a 7-year, prospective, population-based, observational multicenter study." Diabetes Care 27(6): 1454-1457.

Colhoun HM, Otvos JD, et al. (2002). "Lipoprotein subclasses and particle size and their relationship with coronary artery classification in men and women with and without type 1 diabetes " Diabetes 51: 7.

Cundiff DK and Nigg CR (2005). Diet and Diabetic Retinopathy: Insights From the Diabetes Control and Complications Trial (DCCT). Medscape General Medicine. 7.

Daneman D (2006). "Type 1 diabetes." The Lancet 367(9513): 847-858.

Dullaart RP, Beusekamp BJ, et al. (1993). "Long-term effects of protein-restricted diet on albuminuria and renal function in IDDM patients without clinical nephropathy and hypertension." Diabetes Care 16(2): 483-492.

Franz MJ, Bantle JP, et al. (2003). "Evidence-based nutrition principles and recommendations for the treatment and prevention of diabetes and related complications." Diabetes Care 26(1): S51-S61.

Franz, M. J., M. A. Powers, et al. (2010). "The Evidence for Medical Nutrition Therapy for Type 1 and Type 2 Diabetes in Adults." Journal of the American Dietetic Association 110(12): 1852-1889.

Fuchsjäger-Mayrl G, Pleiner J, et al. (2002). "Exercise training improves vascular endothelial function in patients with type 1 diabetes." Diabetes Care 25(10): 1795-1801.

Georgopoulos A, Bantle JP, et al. (2000). "A high carbohydrate versus a high monounsaturated fatty acid diet lowers the atherogenic potential of big VLDL particles in patients with type 1 diabetes." The journal of nutrition 130(10): 2503-2507.

Gunther ALB, Liese AD, et al. (2008). "Association Between the Dietary Approaches to Hypertension Diet and Hypertension in Youth With Diabetes Mellitus." Hypertension 53(1): 6-12.

Hansen HP, Christensen PK, et al. (1999). "Low-protein diet and kidney function in insulin-dependent diabetic patients with diabetic nephropathy." Kidney International 55(2): 621-628.

Hansen HP, Tauber-Lassen E, et al. (2002). "Effect of dietary protein restriction on prognosis in patients with diabetic nephropathy." Kidney International 62(1): 220-228.

Helgeson, V. S. (2006). "Diet of Adolescents With and Without Diabetes: Trading candy for potato chips?" Diabetes Care 29(5): 982-987.

Herbst A, Kordonouri O, et al. (2007). "Impact of Physical Activity on Cardiovascular Risk Factors in Children With Type 1 Diabetes: A multicenter study of 23,251 patients." Diabetes Care 30(8): 2098-2100.

Hovind P (2004). "Predictors for the development of microalbuminuria and macroalbuminuria in patients with type 1 diabetes: inception cohort study." Bmj 328(7448): 1105-1100.

Hu, F. B., J. E. Manson, et al. (2001). "Diet, lifestyle, and the risk of type 2 diabetes mellitus in women." N Engl J Med. 345(11): 790-797.

International Diabetes Federation (IDF). (2010). "IDF Diabetes Atlas: The Economic Impacts of Diabetes." Retrieved 21 March, 2011, from http://www.diabetesatlas.org /content/economic-impacts-diabetes.

Jensen T, Borch-Johnsen K, et al. (1987). "Coronary heart disease in young type 1 (insulin-dependent) diabetic patients with and without diabetic nephropathy: incidence and risk factors." Diabetologia 30(3): 144-148.

Jibani MM, Bloodworth LL, et al. (1991). "Predominantly vegetarian diet in patients with incipient and early clinical diabetic nephropathy: effects on albumin excretion rate and nutritional status. ." Diabetic Medicine 8(10): 949-953.

Klein R, Lee KE, et al. (2010). "The 25-Year Incidence of Visual Impairment in Type 1 Diabetes MellitusThe Wisconsin Epidemiologic Study of Diabetic Retinopathy." Ophthalmology 117(1): 63-70.

Kornerub K, Nordestgaard BG, et al. (2003). "Increased transvascular low density lipoprotein transport in insulin dependent diabetes: a mechanistic model for development of atherosclerosis." Atherosclerosis 170: 163-168.

Kriska AM, LaPorte RE, et al. (1991). "The association of physical activity and diabetic complications in individuals with insulin-dependent diabetes mellitus: the Epidemiology of Diabetes Complications Study." Journal of Clinical Epidemiology 44(11): 1207-1214.

Lee CC, Sharp SJ, et al. (2010). "Dietary Intake of Eicosapentaenoic and Docosahexaenoic Acid and Diabetic Nephropathy: Cohort Analysis of the Diabetes Control and Complications Trial." Diabetes Care 33(7): 1454-1456.

Lehmann R, Kaplan V, et al. (1997). "Impact of physical activity on cardiovascular risk factors in IDDM." Diabetes Care 20(10): 1603-1611.

Liese AD, Bortsov A, et al. (2011). "Association of DASH Diet With Cardiovascular Risk Factors in Youth With Diabetes Mellitus: The SEARCH for Diabetes in Youth Study." Circulation 123(13): 1410-1417.

Möllsten AV, Dahlquist GG, et al. (2001). "Higher intakes of fish protein are related to a lower risk of microalbuminuria in young Swedish type 1 diabetic patients." Diabetes Care 24(5): 805-810.

Moss SE, Klein R, et al. (1992). "Alcohol consumption and the prevalence of diabetic retinopathy." Ophthalmology 99(6): 926-932.

National Institute for Public Health and the Environment (RIVM). (2007). "Diabetes in Nederland. Omvang, risicofactoren en gevolgen, nu en in de toekomst." Retrieved 22 March, 2011, from http://www.rivm.nl/bibliotheek/rapporten/260322001.pdf.

National Institute for Public Health and the Environment (RIVM). (2010). "Nationaal Kompas Volksgezondheid: Diabetes mellitus samengevat." Retrieved 21 March, 2011, from http://www.nationaalkompas.nl/gezondheid-en-ziekte/ziekten-en-aandoeningen/endocriene-voedings-en-stofwisselingsziekten-en-immuniteitsstoornissen/diabetes-mellitus/diabetes-mellitus-samengevat/.

O'Hayon BE, Cummings EA, et al. (2000). "Does dietary protein intake correlate with markers suggestive of early diabetic nephropathy in children and adolescents with Type 1 diabetes mellitus?" Diabetic Medicine 17(10): 708-712.

Øverby NC, Flaaten V, et al. (2006). "Children and adolescents with type 1 diabetes eat a more atherosclerosis-prone diet than healthy control subjects." Diabetologia 50(2): 307-316.

Percheron C, Colette C, et al. (1995). "Effects of moderate changes in protein intake on urinary albumin excretion in type I diabetic patients." Nutrition 11(4): 345-349.

Raal FJ, Kalk WJ, et al. (1994). "Effect of moderate dietary protein restriction on the progression of overt diabetic nephropathy: a 6-mo prospective study." The American Journal of Clinical Nutrition 60(4): 579-585.

Riley MD and Dwyer T (1998). "Microalbuminuria is positively associated with usual dietary saturated fat intake and negatively associated with usual dietary protein intake in people with insulin-dependent diabetes mellitus." The American Journal of Clinical Nutrition 67(1): 50-57.

Roper NA, Bilous RW, et al. (2002). "Cause-specific mortality in a population with diabetes." Diabetes Care 25(1): 43-48.

Sadauskaitė-Kuehne V, Ludvigsson J, et al. (2004). "Longer breastfeeding is an independent protective factor against development of type 1 diabetes mellitus in childhood." Diabetes/Metabolism Research and Reviews 20(2): 150-157.

Sahakyan K, Klein BEK, et al. (2011). "The 25-Year Cumulative Incidence of Lower Extremity Amputations in People With Type 1 Diabetes." Diabetes Care 34(3): 649-651.

Seeger JPH, Thijssen DHJ, et al. (2011). "Exercise training improves physical fitness and vascular function in children with type 1 diabetes." Diabetes, Obesity and Metabolism 13(4): 382-384.

Snell-Bergeon JK, Chartier-Logan C, et al. (2009). "Adults with type 1 diabetes eat a high-fat atherogenic diet that is associated with coronary artery calcium." Diabetologia 52(5): 801-809.

Soedamah-Muthu SS, Fuller JH, et al. (2006). "High risk of cardiovascular disease in patients with type 1 diabetes in the U.K.: a cohort study using the general practice research database." Diabetes Care 29(4): 798-804.

Stampfer, M. J., F. B. Hu, et al. (2000). "Primary prevention of coronary heart disease in women through diet and lifestyle." N Engl J Med. 343(1): 16-22.

Strychar I, Cohn JS, et al. (2009). "Effects of a Diet Higher in Carbohydrate/Lower in Fat Versus Lower in Carbohydrate/Higher in Monounsaturated Fat on Postmeal Triglyceride Concentrations and Other Cardiovascular Risk Factors in Type 1 Diabetes." Diabetes Care 32(9): 1597-1599.

Toeller M: Lifestyle Issues: Diet. In: Textbook of Diabetes. Holt RIG, Cockram CS, Flyvbjerg A, Goldstein BJ (eds). 4th edition, Wiley-Blackwell Chichester U.K. 2010, pp 346-357

Toeller M, Buyken A, et al. (1997). "Protein intake and urinary albumin excretion rates in the EURODIAB IDDM Complications Study." Diabetologia 40(10): 1219-1226. [1]

Toeller M, Buyken AE, et al. (1999). "Prevalence of chronic complications, metabolic control and nutritional intake in type 1 diabetes: comparison between different European regions. EURODIAB Complications Study group." Hormone and Metabolic Research 31(12): 680-685. [2]

Toeller M, Buyken AE, et al. (1999). "Fiber intake, serum cholesterol levels, and cardiovascular disease in European individuals with type 1 diabetes. EURODIAB IDDM Complications Study Group." Diabetes Care 22(2): B21-B28. [3]

Toeller M, Buyken AE, et al. (1999). "Associations of fat and cholesterol intake with serum lipid levels and cardiovascular disease: the EURODIAB IDDM Complications Study." Experimental and Clinical Endocrinology & Diabetes 107(8): 512-521.

Toeller M, Klischan A, et al. (1996). "Nutritional intake of 2868 IDDM patients from 30 centres in Europe. EURODIAB IDDM Complications Study Group." Diabetologia 39(8): 929-939.

Trigona B, Aggoun Y, et al. (2010). "Preclinical Noninvasive Markers of Atherosclerosis in Children and Adolescents with Type 1 Diabetes Are Influenced by Physical Activity." The Journal of Pediatrics 157(4): 533-539.

U.S. National Library of Medicine. (2011). "Type 1 diabetes."   Retrieved 24, 2011, from http://www.nlm.nih.gov/medlineplus/ency/article/000305.htm.

Valerio G, Spagnuolo M, et al. (2007). "Physical activity and sports participation in children and adolescents with type 1 diabetes mellitus." Nutrition, Metabolism and Cardiovascular Diseases 17(5): 376-382.

Watts GF, Gregory L, et al. (1988). "Nutrient intake in insulin-dependent diabetic patients with incipient nephropathy." European Journal of Clinical Nutrition 42(8): 697-702.

Weis U, Turner B, et al. (2001). "Long-term predictors of coronary artery disease and mortallity in type 1 diabetes." QJM 94: 623-630.

World Diabetes Foundation (WDF). (2010). "Diabetes facts "   Retrieved 21 March, 2011, from http://www.worlddiabetesfoundation.org/composite-35.htm.

World Health Organization (WHO). (2008). "Fact sheet N°310 The top 10 causes of death."
    Retrieved 21 March, 2011, from
    http://www.who.int/mediacentre/factsheets/fs310/en/index.html
Yusuf, S., S. Hawken, et al. (2004). "Effect of potentially modifiable risk factors associated
    with myocardial infarction in 52 countries (the INTERHEART study): case-control
    study." Lancet. 364(9438): 937-952.
Zeller K, Whittaker E, et al. (1991). "Effect of restricting dietary protein on the progression of
    renal failure in patients with insulin-dependent diabetes mellitus." The New
    England Journal of Medicine 324(2): 78-84.

4

Prevalence of Type 1 Diabetes Correlates with Daily Insulin Dose, Adverse Outcomes and with Autoimmune Process Against Glutamic Acid Decarboxylase in Adults

Mykola Khalangot[1], Vitaliy Gurianov[2], Volodymir Kovtun[1],
Nadia Okhrimenko[1], Viktor Kravchenko[1] and Mykola Tronko[1]
*[1]Komisarenko Institute of Endocrinology and
Metabolism Academy of Medical Sciences, Kiev
[2]National Medical University, Donetsk,
Ukraine*

1. Introduction

The territorial differences in the prevalence of type 1 diabetes mellitus (T1D) around the world were previously reported (Amos et al., 1997; Green & Patterson, 2001; Lévy-Marchal, 2001), but the data were based on the study of juvenile T1D epidemiology, i.e., in patients diagnosed with T1D before the age of 15 years. These data became the basis for the epidemiological evaluation of the whole T1D patient population. With the relatively limited number of children with T1D within the current territory, less effort is required for data gathering. Besides, as the age increases, it becomes more difficult to relate a diabetic condition to a certain diabetes type (Keen, 1998), thus, making it impossible to directly use the diabetes-type data obtained from Primary Care. In modern epidemiological studies, the key data concern the age at the time of the diagnosis — patients who were diagnosed before the age of 30 years and are insulin-treated, are considered to suffer from T1D.

1.1 T1D epidemiology in adults

European researchers have proved that the epidemiological characteristics of T1D in children significantly differ from that in young adults (Kyvik et al., 2004). Therefore, studying the peculiarities of T1D in adults is a major concern. Furthermore, data on the number of diabetic patients usually found in the reports of the healthcare system are unstructured according to the history of the disease, and cannot be a source of epidemiological information on patients suffering from T1D. Owing to the development of the Diabetes Register in Ukraine, it has become possible to conduct analytical comparisons and further studies on almost all the T1D adult populations.

1.2 Diabetes Register

The Diabetes Register contains individual, structured information on the disease history, and has already been used in some epidemiological studies (Khalangot et al., 2009a;

Khalangot et al., 2009[b]; Vaiserman et al., 2009; Khalangot et al., 2009[d]; Vaiserman & Khalangot, 2008). Until recently there was no evidence on age and gender structure of patients diagnosed with diabetes mellitus in Ukraine. Neither is there any information on risk factors that may influence main aetiological diabetes mellitus type's incidence, as well as development of diabetic complications in Ukraine. Diabetes register is recognized as an important tool of diabetes research: it is a fully functioning diabetes register created in Ukraine. It includes over 620 000 diabetes patients (2010) and gives a unique possibility to analyze the structure of aetiological types, gender and age features, prevalence, trends of incidence, risk factors of non-fatal events and mortality among Ukrainian diabetes patients. Observational cross-sectional (distribution of diabetes types and treatment, trends of life span) and cohort (assessment of mortality risks) epidemiological studies using national patient register based on data provided by primary care doctors became possible. The register included most of Ukraine's insulin treated patients, as well as significant part of patients receiving oral glucose lowering drugs (OGLD). The insulin-treated patient data covers 24 out of 25 Ukrainian regions, meaning that at least nearly all of Ukraine's T1D population is included in the register. According to the Health Ministry data, the total amount of patients with known diabetes is 1 048375 (2006), which means that nearly half of type 2 diabetes (T2D) patients have yet to be included in the register, which consists of 509 933 patients, including 37 406 death cases.

1.3 Register-based diabetes epidemiology studies

Systematic epidemiological study of main diabetes mellitus (DM) types through analysis of electronic population registers has been lasting for over 10 years. Usage of DM population registers has become quite advanced in the UK, in particular in Scotland, where by the end of 2004, 161 946 diabetics have been included into local diabetic registers which is equal to 3.2% of the general population. In Scotland, 14 out of 15 healthcare institutions are involved in controlling treatment of DM patients. An important aspect is that Scottish DM registers include all DM patients, unlike others, that only include patients receiving certain kind of treatment. It seems that at the moment, the most advanced and successful Scottish local register is Tayside (Boyle et al., 2001; Leese et al., 2006; Morris et al., 1997). It should be noted that this relatively small, but constantly functioning register became a source of not just "traditional" epidemiologic information concerning prevalence and annual incidence of T1D and T2D, dynamics of DM complications frequency, and quality of treatment, which is a generalization of routine data from active GPs working in the region, and can be accessed through the register's website (http://www.diabetes-healthnet.ac.uk/), but also of purely scientific fundamental data (Doney et al., 2003, 2005; Evans et al., 2005, 2006; Schofield et al., 2006). A few of these papers have entirely clinically-epidemiological nature, comparing mortality among patients with limb amputations depending on presence of DM (Schofield et al., 2006), or mortality risks depending on certain type of treatment (Evans et al., 2005, 2006), while others use the register to study genetic characteristics among different categories of DM patients (Doney et al., 2003, 2005). One of the researchers of Belgian Diabetic Register (BDR) Prof. Frans K. Gorus (Diabetes Research Center, Vrije Universiteit Brussel) indicated the possibility of such scientific use of diabetic registers (Gorus, 1996). Important epidemiologic, immunologic, and genetic studies of T1D in children and adolescents were carried out using BDR (Gorus, 1996; Vandewalle et al., 1997; Weets et al., 2001, 2002).

Prevalence of Type 1 Diabetes Correlates with Daily Insulin Dose, Adverse Outcomes and with
Autoimmune Process Against Glutamic Acid Decarboxylase in Adults

63

1.3.1 Register-based T2D epidemiology studies

Some results obtanied by means of studying electronic registers may at first seem unusual or paradoxic. In particular our studies of T2D patients (Khalangot et al., 2009[b]) indicate that Hazard Ratios (HRs) of cardiovascular disease (CVD) mortality among extremely obese patients [body mass index (BMI) $\geq$ 35 kg/m²] adjusted for age, smoking and alcohol consumption were higher than for overweight patients [BMI 25-29 kg/m²]: HR=1.54 (95% CI 1.16-2.05) and 1.35 (95% CI 1.15-1.59) among men an women respectively, p<0.01. Furthermore, the graph that shows risks of general and CVD mortality for T2D patients depending on BMI has the shape of an asymmetric parabola: HRs associated with low and normal BMI were significantly higher comparing to those, related to overweight or moderate obesity. The above phenomenon partially corresponds to "obesity paradox" that has been recently discovered among patients suffering from CVD (Gruberg et al., 2002; Curtis et al., 2005) , however in our study this effect concerns T2D patients. An observational study that included 25 361 T2D patients showed that glibenclamide treatment is associated with much higher risk of general and CVD mortality, comparing to treatment with another derivative of sulfonylurea – gliclazide. HRs for total and CVD mortality within the glibenclamide patient cohort were 2.57 (95% CI 1.73–3.82) and 2,93 (95%CI 1.83–4.71) respectively; (p < 0,001). These data correspond to changes of OGLD distribution and trends of life duration among DM patients that we have revealed as well (Khalangot et al., 2009 [e]). Previously, there had been only one study where similar results concerning total mortality associated with the use of glibenclamide or gliclazide in a cohort of 568 T2D patients were obtained (Monami et al., 2007). Our study broadens this tendency onto CVD mortality.

1.3.2 Register-based T1D epidemiology studies

T1D incidence among Ukrainian adults from 1994 till 2004, that we have evaluated retrospectively according to the register data, had a decreasing tendency (Khalangot, 2009). Our assessment of T1D incidence dynamics among adults does not confirm the information about steady increase of global T1D incidence (Green et al., 2001; Gale, 2002), however these studies only concerned child incidence. As Ukraine is also experiencing a rise of DM incidence among children, our data can be easily explained by earlier DM manifestation among people, who carry the genotype predisposing to T1D. Researchers of Danish DM register have recently reported a decrease of DM incidence among young adults. National diabetic register of Denmark has collected data on 359 000 DM cases between 1995 and 2006, and it includes the total population, diagnosed with DM. This register has recorded a clear tendency towards reduction of mortality among DM patients, which has been observed since 2003 (Carstensen et al., 2008). We have recently conducted a series of studies as well that focused on factors influencing mortality and territorial heterogeneity of T1D in Ukraine (Khalangot, 2008; Khalangot et al., 2009 [c]; 2010). The purpose of these studies (Khalangot et al., 2009 [d]) was also to determine whether the insulin requirement can change systematically in T1D patients, and whether this requirement depends on the same factors that determine its prevalence. This chapter is mainly a review of these studies.

2. Methods

A database with 282,988 records of diabetic patients was developed on the basis of epidemiological analysis conducted during the 2005–2006 register verification (01.12.2006). To evaluate the completeness of the register data, we compared it to the official 2005

Ministry of Health statistical data (Anonymous, 2006). The integrity of the register, i.e., the data on the number of patients who have received insulin, was assessed based on the information provided by the primary care doctors (district endocrinologists) to the regional diabetic registers. Consequently, the regional endocrinologists were responsible for updating the data and endorsing it to the central level. Accordingly, by assuming that the data were encoded into the regional registers with various degrees of completeness, significant limitations were noted in the assessment of the prevalence of insulin-dependent diabetes as well as in further epidemiological evaluations. Considering the fact that Ukraine has a national, free-of-charge insulin supply to the patients who require it, the Ministry of Health data reflect the number of these patients to the fullest extent. However, the Ukrainian Ministry of Health receives only non-personalized data that are difficult to verify. A comparison of the data from the 2006 Diabetes Register with the 2005 data on the insulin-treated patients from the Ministry of Health (considered 100%) revealed certain similarities: the fraction of the patients included in the register was 91.1%, based on the number of the patients according to the Ministry of Health data. However, in the Kharkiv region, only 58.6% of the Ministry of Health patients were in the register. It was assumed that the Kharkiv region data in the register could be incomplete, and hence, was not used in the analysis of T1D prevalence among adults.

2.1 T1D cases selection
Therefore, the analysis was carried out using the T1D criteria used by the epidemiologists–researchers for the European diabetes population databases (Kyvik et al., 2004; Soedamah-Muthu, 2006). The patients were selected based on the following conditions: T1D primary care diagnosis; age at the time of being included in the register ≥15 years; place of residence and gender; and data on diagnoses before the age of 30 years.

2.2 T1D prevalence assessment
The prevalence of T1D in the Ukrainian regions was determined as of the end of 2004. The T1D prevalence was calculated using the official data on the adult population of the corresponding regions (Anonymous, 2006), and 95% confidence interval (CI) was determined using arcsine transformation (Altman et al., ed-s., 2003). Multiple comparisons of T1D regional prevalence were subsequently carried out using the modified (Liakh & Gurianov, 2004) L. Marascuilo mathematical procedure (Marascuilo, 1966). The MedStat statistical package was used for the calculations (Liakh & Gurianov, 2004). Logistic regression analysis was used to determine the influence of the explanatory variables on the resulting variable (Bland, 2000). For each input variable, we evaluated the estimated logistic regression coefficient with the standard error, estimated as the odds ratio (OR) with a CI for its actual value and associated p value, and performed a Wald test (testing the null hypothesis on the congruency of the OR of the "disease" associated with the increase of this variable by 1). We used this information to determine whether each variable was related to the outcome of interest, and to quantify the extent of such a relationship (Bland, 2000). The Statistica 5.5 (StatSoft Inc., 1999) package was used in this set of calculations.

2.3 T1D outcomes assessment
We have evaluated the prevalence of proliferative retinopathy (PR), arterial hypertension (AH), and mortality risks in the retrospective cohort of T1D (27,896 patients); these data was

published elsewhere (Khalangot et al., 2009[c] ; 2010). In brief, mortality was assessed using the Cox regression model, determining hazard ratios (HRs) and corresponding 95% confidence intervals (95% CI). We calculated odds ratios (ORs), and used a logistic regression to compare PR and AH.

2.4 Diabetes-associated antibodies and c-peptide measurements

A total of 86 T1D patients (42 males and 44 females), with a mean age of 27.5 years (0.86) and mean diabetes duration of 10.3 (0.72) years (SE), were randomly selected from four regional diabetes-mellitus registers: Chernihivska, Zaporizka; Ivano-Frankivska, and Chernivetska. The glutamic acid decarboxylase 65 antibody (GADA), insulin antibody (IA), and plasma c-peptide levels were determined using radioimmunoassay (RIA) kits (IMMUNOTECH™) after obtaining the patients' informed consent. The model of the logistic regression was used for the multifactor data analysis of GADA, IA, c-peptide persistence, OR, and the 95% CI that were determined. The plasma was considered GADA- or IA-positive, if GADA >1 U/ml or IA >0.4 U/ml, and low c-peptide, if its level was <32.6 pmol/l.

3. Register analysis results and discussion

The analysis of the register of diabetic patients has allowed for the first time to assess the adult prevalence of T1D in Ukraine in comparison with important clinical (daily insulin dose, mortality, and complications) and some paraclinical (GADA) characteristics of the disease (Khalangot et al., 2009 [c]; Khalangot et al., 2009 [d]; 2010).

3.1 T1D territorial dissimilarity and clusterization

The data on adult T1D prevalence in 24 Ukrainian regions (Table 1) indicated territorial dissimilarity: chi-square = 648.30, degree of freedom, k =23 (p< 0.001).

Further multiple comparisons using the modified Marascuilo procedure (Marascuilo, 1966) allowed conducting a pairwise assessment of each region. This assessment enabled clustering of the regions according to T1D prevalence. The flagged regions that did not statistically differ from the minimal level according to prevalence were considered as a cluster. This procedure was repeated for the remaining regions as well. The following regional clusters were distinguished according to the T1D prevalence:

Minimal prevalence cluster = AR Crimea, Ivano-Frankivska, Mykolaivska, Odeska, Chernivetska, and Luganska regions.

Intermediate prevalence cluster = Vinnitska, Volynska, Dnipropetrovska, Donetska, Zhytomyrska, Zakarpatska, Kirovogradska, Lvivska, Rivnenska, Kievska, Sumska, Ternopilska, Poltavska, Khersonska, and Cherkaska regions.

Maximal prevalence cluster = Zaporizka, Khmelnytska, and Chernigivska regions.

Cases of T1D in each regional cluster were unified and the prevalence was calculated for the actual clusters. The T1D prevalence was found to be 6 (5–6), −7 (6–7), and −9 (8–9) per 10,000 adults, for the minimal, intermediate, and maximal prevalence clusters respectively. A comparison of the differences between these groups indicated a high level of confidence (χ^2 = 214.4; p< 0.001), as shown in figure 1.

Region (oblast')	Gender		Number of type1 adult diabetic patients		Total adult population
	males	females	total, n	per 10 000 adults (95 % CI)	
AR Crimea	564	513	1077	5 (5-6)	2 032 600
Vinnitska	600	464	1064	7 (7-8)	1 440 600
Volynska	354	271	625	7 (7-8)	844 300
Dnipropetrovska	1107	1017	2124	7(6-7)	2 992 000
Donetska	1477	1282	2759	7 (6-7)	4 071 100
Zhytomyrska	387	339	726	6 (6-7)	1 122 300
Zakarpatska	354	264	618	6(6-7)	1 000 700
Zaporizka	732	712	1444	9 (8-9)	1 619 200
Ivano-Frankivska	351	274	625	5 (5-6)	1 137 500
Kievska	1476	1514	2990	8 (7-8)	3 804 900
Kirovogradska	334	327	661	7 (7-8)	913 500
Luganska	604	623	1227	6 (5-6)	2 127 900
Lvivska	802	700	1502	7 (6-7)	2 136 000
Mykolaivska	292	279	571	5 (5-6)	1 041 600
Odeska	470	438	908	4 (4-5)	2 037 900
Poltavska	552	464	1016	7 (7-8)	1 345 600
Rivnenska	355	316	671	7 (7-8)	930 000
Sumska	408	321	729	7 (6-7)	1 071 700
Ternopilska	411	297	708	8 (7-8)	925 000
Kharkivska	*597*	*493*	*1090*		*2 479 700*
Khersonska	303	286	589	6 (6-7)	957 000
Khmelnitska	510	468	978	8 (8-9)	1 163 000
Cherkaska	408	366	774	7 (6-7)	1 154 600
Chernivetska	267	177	444	6 (5-6)	746 000
Chernigyvska	473	403	876	9 (8-9)	1 020 300
Total	14188	12608	26796		40 115 000

Table 1. Prevalence of Type 1 Diabetes Mellitus in Adults Diagnosed Before the Age of 30 in Ukrainian Regions (Khalangot et al., 2009d)

3.2 T1D gender assessment

The fraction of males among the 26,796 adults diagnosed before the age of 30 years corresponded to 52.95%, and varied from 49.2% in Luganska to 60.1% in Chernivetska regions. In the majority (23 out of 25) of the regions, this fraction was >50%. Comparison of the 25 regions with the fraction of T1D males revealed a certain variation according to the territorial attribute (chi-square = 67.70, the degrees of freedom, k =24; p <0.001). However, multiple comparisons failed to reveal any distinctions according to the fraction of T1D males between the specific regions. Furthermore, it must be noted that there was no increase in the female fraction among T1D adults, which is common in the general population.

It is possible that an increase in the male fraction in this population reflects the epidemiological peculiarities of this disease, which have not yet been described by the identified (as well as the unknown) factors that could lead to the increase in the mortality among males.

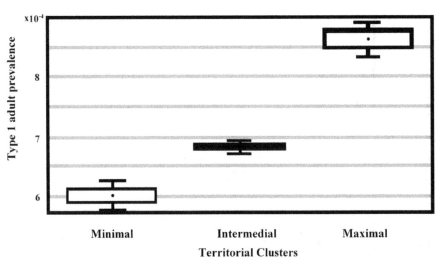

Territorial Clusters

Note: given Means ± SE (the dot within the box and height of boxes respectively), 95% CI (lines that emerge above and below the boxes)

Fig. 1. Prevalence of Type 1 Diabetes Mellitus Diagnosed in Patients Under the Age of 30 in Territorial Clusters of Ukrainian Regions (per 10 000 adults, 95% CI) (Khalangot et al., 2009 [d])

3.3 T1D insulin doses assessment

The data analysis of the 23,633 T1D patients (Table 2) from the register, who were classified according to insulin dose, age, and disease duration, indicated that women have a higher average age and disease duration, but lower daily insulin dose, when compared with men.

Number of T1D patients (n)	Mean age, yrs(SD)	Mean diabetes duration, yrs(SD)	Mean insulin dose, U/day (SD)
Man (12364)	32.48 (11.60)	14.11 (10.47)	52.03 (18.56)
Women (11269)	33.38 (12.43)	15.69 (10.99)	49.50 (17.98)
Total (23633)	32.91 (12,01)	14.86 (10.75)	50.83 (18.33)

Note: P (man/women) < 0.001

Table 2. Average Age, Disease Duration, and Daily Insulin Dose of Type 1 Diabetes Mellitus Patients in Ukraine According to the Diabetes Register data (Khalangot et al., 2009 [d])

3.3.1 T1D insulin doses and diabetes duration

As the average duration of the disease was found to be 14.86 years, the average daily insulin doses were calculated for each year of the duration, from 0 (<1) to 15 years.

The regression analysis (figure 2) indicated that in this range, the insulin dose rises with the increase in the disease duration:

Insulin (units/day) = 0.7326 × duration (years) + 43.74 (coefficient of linear correlation, R = 0.899, $p < 0.001$).

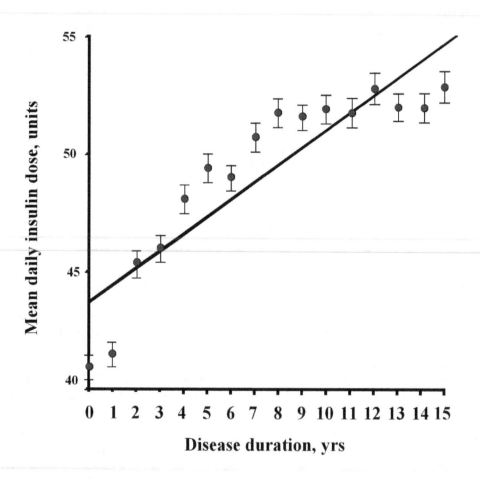

Fig. 2. Average (Mean ± SE) daily insulin doses of type 1 diabetes mellitus patients depending on the disease duration in the range of 0-15 years (Khalangot et al., 2009 [d])

A further increase in the disease duration in the range of 16–31 years was not accompanied by regular changes in the insulin dose. The regular rise of insulin dose, observed with the increase in the duration of T1D in adults diagnosed before the age of 30 years, is still an unknown phenomenon. However, this phenomenon was observed to correspond to the observation that T1D patients have long-standing insulin secretion at times (the study of c-peptide level), which was proven by Bonora (Bonora et al., 1984) and confirmed by the Diabetes Control and Complications Trial (DCCT). These research efforts uncovered the diverse influence of different insulin-therapy patterns on the process described (*The DCCT Research Group*, 1987; 1998). The confirmation of this data with the prospective observation was undertaken in Germany (Linn et al., 2003). Our results could be viewed as an indirect confirmation of the extended continuation of the β-cell secretion, obtained through the cross-sectional treatment data analysis of almost the entire population of T1D patients in Ukraine. The standardization of the daily insulin doses, depending on the disease duration, enables the necessary quantitative comparisons of the treatments for T1D adult patients.

3.3.2 T1D insulin doses in territorial clusters

It would be logical to consider that the rate of decrease in insulin secretion among the T1D patients that differs according to the prevalence of such autoimmune disease, as T1D will also vary. Table 3 presents the comparisons of the daily insulin doses (median) in all the three clusters of the regions selected according to the prevalence of T1D in adults.

Type 1 diabetes prevalence cluster	Insulin doses standardized according to diabetes duration, median, U/day	95%CI	P
1. minimal	45.89	45.28 - 47.19	< 0.01 (1 vs 3)
2. intermediate	52	47.61 - 52.78	< 0.05 (1 vs 2)
3. maximal	56.59	53.33 -57.88	< 0.05 (2 vs 3)

Note: Number of diabetes duration yearly groups (n) in all clusters is 16.

Table 3. Comparison of daily insulin doses standardized for every year of disease duration in the range of 0-15 years in clusters of regions singled out according to prevalence of diabetes mellitus type 1 (Khalangot et al., 2009 [d]).

Insulin doses standardized according to the disease duration within the range of 0–15 years in the minimal prevalence cluster of T1D prevalence were significantly lower, when compared with the intermediate and maximal prevalence clusters. The values in the intermediate prevalence cluster were lower than those in the maximal prevalence cluster (figure 3, table 3).

By evaluating the data presented in table 3, it should be noted that the probability coefficients (*P*), in this case, reflect a relatively small number of the "yearly" groups (*n*=16) in each cluster. If we were to assess the individual data on the insulin dose in each cluster without yearly grouping, then the number of cases (*n*) corresponding to the number of patients would greatly increase: 4,658; 14,712 and 2,879 in the minimal, intermediate, and maximal prevalence clusters, respectively. The unstandardized according to the diabetes duration average doses and their standard deviations (SD) in each of the three clusters, were observed to be 46.62 (19.38); 51.54 (17.57); and 55.94 (19.46) units/day, respectively, which was found to increase ($p < 0.0001$) in the clusters with higher T1D prevalence. However, the correlation of the insulin dose and the T1D prevalence found in this current region needs to be explained. One of the explanations for the difference in the daily insulin doses could be that in different Ukrainian regions, the doctors administer different levels of diabetes control: the lower dose is explained not only by the lower requirement of insulin by patients, but rather by the lower quality of treatment. An alternative explanation could be the higher intensity of the autoimmune process in patients residing in a territory with higher T1D prevalence.

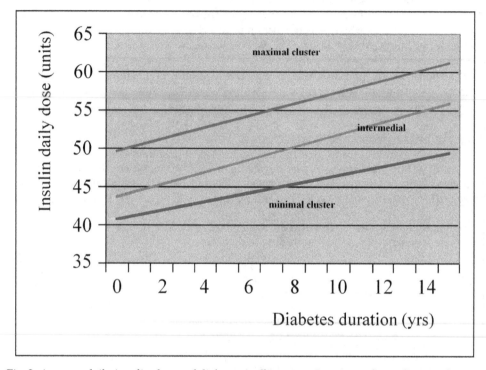

Fig. 3. Average daily insulin doses of diabetes mellitus type 1 patients depending on the disease duration (in the range of 0-15 years) as well as on the territorial cluster, selected according to disease prevalence (Khalangot et al., 2009 [d])

3.3.3 Quality of glucose lowering treatment and mean insulin doses in T1D prevalence clusters

Glycated hemoglobin (HbA1c) is considered as the most evident criteria in determining the quality of glucose-lowering treatment. We have analyzed and compared the levels of HbA1c of 1,288 T1D patients, included in the register. Table 4 shows the average HbA1c levels and the daily insulin doses according to the T1D prevalence clusters.

Type1 diabetes prevalence cluster	N	Mean HbA1c level, % (SD)	Mean insulin dose, U/day (SD)
1. Minimal	111	8.57 (3.29)	40.91(16.24)
2. Intermediate	778	8.24 (2,3)	51.5 (14.8)
3. Maximal	240	9.52 (2.24)	54.79 (18.05)
P (1 vs 3)		< 0.01	< 0.001

Table 4. Average levels of HbA1c (%) and insulin doses (units/day) considering territorial clusters with various diabetes type 1 prevalence (Khalangot et al., 2009 [d])

Prevalence of Type 1 Diabetes Correlates with Daily Insulin Dose, Adverse Outcomes and with
Autoimmune Process Against Glutamic Acid Decarboxylase in Adults

71

The level of HbA1c in the maximal prevalence cluster was significantly greater than that in the minimal prevalence cluster, which does not support the assumption of lower treatment quality in the regions with lower T1D prevalence. Therefore, the alternative explanation using the discovered phenomenon remains rather the most likely one. Its confirmation may include c-peptide determination as well as the determination of antibodies associated with diabetes in patients residing in the Ukrainian territories with different T1D prevalence. However, the reason for the heterogenic prevalence of T1D is still unknown.

3.4 GADA, IA and c-peptide levels in plasma of T1D patients from different prevalence clusters

The GADA and IA levels in children recently diagnosed with T1D are observed to be higher in countries with a greater incidence of this disease, such as Sweden, when compared with those where the T1D incidence is lower, such as Lithuania (Holmberg et al., 2006). In our study, the GADA levels and persistence in patients from the maximal T1D prevalence cluster (n=38), were higher than that in patients from the minimal prevalence cluster (n=48): 14.1±4.6 and 3.2±1.2 U/ml, respectively, mean ± SE = 0.028; OR = 9.66 (3.31–28.17), p< 0.001. Adjusting for age, gender, and duration of diabetes affected the results only slightly: OR = 7.91 (2.44–25.57), p< 0.001. However, the IA and c-peptide levels and their persistence were not observed to be associated with T1D prevalence. It should be noted that persistence of IA is common only for children with T1D (reviewed by Dib & Gomes, 2009), when our study analyzed adults. These data was obtained in 2007 and published earlier elsewhere (Khalangot et al., 2009 [d]). In another series of our studies (unpublished data) conducted in 2010 on T1D patients (11 from Minimal cluster and 18 from Maximal one) selected in the same way, the GADA levels also differed significantly: 0.92 (0.61-3.04) and 24.43 (3.28-61.42) U/l, Me , 95% CI, p = 0.003; adjusted for diabetes duration OR = 8.6 (1.1-65.7), p=0.036.

That is, the chance to have high GADA levels is almost 9 times higher for patients from the Maximal cluster as compared to the Minimal cluster, and this ratio was stable during repeated trials in these populations of T1D. Thus, the phenomenon of stable GADA persistence was discovered among adult T1D patients, residing in Ukraine within the maximal prevalence cluster.

3.5 T1D outcomes assessment in territorial prevalence clusters

The obtained results allow us to assume that there may be differences in the incidence of adverse outcomes of the disease among populations with varying prevalence of T1D. The gathered large cohort (29 708 T1D patients) may be viewed as almost complete data on this category of patients in Ukraine (Khalangot et al., 2009 [c], 2010). It should be noted, that the average duration of T1D is low (17.32 years). According to the data from a cross sectional study of Swedish National Diabetic Register (NDR), in 1997 the duration of T1D was 23.1 years and in 2004 it increased to 26.1 years. The criteria for T1D in the NDR study were treatment by insulin only and diagnosis before the age of 30 (Eeg-Olofsson et al., 2007), which corresponds to criteria used by us. According to the data from one of the regional diabetic registers in the US, the average T1D duration in a cohort of patients who were diagnosed before 19 years of age exceeded 25 years (Nishimura et al., 2001).

3.5.1 Main characteristics of T1D patients from the cohort studied

The number of men in this cohort is greater than the number of women. Men have shorter disease duration (P <0,001) and higher levels of blood pressure (BP) (p <0,001), whereas women have slightly higher levels of fasting glycemia (P <0,05). Blindness, cataracts and proliferative retinopathy more common for women (P <0,001). During 122,656.9 person-years (median observation period 4.7 years) 1958 deaths were recorded. The main cause of death was kidney failure. Cancer was very insignificant among other causes of death (table 5) . Possible reason for this phenomenon may be a short life expectancy of patients with diabetes.

Characteristics	Men	Women	All
Number of patients, n	15738	13970	29 708
Mean age, years (SD)	34.35(12.55)	34.61(13.30)	34.47(12.91)
Body mass index, kg/m² (SD)	23.01(3.84) n=14331	23.34(4.37) n=12729	23.16(4.10)
BP systolic, mm Hg (SD)	126.29(18.75)	125.48(20.81)	125.91(19.75)
BP diastolic, mm Hg. (SD)	78.57(10.53) n=14298	77.66(11.38) n=12654	78.15(10.94)
Fasting blood glucose, mmol/l (SD)	9.23(2.82) n=13747	9.30(2.87) n=12174	9.26(2.85)
HbA1c, % (SD)	8.68(2.53) n=1784	8.83(2.61) n=1789	8.75(2.57)
Smoking, n (%)*	3223 (20.48)	414(2.96)	3637(12.24)
Mean T1D duration, years	16.73	17.98	17.32
Nephropathy treatment, n (%)*	4627(31.42)	4921(37.59)	9548(34.32)
Cataract, n (%) *	1573(10.68)	2041(15.59)	3614(12.99)
Proliferative retinopathy, n (%) *	1187(8.06)	1297(9.91)	2484(8.93)
Blindness, n (%) *	459(3.1)	506(3.9)	965(3.47)
Follow up period, median, years	4.7	4.73	4.71
Total mortality cases, n (%)	1149 (100)	809(100)	1958(100)
CVD mortality, n (%)	266(23.15)	182(22.5)	448(22.88)
Cancer mortality, n (%)	16(1.39)	7(0.87)	23(1.17)
Renal failure, n (%)	295(25.67)	262(32.39)	557(28.45)
DKA and Coma	25(2.18)	36(4.45)	61(3.12)
Other reasons (%)	344(29.94)	174(21.51)	518(26.46)
Unknown	203(17.68)	148(18.29)	351(17.93)

Notes. BP – blood pressure, DKA – diabetic ketoacidosis;
* - data concerned to 14723 man and 13092 women

Table 5. Same characteristics of T1D patients' cohort (Khalangot et al., 2010)

Life expectancy of T1D patients in Ukraine in 2007, assessed according to age at the time of death did not exceed 40.2 yrs (Khalangot, 2008). In UK, according to similar cohort study this value is 55 yrs (Soedamah-Muthu et al., 2006), however the British cohort also included children, which could influence the assessment of average T1D duration and age at the time of death. Renal failure is the leading cause of death (28.4%) in T1D patient cohort, whereas according to a British study of DM patient register containing primary care data, the leading cause of death among T1D patients was CVD (Laing et al., 1999). Similar results were obtained by a European study EURODIAB (Soedamah-Muthu et al., 2008). Comparison of main causes of death according to EURODIAB data and Ukrainian Diabetes Register (UDR) data is shown in figure 4. Apparently death from renal failure among T1D patients in Ukraine prevails several times over other causes, while in other parts of Europe the main cause of death is CVD. It was previously noted by epidemiologists that the main cause of death for T1D patients is renal failure (Dorman et al., 1984), however these data were relevant in 1960s-1970s. Today's experts believe that the shift in mortality structure towards CVD happened due to intensification of hypotensive therapy and insulin treatment (Maahs et al., 2006), therefore the mortality structure of T1D patients that we have revealed when analyzing UDR can be assumed to conform to earlier time period of clinical practice.

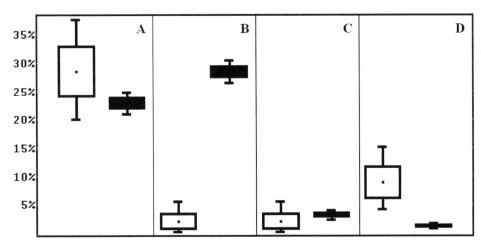

Note: given Means (%) ± SE (the dot within the box and height of boxes respectively), 95% CI (lines that emerge above and below the boxes). Data from Ukrainian Diabetes Register given according to Khalangot et al., 2010; EURODIAB given according to Soedamah-Muthu et al., 2008.

Fig. 4. Interval estimation of structure (%) of the main death causes among T1D patients, diagnosed before 30 years of age according to EURODIAB data (white boxes) and Ukrainian Diabetes Register (black boxes). Death causes: CVD (A); renal failure (B); DKA or coma (C); cancer (D).

3.5.2 Mortality assesment in territorial T1D prevalence clusters

To build the regression model we used 1925 deaths recorded among 27 896 patients. We have found that the patients living on the territory belonging to the maximal T1D prevalence cluster associated with increased risk of total mortality compared with the minimal prevalence cluster. In the minimal territorial cluster mortality was 15.68, and in the maximal -- 22.64 cases per 1000 person-years of follow up, $p < 0.001$. The risk (hazard ratio - HR) of death from all-cause mortality in patients from maximal in relation to the the minimal cluster was 1.5 (95% CI 1.31-1.79). Adjusting for gender had almost no effect on this risk: HRs standardized according to age, gender, and T1D duration for all cause mortality in the maximal T1D prevalence cluster compared to the minimal made up 1.56 (95 % CI 1.33-1.81), p<0.001, whereas the same value for diabetes-related mortality was 1.5 (95 % CI 1.14-1.96), p<0.001. The risk of total mortality for patients from the intermediate cluster did not differ from the minimal one (fig. 5, 6).

During the whole period of observation, 57 cases of death from acute T1D complications among 27510 patients have been recorded. It has been established, that prevalence of T1D is directly associated with the increase of mortality from acute T1D complications (table 6, figure 7). Hazard ratios, determined using Cox model of regression, and standartized according to gender, duration, and age in maximal territorial cluster of T1D prevalence comparing to the minimal cluster, exceeded 5 : HR= 5.25 (95% CI 1.76-15.63), p<0.001.

T1D prevalence cluster	Patients, n	Follow up period, person years	Mean Follow up, years	SD	Death cases, n	Death cases per 1000 person-years
Minimal	5 769	20 079,52	3.48	1.74	4	0.2
Intermedial	17 898	77 323,3	4.3	1.69	36	0.47
Maximal	3 919	17 974,66	4.59	1.79	17	0.95

Table 6. Mortality related to acute T1D complications (Khalangot et al., 2010)

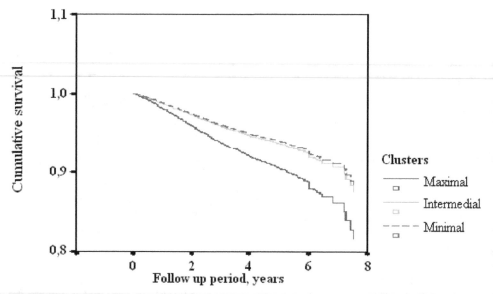

Fig. 5. All cause mortality represented by survival function in minimal, intermediate, and maximal clusters of T1D prevalence (Khalangot et al., 2009c)

3.5.3 Assesment of high blood pressure and proliferative retinopathy prevalence in territorial T1D prevalence clusters

Assessment of arterial hypertension (AH) incidence among patients in regional clusters was performed using the same cohort of 27 896 patients. A total of 4159 hypertension cases, or

Prevalence of Type 1 Diabetes Correlates with Daily Insulin Dose, Adverse Outcomes and with
Autoimmune Process Against Glutamic Acid Decarboxylase in Adults

75

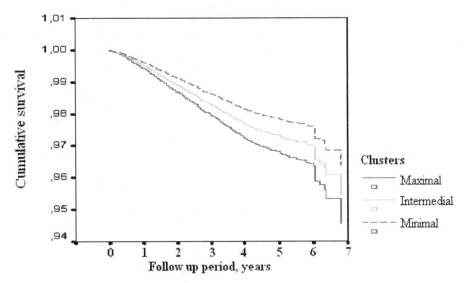

Fig. 6. DM-related mortality represented by survival function in minimal, intermediate, and maximal clusters of T1D prevalence (Khalangot et al., 2009c)

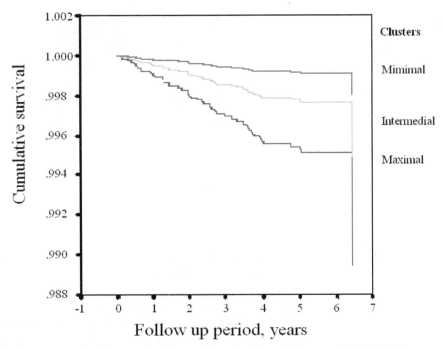

Fig. 7. Mortality related to acute T1D complications (cumulative survival) in different territorial clusters (Khalangot et al., 2010)

14.91%, were recorded. The minimal cluster included 691 AH cases (11.79%), maximal cluster had 570 cases (14.46%), and intermediate cluster included 2898 AH cases (16.02%). The prevalence of AH or proliferative retinopathy (PR) in the maximal or intermediale clusters is greater in relation to the minimal one (Table 7, Fig. 8). Hazard ratios were 1.36 and 1.46 for maximal and intermediale clusters in relation to the minimal cluster, the HR of which was considered as 1. Each year the T1D duration increases the risk of having hypertension. Adjusting according to gender, age and diabetes duration did not significantly change the risk of AH (table 6). Corresponding ORs for AH and PR were 1.36 (95% CI 1.2-1.54), p<0,001 and 2.04 (95 % CI 1.72-2.41), p<0.001. It was revealed that T1D prevalence is directly linked to the increase of all-cause and diabetes-related mortality risks, as well as to PR and AH prevalence.

T1D prevalence cluster	Patients, n	Cases of Arterial Hypertension, n	%	95 % CI
Minimal	5860	691	11.8	11.0-12.6
Intermedial	18095	2898	16.0	15.5-16.6
Maximal	3941	570	14.5	13.4-15.6

Table 7. Prevalence of arterial hypertension in T1D patients in different territorial clusters (Khalangot et al., 2009c)

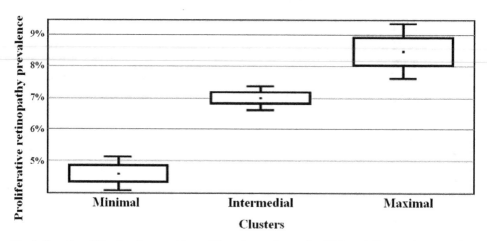

Fig. 8. Fraction (%) of patients with proliferative retinopathy (PR) in different clusters of T1D prevalene. The levels of PR prevalence (the dot within the box), its standart errors (the box height) and 95% CI (lines that emerge) are shown (Khalangot et al., 2009c).

We have found only one study that compared mortality between populations that differ in prevalence of T1D. This was a joint study of epidemiologists from Finland and Japan (Asao et al., 2003). Previously it was known that the incidence and prevalence of T1D in Finland is several times higher than in Japan, however mortality is higher among Japanese patients. The researchers explain this phenomenon by the fact that Finland was "disturbed" by its world's highest incidence of T1D, and because of that the Finnish health care system has long been implementing public programs of relevant quality for treating diabetes (Asao et al., 2003). Comparison of our mortality data among patients with T1D in Ukraine (from 15.7 to 22.6 per 1000 person-years, respectively, in the minimal and maximal prevalence clusters) with mortality among patients with juvenile T1D in Japan and Finland (6.07 and 3.52 per 1000 person-years, respectively), demonstrates a considerably higher mortality in Ukraine and the presense of an opposing relationship between the frequency of T1D in compared countries and mortality in cohorts of patients with juvenile diabetes. Please note that cited Asao et al. study (2003) compared the mortality in cohorts of patients with infantile T1D from different countries, while our study compares T1D that develops in patients before the age of 30 in the same country.

4. T1D sybtype may be responsible for the T1D territorial heterogenity in Ukraine

Currently, researchers (eg. Dib & Gomes, 2009) distinguish such subtypes of T1D, as T1A (characterized by selective destruction of beta-cells by an autoimmune process that quickly leads to absolute insulin deficiency; most common among caucasians), LADA (Latent Autoimmune Diabetes in Adults with an onset usually after 35 years of age and characterized by slowly developing insulin deficit), and T1B, also called idiopathic (clinical course is similar to T1A, but without the autoimmune component). Fulminant diabetes is one of the subtypes of T1B. Its is common in asian countries, such as Japan, China, and Korea. It is characterized by a very quick progression of acute metabolic decompensation, damage of alpha and beta cells of pancreas, and absence of autoimmune disorders. The discovered positive relationship between T1D prevalence, exogenic insulin requirement level, development of diabetes complications, and mortality does not allow us to associate T1D territorial heterogenity with LADA. Furthermore, the increase of GADA persistence in T1D patients who reside in regions with higher prevalence of this disease does not allow to consider T1B as responsible for this phenomenon. Thus, T1A rather than T1B subtype of T1D determines the territorial differences in the risk of developing T1D as well as course severity of this autoimmune disease.

5. Future studies

Causal link between the territorial distribution of autoimmune T1D in adults and the severity of its course and outcomes remains unknown. The recently discovered antibodies to the type 8 zinc transporter (ZnT8As) have substantially improved the clinical stratification of autoimmune diabetes in adults, demonstrating the link to a more severe insulin deficiency (Lampasone et al., 2010). Swedish researchers point out the possibility of low zinc content in drinking water as a possible T1D risk factor in children (Samuelsson et al., 2010; Haglund et al., 1996). Interestingly, in accordance with our preliminary results (unpublished data), there is no shortage of zinc in blood plasma in adults without diabetes, residing on territories with high prevalence of T1D, and we have even observed an increase of plasma zinc levels among adults with T1D comparing to similar patients from the minimal cluster. Plasma zink levels may be low (T2D) or high (T1D), zink supplementation may improve glycemic control in the two major types of diabetes, however the underlying molecular mechanisms have been elucidated very insignificantly (reviewed by Jansen et al. , 2009). It is possible that the study of ZnT8As in comparison to the levels of zinc in the environment and human body will provide new information about the cause of territorial heterogeneity of T1D.

6. Conclusions

We have shown, that the prevalence of T1D in the Ukrainian regions differs substantially. The daily insulin dose was found to increase regularly with the duration of the disease. This study also revealed a positive relation between T1D prevalence and the daily insulin doses, and observed a difference in the blood GADA levels among the T1D adults residing in territories with different T1D prevalence.

A unique feature of this study is that instead of examining the incidence, the prevalence of T1D was examined. This can be attributed to the relatively recent development of the Ukrainian diabetes-mellitus register (Khalangot & Tronko, 2007). Nevertheless, we believe that such an approach enabled us to study virtually the entire Ukrainian T1D population, and reveal a positive correlation between T1D prevalence, intensity of insulin treatment, hyperglycemia (HbA1c), and GADA levels, and its prevalence in adults. However, an earlier study of GADA in children recently diagnosed with T1D did not find any relation between GADA positivity and the clinical parameters of the disease (Holmberg, 2006).

7. Acknowledgements

The authors of this work acknowledge the efforts of all Ukrainian endocrinologists, who have contributed data about their patients to the diabetes mellitus register. Special thanks to Novo Nordisk A/C, Ukraine, for helping to promote the manuscript.

8. References

Altman D.G., Machin D., Bryant T.N., Gardner M.J. (Ed(s)). (2003). Statistics with confidence. Confidence intervals and statistical guidelines. Edited by Bristol.– BMJ Books. Second edition.–240 p.

Amos A.F., McCarty D.J., Zimmet P. (1997). The rising global burden of diabetes and its complications: estimates and projections to the year 2010. Diabet Med. Vol. 14, suppl 5, pp. S1-85.

Anonymous. (2006) Main indicators of endocrinologicalcare of Ukraine for 2005: review. Kiev: V.P. Komisarenko Institute of Endocrinology and Metabolism (Acad Med Sci, Ukraine Ministry of Health) Press Limited, (in Ukrainian).

Asao K., Satri C., Forsen N. et al. (2003). Long-term mortality in nationwide cohorts of childhood-onset type 1 diabetes in Japan and Finland. Diabetes Care. Vol. 26, pp. 2037-2042.

Bland M. (2000). An introdaction to medical statistics. New York. Oxford University Press. Third edition. 405 p.

Bonora E., Coscelli C., Butturini U. (1984). Residual B-cell function in type 1 (insulin-dependent) diabetes mellitus: its relation to clinical and metabolic features. *Acta Diabetol. Lat.* Vol. 21, № 4, pp. 375 – 383.

Boyle D.I., Cunningham S., Sullivan F.M., Morris A. (2001). Technology integration for the provision of population-based equitable patient care: The Tayside Regional Diabetes Network--a brief description. *Diabetes Nutr Metab.* Vol. 14, pp. 100-103.

Carstensen B., Kristensen J.K., Ottosen P., Borch-Johnsen K. (2008). On behalf of the steering group of the National Diabetes Register. The Danish National Diabetes Register: trends in incidence, prevalence and mortality. *Diabetologia*. Vol. 51, pp. 2187-2196.

Curtis J.P., Selter J.G., Wang Y., et al. (2005). The obesity paradox: body mass index and outcomes in patients with heart failure. *Arch Intern Med*. Vol. 165, pp. 55-61.

Dib SA, Gomes MB. (2009). Etiopathogenesis of type 1 diabetes mellitus: prognostic factors for the evolution of residual beta cell function. *Diabetol Metab Syndr*. Vol. 4, № 1, 25 p.

Doney A.S., Fischer B., Cecil J.E., Cohen P.T., Boyle D.I., Leese G., Morris A.D., Palmer C.N. (2003). Male preponderance in early diagnosed type 2 diabetes is associated with the ARE insertion/deletion polymorphism in the PPP1R3A locus. *BMC Genet*. Vol. 4, p.11.

Doney A.S.F., Lee S., Leese G.P., Morris A.D., Palmer C.N.A. (2005). Increased cardiovascular morbidity and mortality in type 2 diabetes is associated with the glutathione S transferase theta-null genotype: A Go-DARTS Study *Circulation*. Vol. 111, pp. 2927-2934.

Dorman J.S., Laporte R.E., Kuller L.H., Cruickshanks K.J., Orchard T.J., Wagener D.K., Becker D.J., Cavender D.E., Drash A.L. (1984). The Pittsburgh insulin-dependent diabetes mellitus (IDDM) morbidity and mortality study. Mortality results. *Diabetes*. Vol. 33, № 3, pp. 271 -276.

Eeg-Olofsson K., Cederholm J., Nilsson P.M., Gudbjörnsdóttir S., Eliasson B. (2007). Steering Committee of the Swedish National Diabetes Register. Glycemic and risk factor control in type 1 diabetes: results from 13,612 patients in a national diabetes register. *Diabetes Care*. Vol. 30, № 3, pp. 496-502.

Evans J.M., Donnelly L.A., Emslie-Smith A.M. et al. (2005). Metformin and reduced risk of cancer in diabetic patients *BMJ*. Vol. 330, pp. 1304-1305.

Evans J.M., Ogston S.A., Emslie-Smith A., Morris A.D. (2006). Risk of mortality and adverse cardiovascular outcomes in type 2 diabetes: a comparison of patients treated with sulfonylureas and metformin. *Diabetologia*. Vol. 49, pp. 930-936.

Gale E.A.M. (2002) The rise of childhood type 1 diabetes in the 20th Century. *Diabetes*. Vol. 51, pp. 3353 - 3361.

Gorus FK. (1996). The importance of diabetes registries and clinical biology for the study and treatment of type1 diabetes mellitus. *Verh K Acad Geneeskd Belg*. V. 58, pp. 539 - 586.

Green A., Patterson C.C. (2001). EURODIAB TIGER Study Group. Europe and Diabetes.Trends in the incidence of childhood-onset diabetes in Europe 1989-1998. *Diabetologia*. Vol. 44, suppl 3, pp. B3-8.

Gruberg L., Weissman N.J., Waksman R., et al. (2002). The impact of obesity on the short-term and long-term outcomes after percutaneous coronary intervention: the obesity paradox? *Am Coll Cardiol*. Vol. 39, pp. 578-584.

Haglund B., Ryckenberg K., Selinus O., Dahlquist G. (1996). Evidence of a relationship between childhood-onset type I diabetes and lowgroundwater concentration of zinc. *Diabetes Care*. Vol. 19, № 8, pp. 873-875.

Holmberg H., Vaarala O., Sadauskaite-Kuehne V., Ilonen J., Padaiga Z., Ludvigsson J. (2006). Higher prevalence of autoantibodies to insulin and GAD65 in Swedish compared to Lithuanian children with type 1 diabetes. *Diabetes Res Clin Pract*. Vol. 72, № 3, pp. 308-314.

Jansen J., Karges W., Rink L. (2009). Zinc and diabetes--clinical links and molecular mechanisms. *J Nutr Biochem*. Vol. 20, № 6, pp. 399-417.

Keen H. (1988). Limitations and problems of diabetes classification from an epidemiological point of view. In: M. Vranic, C. H. Hollenberg, G. Steiner (Ed.) *Comparison of type I and type II diabetes*. New York, Plenum Press.

Khalangot M, Tronko M. (2007). Primary care diabetes in Ukraine. *Primary Care Diabetes*. № 1, pp. 203-205.

Khalangot, 2008 . [Age and sex–related pecularietes of mortality in type 1 diabetes mellitus patients]. (Article in Ukrainian) Problemy starenia I dolgoletia. 2008. 17(1): 75-82. http://www.nbuv.gov.ua/portal/Chem_Biol/PSD/2008_1.

Khalangot M. D. (2009) Epedemiologic characteristics of diabetes mellitus type1 and 2 according to data from national population-based patient register. Manuscript. Thesis for the Degree of Doctor of Medical Sciences. V.P.Komisarenko Institute of Endocrinology and Metabolism AMS of Ukraine, Kiev.

Khalangot M., Hu G., Tronko M., Kravchenko V., Guryanov V. (2009a January-February). Gender risk of nonfatal stroke in type 2 diabetic patients differs depending on the type of treatment. *J Womens Health (Larchmt)*. Vol. 18, № 1, pp. 97-103.

Khalangot M., Tronko M., Kravchenko V., Kulchinska J., Hu G. (2009b, March). Body mass index and the risk of total and cardiovascular mortality among patients with type 2diabetes: a large prospective study in Ukraine. *Heart*. Vol. 95, № 6, pp. 454-560.

Khalangot M. D., Kravchenko V. I., Okhrimenko N. V., Kovtun V.A., Tronko E. M. (2009c). [Analysis of mortality, proliferative retinopathy prevalence, and arterial hypertension among type 1 diabetic patients residing in areas that differ in prevalence of this disease] *Endocrinologia*. Vol. 14 , № 1, pp. 77-85 (Article in Ukrainian).

Khalangot M., Kravchenko V., Tronko M., Gur'ianov V. (2009 d, Octoвer). Correlation between the prevalence of type 1 diabetes with the daily insulin dose and the autoimmuneprocess against glutamic acid decarboxylase in adults. *Eur J Intern Med*. Vol. 20, № 6, pp. 611-615.

Khalangot M., Tronko M., Kravchenko V., Kovtun V. (2009 e, December) Glibenclamide-related excess in total and cardiovascular mortality risks: data from large Ukrainian observational cohort study. *Diabetes Res ClinPract*. Vol. 86, № 3, pp. 247-253.

Khalangot M. D., Tronko M.D., Kravchenko V. I., Kovtun V.A., Okhrimenko N. V., Bolgarska S.V. (2010) [Some mortality risk factors for type 1 diabetes mellitus patients in Ukraine evaluated according to data from National Register] *Endocrinologia*. Vol. 15 , № 1, pp. 62-70 (Article in Ukrainian).

Kyvik K.O., Nystrom L., Gorus F., Songini M., Oestman J., Castell C., Green A, Guyrus E., Ionescu-Tirgoviste C., McKinney P.A., Michalkova D., Ostrauskas R., Raymond N.T. (2004, Mar.) The epidemiology of Type 1 diabetes mellitus is not the same in young adults as in children. *Diabetologia*. Vol. 47, № 3, pp. 377-384.

Laing S.P., Swerdlow A.J., Slater S.D., Botha J.L., Burden A.C., Waugh N.R., Smith A.W., Hill R.D., Bingley P.J., Patterson C.C., Qiao Z., Keen H. (1999). The British Diabetic Association Cohort Study, II: cause-specific mortality in patients with insulin-treated diabetes mellitus. *Diabet Med*. Vol. 16, № 6, pp. 466-471.

Lampasona V., Petrone A., Tiberti C., Capizzi M., Spoletini M., di Pietro S., Songini M., Bonicchio S., Giorgino F., Bonifacio E., Bosi E., Buzzetti R. (2010). Non Insulin

Prevalence of Type 1 Diabetes Correlates with Daily Insulin Dose, Adverse Outcomes and with
Autoimmune Process Against Glutamic Acid Decarboxylase in Adults

81

Requiring Autoimmune Diabetes (NIRAD) Study Group. Zinc transporter 8 antibodies complement GAD and IA-2 antibodies in the identification and characterization of adult-onset autoimmune diabetes: Non Insulin Requiring Autoimmune Diabetes (NIRAD) 4. *Diabetes Care.* Vol. 33, № 1, pp. 104-108.

Leese G., Boyle D., Morris A. (2006). The Tayside Diabetes Network . *Diabetes Research and Clinical Practice* . Vol. 74, suppl. 2, pp. 197 – 199.

Lévy-Marchal C., Patterson C.C., Green A. (2001). EURODIAB ACE Study Group. Europe and Diabetes. Geographical variation of presentation at diagnosis of type I diabetes in children: the EURODIAB study. *Diabetologia.* Vol. 44, suppl. 3, pp. B75-80.

Liakh Yu.E., Gurianov V.G. (2004). Data Analysis of Biomedical Researches and Clinical Trials by Means of Statistical Program MedStat.*Vestn. Hyg. Epid.* Vol. 8, № 1, pp. 155 - 167.

Linn T., Mann M., Mann M., Bretzel R.G., Boedeker R.H. (2003). Randomised prospective study for the effect of therapy on residual beta cell function in type-1 diabetes mellitus. *BMC Endocr. Disord.* Vol. 3, № 1, 5 p.

Maahs DM, Rewers M. Editorial: (2006). Mortality and renal disease in type 1 diabetes mellitus — progress made, more to be done. *J Clin Endocrinol Metab.* Vol. 91, № 10, pp. 3757 – 3759.

Marascuilo, L. (1966) Large-Sample Multiple Comparisons. *Psychological Bulletin.* V. 65, № 4, pp. 289-299.

Monami M., Balzi D., Lamanna C., Barchielli A., Masotti G., Buiatti E., Marchionni N., Mannucci E. (2007). Are sulphonylureas all the same? A cohort study on cardiovascular and cancer-related mortality. *Diabetes Metab Res Rev.* Vol. 23, pp. 479-484.

Morris A.D., Boyle D.I., MacAlpine R. et al. (1997). The diabetes audit and research in Tayside Scotland (DARTS) study: electronic record linkage to create a diabetes register (DARTS/MEMO Collaboration). *BMJ.* Vol. 315, pp. 524–528.

Nishimura R., LaPorte R.E., Dorman J.S., Tajima N., Becker D., Orchard T.J. (2001). Mortality trends in type 1 diabetes. The Allegheny County (Pennsylvania) Registry 1965-1999. *Diabetes Care.* Vol. 24, № 5, pp. 823-827.

Samuelsson U., Oikarinen S., Hyöty H.,Ludvigsson J. (2010). Low zinc in drinking water is associated with the risk of type 1 diabetes in children. *Pediatr Diabetes.*, 7. doi: 10.1111/j.1399-5448.2010.00678.x.

Schofield C.J., Libby G., Brennan G.M., MacAlpine R R., Morris A.D., Leese G.P. (2006). (DARTS/MEMO Collaboration). Mortality and hospitalization in patients after amputation: A comparison between patients with and without diabetes. *Diabetes Care.* Vol. 29, pp. 2252–2256.

Soedamah-Muthu S.S., Fuller J.H., Mulnier H.E., Raleigh V.S., Lawrenson R.A., Colhoun H.M. (2006). All-cause mortality rates in patients with type 1 diabetes mellitus compared with a non-diabetic population from the UK general practice research database, 1992-1999. *Diabetologia.* Vol. 49, № 4, pp. 660-666.

Soedamah-Muthu S.S., Chaturvedi N., Witte D.R., Stevens L.K., Porta M., Fuller J.H. (2008). EURODIAB Prospective Complications Study Group. Relationship between risk factors and mortality in type 1 diabetic patients in Europe: the EURODIAB Prospective Complications Study (PCS). *Diabetes Care.* Vol. 31, № 7, pp. 1360-1366.

The DCCT Research Group. (1987). Effects of age, duration and treatment of insulin-dependent diabetes mellitus on residual beta-cell function: observations during eligibility testing for the Diabetes Control and Complications Trial (DCCT). *J Clin Endocrinol Metab.* Vol. 65, № 1, pp. 30 – 36.

The Diabetes Control and Complications Trial Research Group. (1998). Effect of intensive therapy on residual beta-cell function in patients with type 1 diabetes in the diabetes control and complications trial. A randomized, controlled trial. *Ann Intern Med.* Vol. 128, № 7, pp. 517 – 523.

Vaiserman A., Khalangot M. (2008). Similar seasonality of birth in type 1 and type 2 diabetes patients: a sign for common etiology? *Med Hypotheses.* Vol. 71, № 46, pp. 604-605.

Vaiserman A.M., Khalangot M.D., Carstensen B., Tronko M.D., Kravchenko V.I., Voitenko V.P., Mechova L.V., Koshel N.M., Grigoriev P.E. (2009) Seasonality of birth in adult type 2 diabetic patients in three Ukrainian regions. *Diabetologia.* Vol. 52, № 12, pp. 2665-2667.

Vandewalle C.L., Coeckelberghs M.I., De Leeuw I.H., Du Caju M.V., Schuit F.C., Pipeleers D.G., Gorus F.K. (1997). Epidemiology, clinical aspects, and biology of IDDM patients under age 40 years. Comparison of data from Antwerp with complete ascertainment with data from Belgium with 40% ascertainment. The Belgian Diabetes Registry. *Diabetes Care.* Vol. 20, pp. 1556-1561.

Weets I., Van Autreve J., Van der Auwera B.J., Schuit F.C., Du Caju M.V., Decochez K., De Leeuw I.H., Keymeulen B., Mathieu C., Rottiers R., Dorchy H., Quartier E., Gorus F.K. (2001). Belgian Diabetes Registry. Male-to-female excess in diabetes diagnosed in early adulthood is not specific for the immune-mediated form nor is it HLA-DQ restricted: possible relation to increased body mass index. *Diabetologia.* Vol. 44, pp. 40-47.

Weets I., Siraux V., Daubresse J.C., De Leeuw I.H., Féry F., Keymeulen B., Krzentowski G., Letiexhe M., Mathieu C., Nobels F., Rottiers R., Scheen A., Van Gaal L., Schuit F.C., Van der Auwera B., Rui M., De Pauw P., Kaufman L., Gorus F.K. (2002). Belgian Diabetes Registry. Relation between disease phenotype and HLA-DQ genotype in diabetic patients diagnosed in early adulthood. *Clin Endocrinol Metab.* Vol. 87, pp. 2597-2605.

Part 2

Psychological Aspects of Diabetes

5

Type I Diabetes in Children and Adolescents

Laura Nabors[1], Phillip Neal Ritchey[2],
Bevin Van Wassenhove[3] and Jennifer Bartz[3]
*[1]School of Human Services, College of Education, Criminal Justice, and
Human Services, University of Cincinnati,
[2]Department of Sociology, College of Arts and Sciences, University of Cincinnati,
[3]Department of Psychology, College of Arts and Sciences, University of Cincinnati,
Cincinnati, Ohio
USA*

1. Introduction

Type I Diabetes is characterized by pancreatic failure. Daily exogenous insulin replacement is necessary for the child's survival. Insulin typically is administered by injections before lunch and dinner. Type I diabetes affects approximately 1 in every 400 to 600 children (Centers for Disease Control and Prevention, 2003). Rates of Type I diabetes are increasing (Chisholm et al., 2007). This is concerning as this disease has long-term health care consequences including problems with circulation, vision, and cardiovascular issues (Frey et al., 2006). The care of children with Type I diabetes involves complex procedures including daily blood glucose testing, dietary monitoring, intensive insulin therapy, and increased physical activity to maintain metabolic control (Anderson et al., 2007). Several studies have shown that children as well as adolescents have difficulty adhering to diet, exercise, blood glucose testing, and insulin regimens (e.g., Chang et al., 2007; Frey et al., 2006). Patterns of diabetes care are established early in the disease course, and therefore understanding factors related to child adherence is a mechanism for generating strategies to improve diabetes management for children. This, in turn, may positively influence health outcomes in adolescence and adulthood (Bui et al., 2005).

Children's management of their diabetes is often measured by assessment of blood glucose or HbA1c levels (i.e., measure of diabetic control). Monitoring blood glucose levels has become an increasingly important self-management task for children who have diabetes (Bui et al., 2005). Psychosocial factors, such as attitudes about one's diabetes, support from others, and stress, have been related to HbA1c levels or other factors serving as proxy variables for diabetes management (Chisholm et al., 2007; Nabors et al., 2010). This chapter reviews the relationship between psychosocial factors, chiefly children's attitudes, support from others, stress, and diabetes management. This chapter will provide suggestions for improving children's attitudes and reducing their stress to improve their diabetes management. The next section of this chapter reviews ways in which children's attitudes, namely health locus of control and stress, influence children's diabetes management.

2. Diabetes management and children

2.1 Attitude and diabetes

Health locus of control, a concept originating from Rotter's (1966) theory, is a belief about whether an individual might receive positive outcomes resulting from a particular health behavior. Thus, a child may estimate that eating "healthy" (e.g., "low carbohydrate" foods), drinking water, engaging in mild exercise, and reducing his or her stress will result in good diabetes management. The relations among beliefs, such as locus of control, and health actions have been illustrated in theoretical models, including the Health Belief Model (Rosenstock, 1974). Research supports relationships between locus of control beliefs and diabetes management (Bennett-Murphy et al., 1997). Locus of control may influence self-confidence, such that children with an internal locus of control, or an "I can do it" attitude, may do a better job of assisting with their diabetes management (Nabors et al., 2010).

Children's perceptions of their diabetes are related to regimen adherence and their HbA1c levels (Edgar & Skinner, 2003). For example, Lehmkuhl and Nabors (2008) found that feelings of sadness and feeling that having the disease was unfair were related to higher HbA1c levels for children. Others have reported that confidence in the ability to improve one's health was an indicator of good diabetes management for children (Skinner & Hampson, 1998). Similarly, Nabors et al. (2010) found that children with a higher level of an internal locus of control over (their health) disease were more likely to have lower HbA1c levels, indicating better glycemic control, than children with lower levels of an internal locus of control. Consequently, it may be that a myriad of attitudinal factors, including locus of control (Nabors et al., 2010), beliefs about the seriousness of one's illness (Edgar & Skinner, 2003), and beliefs about being able to compensate for different behaviors that might negatively influence diabetes management (Rabiau et al., 2009) contribute to self-management behaviors.

2.2 Stress and diabetes

Another psychological factor influencing diabetes management is stress (Beveridge et al., 2006; Seiffge-Krenke & Stemmler, 2003). Research has demonstrated that stress is indirectly related to HbA1c levels (Aiken et al., 1992). Balfour and colleagues (1993) proposed that stress is directly related to dietary control, which then influences glycemic control. Likewise, Helgeson et al. (2010) reported that stress may be related to poor self-care, which in turn negatively influences metabolic control. One type of stress that might be particularly salient for children with Type I Diabetes is fear of hypoglycemic episodes. These episodes can cause seizures, resulting in a coma and even death (Green et al., 1990). When a child is fearful of hypoglycemic episodes, he or she may ignore a medical regimen and administer insulin as he or she deems necessary. This can result in poor control. Over time, this can lead to negative health outcomes and elevated stress for the child. Then again, this "worry" is not a universal experience for all children who have diabetes. Marrero et al. (1997) assessed parent perceptions of child reactions to hypoglycemic episodes. Their results indicated that youth who had experienced a hypoglycemic event were experiencing higher levels of worry and anxiety. This was not necessarily related to diabetes management, however, which is a positive finding in that the worry was not appearing to translate into poor disease management. On the other hand, these authors have found that children also can worry about experiencing hyperglycemia or feeling "high." Thus, the medical team should carefully assess child or parent fears about these types of episodes and explain ways to treat these episodes and make referrals for counseling as necessary.

Children may experience stress related to feeling different from peers due to having Type I Diabetes. They also may have difficulty talking to teachers about how to manage their disease at school (Nabors et al., 2003). Coaching for these children, in addition to written care plans may assist them in communicating important information to teachers and other professionals in the school setting. But, not all children and adolescents with diabetes may face significant diabetes-related stressors. For example, Hema et al. (2009) discovered that children and adolescents with diabetes reported daily stressors similar to youth without chronic illnesses; interestingly, they did not report significant diabetes-related stressors as being hassles. Consequently, health care professionals need to consider the social and emotional needs of children with diabetes to determine whether recommendations for stress management or referral for counseling is appropriate (Chisholm et al., 2007).

Children with diabetes also can experience stress related to negative school experiences. Storch et al. (2006) found a link between bullying of children with diabetes and self-management behaviors. If children with diabetes experienced teasing or negative reactions from peers for testing their blood glucose or other self-management behaviors, they were less likely to engage in self-care. In addition, these researchers proposed that children who are depressed because of having diabetes may be less likely to monitor their glucose levels. They concluded that assessment of bullying experiences by peers is an important component of clinical interviews with school-age children, because bullying can be an indicator of poor self-management and higher HbA1c levels.

In another study, Peters et al. (2008) assessed the relationship between experiences of teachers being unsupportive and adherence and self-management in one hundred and sixty-seven children, between the ages of eight to seventeen years, with Type 1 Diabetes. Their findings indicated that perceptions of teachers as being unsupportive of the child's self-management were related to poorer adherence behaviors for younger children, between the ages of eight and eleven years, but not for older children (ages twelve through seventeen). Thus, a poor teacher-student relationship, often characterized by teachers misunderstanding the importance of adherence to the medical regimen, may be detrimental to diabetes management for elementary or primary school-age youth, who depend on teacher support and guidance to facilitate their efforts at managing their diabetes at school.

3. Systems-level factors and diabetes management

3.1 Support from others

Diabetes management can be very difficult and children may not be able to independently manage their treatment regimen (Allen et al., 1983). Additionally, children have reported that they benefit from support from teachers, peers, and nurses in school settings (Nabors et al., 2003). A key factor influencing diabetes management is support from friends and family. LaGreca et al. (1995) reported that support from parents and friends were protective factors for adolescents with diabetes. Greco and her colleagues (2001) found that support from a best friend was perceived as beneficial for diabetes management by adolescents. Skinner and Hampson (1998) also discovered that family support is a critical component of diabetes management for adolescents.

Arguably, the most important support for diabetes management may come from children's parents. Hanna and Guthrie (2001) reported that when parents acted as supervisors, providing guidance to assist their child in diabetes management, both parents and their child who had diabetes felt more comfortable about managing the child's disease. Guidelines of the American Diabetes Association (Silverstein et al., 2005) suggest that parent and child teamwork, or shared responsibility, for diabetes management tasks facilitates diabetes management. Thus, a partnership between the child and parent, synonymous with joint ownership of diabetes management and care, may be one strategy that doctors can emphasize to promote child wellness (Beveridge et al., 2006). We believe that the supportive role of parents can be influenced by other family and disease related factors; consequently, these factors also are an area of inquiry for clinical interviews and possible intervention.

3.2 Family adjustment model

John Rolland (1987) presented a conceptual framework for viewing family adjustment to a child's chronic illness. He suggested that the family's developmental stage, the child's own developmental stage, and factors related to the child's illness influence family members' adjustment to a child's chronic illness. Rolland proposed that these factors interact and influence child and family adjustment at different points in the child's life. This theory has explanatory "validity" when one reviews literature on parents' and children's adjustment to childhood diabetes. For example, literature reviewed for this chapter indicated that parents respond differently, in terms of helping the child manage his or her diabetes, based on the child's age or the duration of his or her diabetes (Fielding & Duff, 1999; Hanna & Guthrie, 2001). Others have shown that child age and health status (e.g., diabetes "control") can have a significant influence on diabetes management (Lewin et al., 2006). Furthermore, parents' roles change based on whether the child has good "control" (i.e., glycemic control) of his or her diabetes (Davis et al., 2000). Thus, the supportive role of parents and family is influenced by parent or family factors, disease-related factors, and the stage of the child's development.

Different points in the child or family lifecycle may influence adherence behaviors, such that education or counseling may be needed at various phases of the child's life (Rolland, 1987). For this reason, we recommend that mental health professionals play a supportive role. The analogy of a "band of support" may illuminate this role. The mental health professional plays an educational or counseling role as needed and offers more or less support based on an assessment of child and family stress as well as anxiety. Because both parents and children often experience stress related to disease management, collaboration between counselors and the child's medical team remains an important part of clinical practice. This collaboration can provide critical information for the child's doctor and other members of their medical team, who also can support the use of stress management techniques, education and therapy to decrease parent or child stress, and dietary and medication changes to manage the waxing and waning symptoms of this disease.

Thus far, we have presented literature highlighting issues for children. Nevertheless, as mentioned, parents experience significant stress too. Consequently, the next section of our chapter presents research related to parental stress and adjustment to a child's diabetes. We begin with a discussion of the association between parenting style and diabetes management. Next, we highlight adolescence as a critical period, as this is a time in the child's life where parental care and support often play a pivotal role in diabetes management. At the same time, due to the developmental changes and struggles experienced by some adolescents, this may be a time of heightened stress for parents. We conclude this section with a review of research related to parental adjustment and needs for counseling and education.

4. Diabetes management and parents

4.1 Parental interactions

Parental "style" or method of interacting with their child may be related to positive diabetes management and adherence to the child's medical regimen. For example, studies have shown that parental warmth and supportiveness are related to "good" glycemic control and adherence to diabetes regimens and fewer instances diabetic ketoacidosis (DKA; Geffken et al., 2008). Davis et al. (2000) assessed parenting styles of parents whose children had diabetes. They discovered that parental warmth and an emphasis on child self-management were related to positive health outcomes. They also reported that a more restrictive parenting style was correlated with relatively poorer management and higher stress levels for children.

Geffken and colleagues (2008) found that negative parental attitudes were related to instances of DKA in children with Type I Diabetes. These researchers assessed the relationship between child and caregiver opinions about family behavior and they also assessed episodes of diabetic ketoacidosis. Participants were one hundred children with Type I Diabetes and their caregivers. Study results indicated that children who perceived their parents attitudes toward them as being warm and caring were less likely to have reported episodes of ketoacidosis and were more likely to have better diabetes management than those who thought that their parents did not use warm and caring parenting styles.

Parenting style may change, based on child and parent/family stage of development (Rolland, 1987). Parents of young children may exhibit higher levels of control to assist the child in following his or her treatment regimen. As children enter adolescence and become more autonomous, parents often become more non-directive and are "available as needed" to provide guidance (Hanna & Guthrie, 2000; 2001). This non-directive stance may change, if the adolescent is managing his or her disease in a manner that results in *poor* glycemic control. If this occurs parent-adolescent conflict can ensue, as parents begin to provide more direct assistance and move away from an advisory role (Nabors et al., 2010). Being able to move between a supportive and directive stance based on the situation and the adolescent's needs may be particularly important as parents provide assistance to their teenager.

4.2 Parental adjustment

Parents may experience significant stress and anxiety related to their child's disease and its management (Driscoll et al., 2010). Parents may experience symptoms of stress similar to those experienced by individuals with Post-traumatic Stress Syndrome (PTSD). These symptoms can include hypervigilance, resulting in an over-monitoring of their child's disease management or conversely, avoidance resulting in under-monitoring. Research has demonstrated that 10% of mothers of children who had diabetes met criteria for a diagnosis of PTSD, while another 15% of mothers displayed some of the symptoms, partially meeting the criteria for this diagnosis (Horsch et al., 2007). Symptoms related to parental experiences of "PTSD" may increase, when the child has mental health problems in addition to his or her diabetes. Researchers have found that parents of children who have diabetes experience increased anxiety and depression if their children are experiencing mental health problems (Driscoll et al., 2010).

Parents may have a difficult time adjusting to their child's diabetes if they or their child do not feel confident about being able to manage the child's diabetes. Similarly, parents whose children have recently been diagnosed or are "newly" diagnosed also may experience high stress. Often a diagnosis occurs with little forewarning and parents may feel shock and grief related to learning about their child's illness. Parents in either of the aforementioned situations may benefit from education about disease management and counseling to improve their abilities to cope with stress as well as co-occurring symptoms of depression or anxiety (Streisand et al., 2008).

Poor parental adjustment and parental stress may be related to becoming overwhelmed with caretaking responsibilities and disease management for a significant period of time, leading to classic symptoms of "burnout. " Parents who are "burned out" may not assist their child with disease management, and feel apathetic about assisting their child in coping with his or her diabetes (Lindstrom et al., 2010). Other variables that may be related to parental stress are uncertainty about the treatment of the child's diabetes and uncertainty about health outcomes related to diabetes (Carpentier et al., 2006). Health care providers should informally assess parental stress and uncertainty associated with their child's illness on a regular, ongoing basis. Counseling should be recommended when parental stress is high, as lowering parental stress can have a positive influence on parents, which leads to improved diabetes management for their child. Parents experiencing high levels of trauma because their child has diabetes may require counseling to avoid symptoms of depression and anxiety (Horsch et al., 2007; Streisand et al., 2008).

5. Adolescence: A critical period

Parental support may be critical to diabetes management during adolescence, as children begin to take a more active role in managing their diabetes (Silverstein et al., 2005). Adherence is a very important area of study for adolescents with diabetes because managing IDDM involves multiple strategies including, diet, exercise, and glucose monitoring as well as administering medication (Helgeson et al., 2010). The early teenage years are a difficult time to manage insulin levels, because adolescents may have decreased insulin sensitivity and poor self-management skills (Shroff-Pendley et al., 2002). Difficulties in managing diabetes may also occur in late adolescence, especially when adolescents experience stressful life events (e.g., change in a romantic relationship, parental divorce; Helgeson et al., 2010). Self-care may be compromised for a period of time as the child copes with the event, and during this period the adolescent may require counseling or additional support from family or friends to manage his or her diabetes. Previous research (Weissberg-Benchell, 2007) and guidelines of the American Diabetes Association (Silverstein et al., 2005) suggest that parent and child teamwork, or shared responsibility, for diabetes management tasks facilitates diabetes management. Thus, a partnership between the adolescent and his or her parents may be one strategy that doctors can emphasize to promote the development of a relationship that is supportive and allows parents to move between doing more to assist with diabetes management when needed and doing less when the adolescent is doing a good job managing on his or her own.

Skinner and Hampson (1998) found that family support, such as high levels of connectedness among family members, is a critical component of diabetes management for teenagers. On the other hand, family conflict and a lack of cohesion in family relationships has been related to with poor metabolic control (higher glycosated hemoglobin levels or HgbA1C levels; Hauser, Jacobson, Lavori, et al., 1990). Strong, constructive family relationships may have a positive influence on adherence (Skinner at al., 2000; Lewin et al., 2006). Family functioning is related to adolescents' adherence, management, and metabolic control (Wysocki et al., 2001). In general, we believe that a positive parent-teenager relationship will lead to family cohesion and will improve diabetes management. For this reason, we recommend that members of the child's medical team encourage a team-based approach to diabetes management and in other aspects of the child's life as a "family-level" intervention when an adolescent is having difficulty with diabetes management.

6. Conclusion

Our review of the literature indicated that child and parent adjustment influence diabetes management. Moreover, the phase of the child's life and phase in the family's own life-cycle impacts disease management and glycemic control (Chisholm et al., 2007; Rolland, 1987). We recommend that health and mental health professionals provide support as needed to children and parents, providing education based on child and parent needs. This type of patient- and family-centered approach may improve child and parent efficacy for disease management. A child- or patient-focused approach to adherence will ensure that health care professionals and school personnel "meet children where they are" and offer patient-centered care that will promote diabetes management and wellness for youth (Bauman, 2000). Counseling for children may improve their ability to cope with difficult psychosocial and developmental issues. Existing studies (e.g., Cohen et al., 2004) indicate that children's emotional and behavioral problems and low family cohesion are related to regimen adherence as well as glycemic control. Interventions which provide education about stress management and increase peer support (i.e., support from close friends) may improve adjustment to diabetes (Boardway et al., 1993; Greco et al., 2001). Health and mental health professionals working with children with diabetes should also work with children and their parents to reduce barriers, such as a lack of support from teachers or friends, to child illness management. Working to strengthen positive attitudes about disease management and illness trajectories and reduce stress also may be related to patient and parent satisfaction with the child's medical care and adherence to the child's medical regimen. More research on ways that group and individual counseling can assist children with diabetes and their parents and other family members will provide more information about the success of these support-based interventions. In conclusion, strengthening child and parent resilience, working with children and parents to develop strategies to facilitate diabetes management, and helping children and parents adjust to diabetes-related stress are elements of successful care that will optimize care and health outcomes for children with diabetes.

7. References

Aiken, J., Wallender, J., Bell, D., & Cole, J. (1992). Daily stress variability, learned resourcefulness, regimen adherence, and metabolic control in Type 1 diabetes mellitus: Evaluation of a path model. *Journal of Consulting and Clinical Psychology,* Vol.60, pp. 113-118, ISSN 0022-006X

Allen, D. A., Tennen, H., McGrade, B. J., Affleck, G., & Ratzan, S. (1983). Parent and child perceptions of the management of juvenile diabetes. *Journal of Pediatric Psychology,* Vol.8, pp. 129-141, ISSN 0146-8693

Anderson, B. J., Svoren, B., & Laffel, L. (2007). Initiatives to promote effective self-care skills in children and adolescents with diabetes mellitus. *Disease Management and Health Outcomes,* Vol.15, pp. 101-108, ISSN 1173-8790

Balfour, L., White, D., Schiffrin, A., Daugherty, G., & Dufresne, J. (1993). Dietary disinhibition, perceived stress, and glucose control in young Type I diabetic women. *Health Psychology,* Vol.12, pp. 33-38, ISSN 0887-0446

Bauman, L. J. (2000). A patient-centered approach to adherence: Risks for non-adherence. In D. Drotar (Ed.). *Promoting adherence to medical treatment in chronic childhood illness: Concepts, methods, and interventions.* Mahwah, N.J.: Lawrence Erlbaum, ISBN 978-8058-3348-5

Bennett-Murphy, L. M., Thomson, R. J., & Morris, M. A. (1997). Adherence behavior among adolescents with type 1 insulin-dependent diabetes mellitus: The role of cognitive appraisal processes. *Journal of Pediatric Psychology*, Vol.22, pp. 811-825, ISSN 0146-8693

Beveridge, R. M., Berg, C. A., Wiebe, D. J., & Palmer, D. L. (2006). Mother and adolescent representations of illness ownership and stressful events surrounding diabetes. *Journal of Pediatric Psychology*, Vol.31, pp. 818-827, ISSN 0146-8693

Boardway, R. H., Delamater, A.M., Tomakowsky, J., & Gutai, J. P. (1993). Stress management training for adolescents with diabetes. *Journal of Pediatric Psychology*, Vol.52, pp. 685-716, ISSN 0146-8693

Bui, H., Perlman, K., & Daneman, D. (2005). Self-monitoring of blood glucose in children and teens with diabetes. *Pediatric Diabetes*, Vol.6, pp. 50-62, ISSN 1399-543X

Carpentier, M. Y., Mullins, L. L., Chaney, J. M., & Wagner, J. L. (2006). The relationship of illness uncertainty and attributional style to long-term psychological distress in parents of children with type 1 diabetes mellitus. *Children's Health Care*, Vol.35, No.2, pp. 141-154, ISSN 0273-9615

Centers for Disease Control and Prevention. (2003). *National diabetes fact sheet: General information and national estimates on diabetes in the United States, 2002.* Atlanta, GA. U.S. Department of Health and Human Services, Centers for Disease Control and Prevention, Government Doc. No. HE 20.7002:D 54/6

Chang, C.-W., Yeh, C.-H., Lo, F.-S., & Shih, Y.-L. (2007). Adherence behaviors in Taiwanese children and adolescents with type 1 diabetes mellitus. *Journal of Nursing and Healthcare of Chronic Illness* in association with *Journal of Clinical Nursing*, Vol.16, No.7b, pp. 207-214, ISSN 0962-1067

Chisholm, V., Atkinson, L., & Donaldson, C., Noyes, K., Payne, A., & Kelnar, C. (2007). Predictors of treatment adherence in young children with Type I diabetes. *Journal of Advanced Nursing*, Vol.57, pp. 482-493, ISSN 0309-2402

Cohen, D. M., Lumley, M. A., Naar-King, S., Partridge, T., & Cakan, N. (2004). Child behavior problems and family functioning as predictors of adherence and glycemic control in economically disadvantaged children with type 1 diabetes: A prospective study. *Journal of Pediatric Psychology*, Vol.29, No.3, pp. 171-184, ISSN 0146-8693

Davis, C., Delameter, A., Shaw, K., La Greca, A., Edison, M., Perez-Rodriguez, J., & Nemery, R. (2000). Parenting styles, regimen adherence, and glycemic control in 4- to 10-year-old children with diabetes. *Journal of Pediatric Psychology*, Vol.26, No. 2, pp. 123-129, ISSN 0146-8693

Driscoll, K. A., Johnson, S. B., Barker, D., Quittner, A. L., Deeb, L. C., Geller, D. E. (2010). Risk factors associated with depressive symptoms in caregivers of children with type 1 diabetes or cystic fibrosis. *Journal of Pediatric Psychology*, Vol.35, No.8, pp. 814-822, ISSN 0146-8693

Edgar, K. A., & Skinner, T. C. (2003). Illness representations and coping as predictors of emotional well-being in adolescents with type 1 diabetes. *Journal of Pediatric Psychology*, Vol.28, pp. 485-493, ISSN 0146-8693

Fielding, D., & Duff, A. (1999). Compliance with treatment protocols: Interventions for children with chronic illness. *Archives of Disease in Childhood*, Vol.80, pp. 196-200, ISSN 0003-9888

Frey, M. A., Ellis, D., Templin, T., Naar-King, S., & Gutai, J. P. (2006). Diabetes management and metabolic control in school-age children with Type 1 diabetes. *Children's Health Care*, Vol.35, pp. 349-363, ISSN 1532-6888

Geffken, G. R., Lehmkuhl, H., Walker, K.N., Storch, E., A., Heidgerken, A. D., Lewin, A. et al. (2008). Family functioning processes and diabetic ketoacidosis in youths with Type I Diabetes. *Rehabilitation Psychology*, Vol.53, No.2, pp. 231-237, ISSN 0090-5550

Greco, P., Pendley, J. S., McDonell, K., & Reeves, G. (2001). A peer group intervention for adolescents with type 1 diabetes and their best friends. *Journal of Pediatric Psychology*, Vol.26, pp. 485-490, ISSN 0146-8693

Green, L., Wysocki, T., & Reineck, B. (1990). Fear of hypoglycemia in children and adolescents with diabetes. *Journal of Pediatric Psychology*, Vol.15, pp. 633-641, ISSN 0146-8693

Hanna, K. M., & Guthrie, D. (2000). Adolescents' perceived benefits and barriers related to diabetes self-management – part 1. *Issues in Comprehensive Pediatric Nursing*, Vol.23, pp. 165-174, ISSN 0146-0862

Hanna, K.M., & Guthrie, D. W. (2001). Health-compromising behavior and diabetes management among adolescents and young adults with diabetes. *Diabetes Educator*, Vol.27, No.2, 223- 230, ISSN 0145-7217

Hauser, S. T., Jacobson, A. M., Lavori, P., Wolfsdorf, J. I., Herskowitz, R. D., Milley, J. E., Bliss, R., & Gelfand, E. (1990). Adherence among children and adolescents with insulin dependent diabetes mellitus over a 4-year longitudinal follow-up: II. Immediate and long-term linkages with family milieu. *Journal of Pediatric Psychology*, Vol.15, pp. 527-542, ISSN 0146-8693

Helgeson, V. S., Escobar, O., Siminerio, L., & Becker, D. (2010). Relation of stressful life events to metabolic control among adolescents with diabetes: 5-year longitudinal study. *Health Psychology*, Vol.29, pp. 153-159, ISSN 0887-0446

Hema, D. A., Roper, S. O., Nehring, J. W., Call, A., Mandleco, B. L., & Dyches, T. T. (2009). Daily stressors and coping responses of children and adolescents with Type I diabetes. *Child Care, Health and Development*, Vol.35, pp. 330-339, ISSN 1365-2214

Horsch, A., McManus, F., Kennedy, P., & Edge, J. (2007). Anxiety, depressive, and posttraumatic stress symptoms in mothers of children with type 1 diabetes. *Journal of Traumatic Stress*, Vol.20, No.5, pp. 881-891, ISSN 1573-6598

LaGreca, A. M., Auslander, W. F., Greco, P., Spetter, D., Fisher, E. B., & Santiago, J. V. (1995). I get by with a little help from my family and friends: Adolescents support for diabetes care. *Journal of Pediatric Psychology*, Vol.20, pp. 449-476, ISSN 0146-8693

Lehmkuhl, H. D., & Nabors, L. A. (2008). Children with diabetes: Satisfaction with school support, illness perceptions, and HbA1C levels. *Journal of Developmental and Physical Disabilities*, Vol.20, pp. 101-114, ISSN 1573-3580

Lewin, A.B., Heidgerken, A. D., Geffken, G. R., Williams, L. B., Storch, E. A., Gelfand, K. M. et al. (2006). The relation between family factors and metabolic control: The role of diabetes adherence. *Journal of Pediatric Psychology*, Vol.31, No.2, pp. 174-183, ISSN 0146-8693

Lindstrom, C., Aman, J., & Norberg, A. L. (2010). Increased prevalence of burnout symptoms in parents of chronically ill children. *Acta Paediatrica*, Vol.99, No.3, pp. 427-432, ISSN 1651-2227

Marrero, D. G., Guare, J. C., Vandagriff, J. L., & Fineberg, N. S. (1997). Fear of hypoglycemia in the parents of children and adolescents with diabetes: Maladaptive or healthy response? *Diabetes Educator*, Vol.23, No.3, pp. 281-286, ISSN 0145-7217

Nabors, L. A., McGrady, M. E., & Kichler, J. (2010). Children's attitudes toward their diabetes, locus of control, and HbA1c levels. *Journal of Developmental and Physical Disabilities*, Vol.22, pp. 475-484, ISSN 1056-263X

Nabors, L., Lehmkuhl, H., Christos, N., & Andreone, T. L. (2003). Children with diabetes: Perceptions of supports for self-management at school. *Journal of School Health*, Vol.73, pp. 216-221, ISSN 1746-1561

Peters, C. D., Storch, E. A., Geffken, G. R., Heidgerken, A. D., & Silverstein, J. H. (2008). Victimization of youth with type-1 diabetes by teachers: Relations with adherence and metabolic control. *Journal of Child Health Care*, Vol.12, No.3, pp. 209-220, ISSN 1367-4935

Rabiau, M. A., Knuper, B., Nguyen, T-K, Sufrategui, M., & Polychronakos, C. (2009). Compensatory beliefs about glucose testing are associated with low adherence to treatment and poor metabolic control in adolescents with Type I diabetes. *Health Education Research*, Vol.24, pp. 890-896, ISSN 0012-3692

Rolland, J. S. (1987). Chronic illness and the life cycle: A conceptual framework. *Family Process*, Vol.26, pp. 203-221, ISSN 0014-7370

Rosenstock, I. M. (1974). Historical origins of the Health Belief Model. *Health Education Monographs*, Vol.2, pp. 328-335, ISSN 0073-1455

Rotter, J. B. (1966). Generalized expectancies of internal versus external control of reinforcements. *Psychological Monographs*, Vol.80 (whole no. 609), ISSN 0096-9753

Shroff-Pendley, J., Kasmen, L. J., Miller, D. L., Donze, J., Swenson, C., & Reeves, G. (2002). Peer and family support in children and adolescents with type I diabetes. *Journal of Pediatric Psychology*, Vol.27, No.5, pp. 429-438, ISSN 0146-8693

Seiffge-Krenke, I., & Stemmler, M. (2003). Coping with everyday stress and links to medical and psychosocial adaptation in diabetic adolescents. *Journal of Adolescent Health*, Vol.33, pp. 180-188, ISSN 1054-139X

Silverstein, J., Klingensmith, G., Copeland, K., Plotnick, L., Kaufman, F., Laffel, L., et al.(2005). Children and adolescents with Type 1 diabetes. *Diabetes Care*, Vol.28, pp. 186-212, ISSN 0149-5992

Skinner, T. C., John, M., & Hampson, S. E. (2000). Social support and personal needs models of diabetes as predictors of self-care and well-being: A longitudinal study of adolescents with diabetes. *Journal of Pediatric Psychology*, Vol.25, pp. 257-267. ISSN 0146-8693

Skinner, T. C., & Hampson, S. E. (1998). Social support and personal models of diabetes in relation to self-care and well-being in adolescents with type 1 diabetes mellitus. *Journal of Adolescence*, Vol.21, pp. 703-715, ISSN 0140-1971

Storch, E.A., Heidgerken, A.D., Geffken, G.R., Lewin, A.B., Ohleyer, V., et al. (2006). Bullying, regimen self-management, and metabolic control in youth with Type I Diabetes, *Journal of Pediatrics*, Vol.148, No.6, pp. 784-787, ISSN 0022-3476

Streisand, R., Mackey, E. R., Elliot, B. M., Mednik, L., Slaughter, I. M., Turek, J. et al. (2008). Parental anxiety and depression associated with caring for a child newly diagnosed with type 1 diabetes: Opportunities for education and counseling. *Patient Education and Counseling*, Vol.73, pp. 333-338, ISSN 0738-3991

Weissberg-Benchell, J., Goodman, S. S., Lomaglio, J. A., & Zebracki, K. (2007). The use of continuous subcutaneous insulin infusion (CSII): Parental and professional perceptions of self-case mastery and autonomy in children and adolescents. *Journal of Pediatric Psychology*, Vol.32, No.10, pp. 1196-1202, ISSN 0146-8693

Wysocki, T., Greco, P., Harris, M. A., Bubb, J., & White, N. H. (2001). Behavior therapy for families of adolescents with diabetes: Maintenance of treatment effects. *Diabetes Care*, Vol.24, pp. 441-446, ISSN 0149-5992

6

Predictors of Adherence, Metabolic Control and Quality of Life in Adolescents with Type 1 Diabetes

M. Graça Pereira[1], A. Cristina Almeida[2],
Liliana Rocha[1] and Engrácia Leandro[2]
[1]University of Minho, School of Psychology
[2]University of Minho, Social Sciences Institute
Portugal

1. Introduction

Diabetes Mellitus Type I (DM1) is a diagnosed disease that appears before age 35 (Hanas, 2007) and is well known, in the pediatric population, as one of the most common diseases (Serafino, 1990). The diagnosis occurs mostly in childhood and adolescence, often between ages 5 and 11 (Eiser, 1990).

The definition of adolescence is a bit controversial but OMS (1965) establishes adolescence between 10 and 19 years old. The beginning of adolescence starts with the appearance of the first biological changes of puberty. According to Erikson's theory of psychosocial development (Erikson, 1968), the central task of adolescence is the development of autonomy, identity and self integration (Barros, 2003). In fact, identity formation, in adolescence, requires a reorganization of capacities, desires, needs and interests in the adolescent, as well as a quest for more independence towards parents. Nevertheless, the difficulties, even in the well succeeded resolution of the psychosocial tasks, may result in "identity confusion" (Erikson, 1968). In adolescents with diabetes, the disease can be an additional stressor functioning as another factor that requires acceptation and self integration. Diabetes exposes adolescents to potentially unpleasant experiences (having to explain others about the disease, medical exams, etc.) that can limit or prevent normal development and life experiences in adolescence (Close et al., 1986). On the other hand, physiological and hormonal changes that take place in adolescence may increase insulin resistance contributing to a weak control of diabetes (Duarte, 2002). In short, adolescence is a developmental phase, marked by changes and identity formation ,that requires a permanent and dynamic adaptation of the adolescent, ranging from feelings of acceptation to anger/anxiety and even depression (Leite, 2005) that can affect adherence to therapy and adaptation to illness. It is important to keep in mind that *being adolescent* is more important than *being diabetic* (Burroughs et al., 1997).

1.1 Adherence and metabolic control

Adherence to therapy in chronic disease is considered one of the main problems that may end in treatment failure (Leite, 2005). Kristeller and Rodin, in 1984, suggested that adherence to treatment was built on three dimensions: 1) Adherence (compliance) that refers to the degree of acceptance of the individual towards prescriptions and medical recommendation; 2) Adherence towards keeping and following the treatment that was agreed in the previous phase, and 3) Adherence (maintenance) to diabetes' self care tasks that have been integrated in the person's life style. Throughout these phases, the diabetic acquires control and develops the autonomy necessary in the maintenance phase.

Any detour from the treatment plan is defined as non adherence to therapy (Bishop, 1994) and can range from missing appointments, forgetting to take insulin (or take more or less than the prescribed amount) to not following the nutritional or the exercise plan. In DM1, adherence is often assessed through hemoglobin levels (HbA1c), (Sperling, 1996). The relationship between therapy adherence and metabolic control is complex and probably bidirectional i.e. low adherence to therapy is often preceded by a weak metabolic control and vice versa (Kakleas et al., 2009). However, there is some controversial regarding this issue. For some, HbA1c is the most valid indicator of adherence to therapy (DCCT, 1994) for others, there isn't a direct relationship between HbA1c and adherence (Silva et al., 2002).

The weak adherence to self-care in diabetes seems to result from a multifactor combination (Fagulha et al., 2004). Warren and Hixenbaugh, in 1998, found demographic variables to weakly predict adherence to self care in diabetes. Some studies have revealed that adolescents typically are less adherent to therapy than children, regarding insulin administration, exercise, nutrition and self monitoring of glucose (Hirschberg, 2001). Each adolescent apprehends and creates meanings about diabetes and its treatment's demands and how (s)he deals with them, in the social context, influences adherence to diabetes (Barros, 2003). Moreover, puberty changes, psychological dilemmas characteristic of adolescence (La Greca, 1992) and cognitive development may also contribute to an increase in non-adherence. Also, immaturity of thought, in adolescence, based on invulnerability may be one of the main causes of low adherence to diabetes treatment (Santos, 2001; Elkind, 1984), in adolescence.

In children and adolescents with diabetes, adherence is higher after diabetes diagnosis and deteriorates over time (Jacobson et al., 1987). On the other hand, non-adherence happens in average 3,5 years after the diagnosis and around age 15 (Anderson & Laffel, 1997). Compared to younger children and adults, adolescents exhibit poorer self-care behavior (Anderson et al., 1990) and poorer metabolic control (Kovacs et al., 1989).ADA (American Diabetes Association, 2003) recommends, as a therapeutic goal, that HbA1c stays below 7%.

Diabetics between 11 and 18 years old show a weak metabolic control (Mortensen et al., 1998; Fagulha et al., 2004). In the first years of diagnosis, lack of knowledge about the disease can affect metabolic control in children and adolescents (Butler et al., 2008) and, after this first phase, adolescents' compliance with treatment depends on adherence to self care tasks and to the degree of parenting supervision regarding disease management (Anderson et al., 1997). According to the authors, in an early phase, parents show more involvement in tasks related to treatment, particularly insulin administration, that best predicts metabolic control. However, throughout adolescence, parental involvement diminishes resulting in a decrease of adherence to therapy and, therefore, in a weak metabolic control.

Differences in adherence and metabolic control, in DM1, by gender, have been reported in the literature (Mortensenn & Hougaard, 1997). Girls tend to present a weaker adherence and poor metabolic control compared to boys. Girls enter puberty earlier than boys and a poor metabolic control is associated to normal physiological changes, in adolescence, such as increased levels of hormones responsible for insulin resistance (Carroll & Shade, 2005). However, other behavioral and psychosocial factors also tend to contribute to non-adherence in diabetes such as feeling reluctant in doing self monitoring of blood glucose, having irregular meals and not complying with the correct insulin doses.

Some studies show a relationship between bad metabolic control and family dysfunction, namely conflict in the family and low family cohesion, although this relationship has not been found in other studies. In fact, higher levels of cohesion and family stability have been related to better boundary definition between family subsystems and, as a result, more incentive to autonomy, more effective family communication and better metabolic control in diabetic adolescents (Fisher et al., 1982). Also, poor social support was found to predict bad metabolic control and low adherence to self care in diabetic adolescents (Fukunishi et al., 1998). In order to overcome the difficulties, related to adherence and metabolic control, it's important to concentrate on the adolescents' social competencies, family support and friends' support (Pereira & Almeida, 2008). There are several factors, that go beyond adherence to self care in diabetes, that can influence metabolic control. Therefore, a lack of a relationship between adherence and metabolic control may be due to insufficient rigorous efforts in adherence 's evaluation (McNabb, 1997).

1.2 Family functioning

The presence of a chronic disease, in a family's member, is a stressor for the entire family limiting the family's ability to go on with usual tasks and psychosocial roles requiring, as a result, flexibility in the family's system (Northam et al., 1996). Family functioning and a supportive parental style have been associated to better adherence to treatment (Manne et al., 1993). Conflict and family dysfunction predicted low adherence to self care in diabetes (Miller-Johnson et al., 1994) while higher levels of social support, cohesion and organization were associated to better metabolic control and adherence. Adolescents with better metabolic control seem to have parents that encourage independence, express feelings openly and communicate directly. On the other hand, adolescents with poor metabolic control have parents that are more critical, suspicious or indifferent to treatment (Anderson et al., 1981). However, the relationship between family functioning (cohesion, good communication, no conflict) and metabolic control is controversial since some studies found this association (Wysocki, 1993; Seiffge-krenke, 1998; La Greca & Thompson, 1998) but others have failed (Kovacs et al., 1989; Wysocki et al., 2001).

1.3 Family social support

Low adherence in diabetes has been associated to low family support and less parental supervision (Beveridge et al., 2006). In an initial phase, after diagnosis, adolescents receive more supervision from parents and adherence is stronger compared to late adolescence, when there is an increasing worry with body image, sexuality and independence from parental and authority figures (Jacbson et al., 1987). Relationships with others, at home or at school, play an important role in adolescence (Papalia et al., 2001). In an attempt to prove they belong and are like their peers, adolescents may abandon the therapeutic regimen (Fagulha et al., 2004). In fact, diabetes treatment does not help adherence i.e. daily insulin administration and the fact that diabetes treatment only avoids negative repercussions in the long term without bringing positive consequences, creates difficulties regarding adherence (Hanson et al., 1989).

Research has shown a relationship among social support, adolescents/family's characteristics and metabolic control in DM1 (Hanson et al., 1989; Wysocki, 1993). A family that provides warmth, advice, and adequate problem solving's strategies promotes adherence (Ellerton et al., 1996). From a developmental perspective, during childhood, parents assume the responsibility for the treatment regimen, however, in adolescence, the responsibility tends to be transferred to the adolescent and often, one or more treatment's components may not be followed. Family support is considered more important for younger adolescents or for those with a shorter duration of the disease (Stern & Zevon, 1990). Parents are the bigger suppliers of social support (more than friends) in diabetes treatment (Hanson et al., 1989) and, as a result, adolescents with parents less involved or with parents that provide poor support show less adherence to therapy and show a lower metabolic control. Nevertheless, in some studies, parental support has been positivity associated to adolescent's adherence but not to metabolic control (Hanson et al., 1989). The authors defend the hypothesis that family support may have a direct effect on adherence given parent's supervision over treatment's tasks.   Due to the need for autonomy and independence, parents' support to deal with diabetes' psychosocial tasks may not always be desirable and adolescents may prefer to solve their problems alone or with friends' help.

1.4 Parental coping

There are few studies regarding parents' coping strategies towards diabetes. Some studies reveal that parents cope well with their children' diabetes (Macrodimitris & Endler, 2001) but others have problems adapting to the disease (e.g. Kovacs & Feinberg, 1982). Adequate coping strategies to deal with diabetes include family involvement and/or sharing tasks, participation of adolescent and family in support groups, knowledge about the disease, use of assertive behaviors in social environment and reorganization of meals. Recently, a study revealed differences between fathers and mothers regarding the use of coping strategies (Correia, 2010). Mothers show greater responsibility, in the daily care tasks of the diabetic adolescent, being responsible for blood glucose records, meals plan and insulin administration (Zanetti & Mendes, 2001). In fact, mothers often seek information regarding the onset and course of diabetes (Nunes & Dupas, 2004).

The strategies used by caregivers may create potential difficulties and obstacles to adherence and metabolic control in diabetes. Sometimes, when confronted with chronic disease, parents' response to stressful situations may lead to a family rupture influencing, as a result, the adolescent and family's adaptation to illness (Trindade, 2000). Some parents, after the diagnosis, cease participating in social parties and forbid the adolescent to eat sweets, transforming social interactions that involve food, in uncomfortable situations for the adolescent, particularly when related to peers (Nunes & Dupas, 2004). This type of coping strategies exacerbate dependency in the adolescent with diabetes increasing parent's stress since they feel they need to protect and control the adolescent in all situations and, as a result, family life needs to be organized and centered on the illness (Brito & Sadala, 2009).

1.5 Illness representations

The self regulation behavior model (Leventhal et al., 1992) emphasizes the importance of beliefs regarding adherence to treatment. In fact, illness representations play a role in personal decisions towards adherence to treatment, in diabetes' self care (Gonder-Frederick et al., 2002). In adults, recent research found that illness representations regarding diabetes accounted for the diversity in disease-related functioning (Petrie et al., 1996). Illness representations are concerned with those variables that patients themselves believe to be central to their experience of illness and its management. Edgar and Skinner, in 2003, described Leventhal's five dimensions of illness representations (Leventhal et al, 1980; Leventhal et al., 1984): *identity*, the label and symptoms associated with the illness (e.g., thirst); *cause*, beliefs about the factors responsible for the onset of illness; *timeline*, perceptions about the duration of illness; *consequences*, illness expected outcomes regarding physical, psychological, social, and economic functioning on a daily basis and in the long term; and *control/cure/treatment*, beliefs regarding the cure of the disease and patient's control over it. Later research, extended the original model adding more items by splitting the control dimension into personal control and treatment control; including also a cyclical timeline dimension; an overall comprehension of illness, and finally, an emotional representation of the illness (Moss-Morris et al., 2002).

In adolescents with diabetes, illness representations have been associated to medical and psychological outcomes. In particular, treatment effectiveness' beliefs have been associated to self-care (Griva et al., 2000; Skinner & Hampson, 2001; Skinner et al., 2002) and perceived consequences to lower levels of emotional well-being (Skinner et al., 2000; Skinner & Hampson, 2001). Illness representations, particularly consequences and emotional representations have been found to predict quality of life (Paddison et al., 2008). The belief that diabetes was a temporary disease, than a lifelong condition, and the perception that diabetes had serious consequences predicted poor metabolic control. Also a perception of control, over the course of illness, has been positively associated to quality of life (Paddison et al., 2008).

1.6 School support

Most of the research on DM1 focused on family support and its implications on adherence, as previously described and did not take in consideration school's support. However, managing a chronic illness in adolescents, who are trying to become independent from their families and integrate in their peer group, is not easy (Holmbeck et al., 2000). In fact, as the adolescent grows, peer relationships become paramount and an important source of emotional support (Wysocki & Greco, 2006). However, research on the implications of peers support on adherence, metabolic control and quality of life is scarce. Peer conflict has been associated to poor metabolic control in girls (Hegelson et al., 2009) and friend support has been related to adherence to blood glucose testing (Bearman & La Greca, 2002). Regardless of whether support from friends is associated to diabetes self-care and metabolic control, support from friends may always help adolescents to better adjust psychologically to diabetes (La Greca et al., 1995).

When faced with the choice of appropriate self-care behavior, older adolescents have better problem solving skills but are more vulnerable to non-adherence in the face of peer pressure (Thomas et al., 1997). Another study showed that adolescents, who perceive their friends reacting negatively to their diabetes' self-care behavior, report more stress which, in turn, is associated to poor metabolic control (Hains et al., 2007).

Research examining the positive and negative aspects of friends and peers, on diabetes outcomes and psychological well-being, is not clear. There seems to be more evidence that conflictual relationships are more harmful than supportive relations are beneficial, which is consistent with the literature on healthy adults (Helgson, 2006). Besides peers' support, teachers' support is also important. A study found that 9 % of parents had to change glucose monitoring and 16% changed treatment administration because of lack of support from teachers (Amillategui et al., 2007). In fact, teachers in general need to be knowledgeable of hyperglycemia and hypoglycemia's episodes in order to assist the adolescent if needed. Support from friends and peers are key factors that help the integration of the adolescent teenager in the school setting, facilitating adaptation to diabetes.

Although diabetes does not cause pain on adolescents, impacts nonetheless, the adolescent and family's daily living and, therefore, the quality of life of all involved (Hanas, 2007) at physical, emotional, social and family 's levels (Pereira et al., 2008).

1.7 Quality of Life (QOL)

Girls perceived lower levels of QOL compared to boys. Worries about metabolic control increase with age but, regardless of gender, as age increases QOL decreases (Hoey et al., 2001). Adolescents who monitor their glucose levels, several times a day, reported better quality of life (Novato, 2009). The monitoring of blood glucose levels allows the teenager to know the variation of blood sugar, over time, perceiving what behaviors impact metabolic control, resulting in better quality of life (Novato, 2009). Regarding the association between quality of life and adherence to self-care in diabetes, literature is contradictory. Diabetes treatment has adverse effects on quality of life (Watkins et al., 2000). In fact, adolescents with diabetes need to follow a set of requirements that can negatively impact the perception of their quality of life and interaction with others. However, other studies conclude that adherence to diabetes care is not related to quality of life (e.g. Snoek, 2000). Diabetics with good metabolic control (measured through glycated hemoglobin) show better quality of life (e.g Glasgow et al., 1997; Silva, 2003) however, in some studies, this relationships has not been found and, in other studies, this relationship is very weak or does not exist (e.g. Grey et al., 1998; Laffel et al., 2003). Family also plays an important role in the perception of adolescents' QOL because QOL is affected by how the family deals with the disease (Hanson, 2001). Family conflict predicts lower QOL in adolescents (Dickenson et al., 2003). Family environment was shown to influence QOL as well as adherence and metabolic control in adolescents with diabetes (Pereira et al., 2008).

While there is a growing interest in psychological issues in diabetes, it is important to identify which variables predict better outcomes. The present study aims to answer this question namely understanding the relationship between psychological variables and diabetes outcomes. The purpose is to find the best predictors of adherence, metabolic control and quality of life in adolescents with type 1 diabetes taking in consideration adolescent variables and family variables. Due to the fact that research on adolescents and chronic illness have failed to incorporate gender (Miller & La Greca, 2005), the present study considers gender in the regression models.

2. Methods

2.1 Sample characteristics

A convenient sample of 170 subjects participated in the study: 85 adolescents and 85 family members that accompanied the teenager to their routine medical appointments, in a diabetes pediatric unit in two central Hospitals, and in a Diabetics Association. All teens received treatment in the hospital and therefore no differences were present between the sample from the Diabetics Association versus Hospitals.

All participants (teenagers and family members) were volunteers. Adolescents' criteria for inclusion were: age between 12 and 19 years, fulfilling ISPAD (1995) criteria for the diagnosis of type 1 diabetes, having a diagnosis longer than a year, being in ambulatory treatment, absence of another chronic and/or mental disease, not being pregnant and having normal cognitive development.

2.2 Procedure

Questionnaires were answered separately by adolescents and family members after they had been informed of the study's goals and filled the informed consent. The value of glycated hemoglobin (HbA1c) was determined by a nurse who collected a drop of blood from the adolescent before the medical appointment. Criteria of good metabolic control was based on ISPAD (2009) i.e. smaller than 7,5% is considered optimal, 7,5% - 9,0% suboptimal and higher than 9%, high risk.

2.3 Instruments

2.3.1 Adolescents and parent

Clinical, Socio-Demographic Questionnaire (Pereira et al., 2010) that reports gender and age in adolescents and their family members as well as metabolic control (glycated hemoglobin) and duration of disease, in the adolescent.

Brief Illness Perception Questionnaire – Brief-IPQ – Broadbent et al. (2006), (Portuguese version of Figueiras & Alves, 2007). The Brief-IPQ is a 9 items questionnaire, measuring cognitive and emotional representations of illness, that includes nine dimensions of illness perceptions: consequences, timeline, personal control, treatment control, identity, concern, coherence, emotional representation and causal representations. Both adolescents and parents answered the questionnaire. *Higher results indicate a more threatening perception of illness.* Due to the fact that each subscale includes only one item, it is not possible to calculate an alpha. As a result, like in the original version, pearson correlations between dimensions were calculated. In adolescents, significant correlations were present between consequences and emotional representation (r=.635), personal control and coherence (r=.511) and personal control and treatment control (r=.371). In the family sample, significant correlations were obtained between consequences and emotional representation (r=.558), personal control and coherence (r=.522) and between concern and coherence (r=.324).

2.3.2 Adolescents

Self Care Inventory – SCI - La Greca, A. (1992), (Portuguese version of Almeida & Pereira, 2010). It´s a 14 items questionnaire assessing adherence to diabetes treatment's recommendations regarding self care that includes four subscales: blood glucose regulation, insulin and food regulation, exercise and emergency precautions. *Higher results indicate more adherence.* Only the full scale was considered in the present study. Internal consistency in the original version was .80 and in this sample was .73.

Diabetes Family Behaviour Scale – DFBS – McKelvey et al., (1993), (Portuguese version of Almeida & Pereira (in press). DFBS is a 47 items questionnaire that assesses family support given to the adolescent in diabetes self care. It is composed of two subscales: Guidance-Control (15 items) and Warmth-Caring (15 items). The remaining 17 items do not belong to any of the subscales. *High results indicate less social support.* Internal consistency, in the original version, was .86, .81 and .79 for the full scale, guidance-control and warmth-caring, respectively. The Portuguese version showed an alpha of .91 (total scale), .76 (guidance-control) and .81 (warmth-caring.). In this study only the full scale was considered (alpha of .75).

Diabetes Quality of Life – DQoL - Ingersoll & Marrero (1991), (Portuguese version of Almeida & Pereira (2008). DQol is a 52 items questionnaire that assesses quality of life in patients with diabetes that includes three subscales: impact of diabetes (23 items); worries towards diabetes (11 items) and satisfaction (towards treatment: 7 items; towards life in general: 10 items) and one item that assesses health and quality of life. Higher results indicate lower quality of life. In the original version, the alpha for the total subscale was .92, followed by .86 (satisfaction), .85 (impact of diabetes) and .82 (worries towards diabetes). In this sample alphas were .89 (total scale), .71 (impact on diabetes), .82 (worries towards diabetes) and .87 (satisfaction). All the subscales were considered in the hypothesis testing.

School Support (Pereira & Almeida, 2009). School Support is a 6 items questionnaire that measures school support (e.g. healthy snacks available in cafeteria) and peer support regarding daily diabetes' management (e.g. feeling supported by fiends regarding diabetes). *Higher results indicate more school support.* The alpha in this sample was .81.

2.3.3 Parent

Family Assessment Device – FAD – Epstein et al., (1983), (Portuguese version provided by Ryan et al., 2005). It´s a 60 items questionnaire distributed by seven subscales: Problems Solving, Communication, Roles, Affective Responsiveness; Affective Involvement; Behavior control and General Functioning. *Higher results indicate low family functioning.* In the original version, Epstein, Baldwin and Bishop (1983) found the following results: Problem solving: .74; Communication: .75; Roles: .72; Affective responsiveness: .83; Affective involvement: .78; Behavior Control: .72 and General Functioning: .92. Only the full scale was used in the present study and the alpha, in the present sample, was .93.

Coping Health Inventory for Parents – CHIP – McCubbin et al., (1983), (Portuguese version of Pereira & Almeida, 2001). CHIP is a 45 items questionnaire that measures parents' response to management of family life when they have a child who is seriously and/or chronically ill. It includes three subscales: 1) Maintaining family integration, cooperation and an optimist definition of the situation; 2) Maintaining social support, self-esteem and psychological stability; and 3) Understanding the medical situation through communication with other parents and consultation with medical staff. *Higher results indicate better coping.* In the original version, the alpha for the first and second subscale was .79 and .71 for the third. In this sample, alphas were: .65 for the first subscale, .79 for the second and .71 for the last subscale.

3. Data analysis

First, descriptive statistics were performed to find the rate of adherence to self-care, metabolic control and quality of life. Hierarchical regression analyses were later performed to identify the best predictors of adherence to self-care, metabolic control and quality of life. Due to the size of the sample, regression analysis were first performed taking in consideration all variables ,except illness perceptions, and later including only them in the regression equation. The first regression was performed using the method *enter* since the selection of variables was based on previous research. The second regression, due to its exploratory nature, was performed using the stepwise method.

For both regressions, the variables considered in the first step were socio-demographic and clinical variables i.e. gender of the adolescent, duration of disease and values of glycated hemoglobin. In the first regression analysis, the second step included adolescents' psychosocial variables i.e. family support, quality of life, adherence and school support. The third step included family variables i.e. family functioning and coping. In the second regression analysis, the second step included adolescents' illness perceptions and the third step included family member's illness perceptions.

4. Results

4.1 Sample caracteristics

The sample consisted of 85 adolescents, 51% males and 49% females. Their age ranged from 12 to 19 with an average of 15.13 (SD=1.97), 15.12 for males (SD=2.00) and 15.14 for females (SD=1.96). Glycated hemoglobin in the sample was, in average, 9.06 (SD=1.58) specifically 9.00 (SD=1.72) for boys and 9.13 (SD=1.44) for girls. Therefore, girls had a poor metabolic control than boys but they were all at high risk. Average of duration of diabetes was 6.61 years (SD=3.68) with boys being diagnosed longer (M=7.05 years; SD=4.10) than girls (M=6.17 years; SD=3.19). In our sample, girls reported better adherence to self-care, less social support, higher school support and family social support when compared to boys but differences were non-significant. Girls showed less quality of life than boys and this difference was significant (t(83)=-2.004; p=.048) (table 1).

Variables	Duration of Diabetes		Adherence		Metabolic Control		Quality of Life		Family Support		School Support	
	M	SD	M	SD	M	SD	M	SD	M	SD	M	SD
Male	7.05	4.10	4.00	0.59	9.00	1.72	75.91	16.96	106.63	13.15	27.93	6.34
Female	6.17	3.19	4.13	0.40	9.13	1.44	83.55	18.19	107.81	11.73	28.21	5.92

Statistics: M (mean), SD (standard deviation)

Table 1. Characteristics of the Adolescents' Sample by Clinical, Socio-demographic and Psychosocial variables

74% of adolescents lived with their nuclear families, 15% belonged to monoparental families, 9.4% to stepfamilies and, only, 1.2% lived in an extended family. 20% of family members, who participated in the study, were fathers and 80% mothers. Average age for fathers was 46 years (SD=4.55) and for mothers was 44 years (SD=6.19).

4.2 Predictors of adherence, metabolic control and quality of life in adolescents on gender, duration of disease, glycated hemoglobin, family support, school support and parental coping

When all variables were included in the model, adherence was predicted by gender of adolescent (p<.05), glycated hemoglobin (p<.05) and family support (p<.001), explaining 30% of the total variance. None of the family variables predicted adherence. Taking in consideration what a high score means, in each instrument, results showed that low perception of family support, gender (being male) and high glycated hemoglobin (bad metabolic control) predicted lower adherence to diabetes self-care.

Metabolic Control was predicted by family support (total) (p<.05), adherence (total) (p<.05), quality of life (total) (p<.05) and parental coping (understanding the medical situation) (p<.05), explaining 15.9% of total variance. As a result, higher adherence of adolescent to self-care and parental understanding of the medical situation predicted lower levels of glycated hemoglobin (better metabolic control). On the other hand, low quality of life and low perception of family support predicted high values of glycated hemoglobin (poor metabolic control).

Quality of life was predicted by gender (p<.05), glycated hemoglobin (p<.05) and school support (total) (p<.01) explaining 26.5% of the total variance. Higher values of glycated hemoglobin (poor metabolic control) predicted lower quality of life. On the other hand, higher adherence and a higher school support predicted better quality of life. Like in adherence, none of the family variables predicted quality of life, in adolescents. Table 2 shows the results.

4.3 Predictors of adherence, metabolic control and quality of life in adolescents on glycated hemoglobin and illness representations

Overall, adherence was predicted by personal control of adolescent's illness representations (p<.001) and family's representation of timeline (p<.05) explaining 20.3% of the total variance. Thus, lower adolescents' perception of personal control predicted lower adherence to self care and higher family perception of diabetes duration (timeline) predicted higher adherence to self care, in adolescents.

Metabolic control, in adolescents, was predicted by emotional representation of adolescents' illness perceptions (p<.001) and by family's perceptions of illness coherence (p<.05), explaining 16.6% of the total variance. Therefore, higher adolescents' perception of emotional representation (diabetes seen as a threatening disease) predicted higher values of glycated hemoglobin (poor metabolic control) and lower family's comprehension of diabetes predicted higher values of glycated hemoglobin.

Quality of life was predicted by glycated hemoglobin (p<.05), adolescent's perception of consequences (p<.05) and emotional representation (p<.05) explaining 31.6% of the total variance. Higher perception of the consequences of diabetes by adolescents and higher perception of emotional representation (diabetes seen as a threatening disease) predicted lower quality of life. None of the family variables predicted adolescent's quality of life. Table 3 shows the results.

Variables	Adherence				Hemoglobin (Metabolic Control)				Quality of Life			
	ΔR²	B	SE B	β	ΔR²	B	SE B	β	ΔR²	B	SE B	β
Step 1	.071				-.023				.129			
Gender		-.133	.108	-.131		-.088	.350	-.028		-6.03	3.55	-.175
Duration of disease		-.011	.015	-.081		-.009	.048	-.020		-.369	.487	-.078
Glycated Hemoglobin		-.092	.034	-.286**		—	—	—		3.745	1.12	.340***
Step 2	.312				.132				.258			
Gender		-.207	.096	-.204*		-.123	.342	-.039		-7.91	3.36	-.229*
Duration of disease		.001	.013	.005		.014	.046	.033		-.295	.464	-.062
Glycated Hemoglobin		-.077	.032	-.239*		—	—	—		2.35	1.128	.214*
Family Support		-.019	.004	-.466***		-.029	.015	-.232		-.104	.159	-.075
School Support		-.003	.009	-.030		-.018	.030	-.070		-.937	.287	-.325**
Adherence		—	—	—		-.932	.381	-.301*		-7.89	3.92	-.232*
Quality of Life		-.006	.003	-.215*		.023	.011	.250*		—	—	—
Step 3	.300				.159				.265			
Gender		-.214	.097	-.211*		-.160	.338	-.051		-6.97	3.389	-.202*
Duration of disease		.001	.013	.006		.018	.045	.042		-.211	.465	-.045
Glycated Hemoglobin		-.085	.033	-.262*		—	—	—		2.34	1.16	.213*
Family Support		-.019	.004	-.459***		-.032	.015	-.251*		-.146	.161	-.105
School Support		-.000	.009	-.008		-.015	.030	-.058		-.958	.292	-.332**
Adherence		—	—	—		-.976	.378	-.315*		-6.865	3.976	-.202
Quality of Life		-.006	.003	-.192		.022	.011	.244*		—	—	—
Family Functioning		-.099	.162	-.060		.146	.549	.029		9.008	5.554	.162
Coping –Medical Situation		-.019	.016	-.124		-.116	.052	-.248*		.414	.547	.080
Coping – Social Support		.002	.007	.026		.018	.023	.086		-.274	.238	-.119

* p < .05; ** p < .01; *** p < .001

Table 2. Predictors of Adherence, Metabolic Control and Quality of Life in Adolescents on Gender, Duration of Disease, Glycated Hemoglobin, Family Support, School Support and Parental Coping (N=85 adolescents; N= 85 family members)

Variables	Adherence				Hemoglobin (Metabolic Control)				Quality of Life			
	ΔR^2	B	SE B	β	ΔR^2	B	SE B	β	ΔR^2	B	SE B	β
Step 1	.070				n.s.				.121			
Glycated Hemoglobin		-.092	.034	-.285**						4.117	1.160	.363***
Step 2	.169				.126				.288			
Glycated Hemoglobin												
Consequences - IPQ Adol.										2.820	1.083	.249*
Personal Control - IPQ Adol.		-.081	.024	-.350***						2.762	.612	.431***
Emotional Representation - IPQ Adol.						.180	.050	.369***				
Step 3	.203				.166				.316			
Glycated Hemoglobin												
Consequences - IPQ Adol.										2.197	1.102	.194*
Personal Control - IPQ Adol.		-.084	.024	-.364***						1.822	.749	.284*
Emotional Representation - IPQ Adol.		.046	.022	.206*		.173	.049	.356***				
Timeline - IPQ Family										1.402	.670	.254*
Coherence - IPQ Family						.154	.069	.224*				

* p < .05; ** p < .01; *** p < .001

Table 3. Predictors of Adherence, Metabolic Control and Quality of Life in Adolescents on Glycated Hemoglobin and Illness Representations (N=85 adolescents; N= 85 fam. members)

5. Discussion

In this study, adolescent's gender (i.e. being male) predicted lower adherence to diabetes self-care and higher quality of life. An association between gender and low adherence to diabetes, in adolescents girls, particularly regarding exercise, has been found in the literature (Patino et al., 2005). Girls with diabetes show lower quality of life than boys because they seemed to worry more regarding their illness (Grey et al., 1998; Rocha, 2010; Hoey et al., 2001). In fact, low quality of life, in girls, has been associated to more difficulties and worries regarding diabetes and less satisfaction with metabolic control. Girls enter puberty earlier than boys and a weak metabolic control may be associated to physiological changes, normal to adolescence, such as increased levels of hormones responsible for insulin resistance (Carroll & Shade, 2005).

In terms of predictors of adherence, taking in consideration the final model, higher values of glycated hemoglobin (poor metabolic control) predicted lower adherence to diabetes self-care and lower quality of life. These results are in accordance with the literature. Adolescents have more difficulties with metabolic control suggesting that hormonal changes, associated with puberty and the decline on adherence to self-care, were responsible for these results (Helgeson et al., 2009). In another study, glycated hemoglobin explained a small variance of quality of life in adolescents with diabetes suggesting that higher levels of glycated hemoglobin (poor metabolic control) had negative effects on the adolescent's perception of quality of life (Malik & Koot, 2009). In a study that addressed metabolic control and quality of life, good metabolic control (measured by glycated hemoglobin) was a predictor of better quality of life (Hoey et al.,2005).

Higher family support predicted higher adherence and better metabolic control (lower levels of glycated hemoglobin). These results are in accordance with the literature. Family support has been found to be a predictor of good metabolic control (Lewin et al., 2006). In fact, low family support was associated to low adherence to diabetes self-care and, indirectly, to a poor metabolic control. La Greca and Bearman, in 2002, suggested that family support predicts adolescents' adherence to diabetes self-care because family support is an important factor on the daily management of diabetes' self-care tasks in adolescents. Higher family support was found to be a predictor of higher adherence to self-care and good metabolic control suggesting the direct impact of parental support on diabetes' management tasks influencing , as a result, adherence and metabolic control, in the adolescent (Duke et al., 2008; Ellis et al., 2007). In a Portuguese sample of adolescents, family support was found to predict adherence in adolescents with type 1 diabetes (Pereira et al., 2008).

In the present study, a lower perception of personal control predicted lower adherence to diabetes self-care in adolescents. Beliefs in the effectiveness of treatment (control over the illness) were found to predict adherence to dietary self-care (Delamater, 2009). When the benefits, compared to costs of following the diabetes regimen were considered lower, diabetes was perceived as a less threatening disease and adherence to self care in diabetes , as a result, was poor (Patino et al., 2005).

Higher family perception of diabetes' duration, as an illness, predicted higher adherence of adolescents to diabetes self-care. In an attempt to understand if there were differences between illness representations in adults with type 2 diabetes and their partners, a relationship was found between partner's perceptions of the duration of diabetes (timeline) and treatment suggesting that partners' perceptions could influence positively patients' adherence to diabetes self-care (Searle et al., 2007). Based on these result, the same may be true for the dyads parent-adolescent. In fact, parent's perception as a long last condition in adolescent's life may be associated to more parental support regarding diabetes' management tasks in order to decrease future complications in the adolescent.

In terms of predictors of metabolic control, higher adherence to diabetes self-care predicted better metabolic control (lower levels of glycated hemoglobin). In fact, higher adherence to diabetes self-care has been found to predict good metabolic control in adolescents with type 1 diabetes, and lower quality of life, on the other hand, to predict poor metabolic control (Lewin et al., 2009). Higher levels of glycated hemoglobin have been associated to more worries regarding diabetes having, therefore, a negative impact on quality of life (Guttmann-Bauman et al., 1998).

Parents' understanding of the medical situation (coping with diabetes) predicted lower levels of glycated hemoglobin (better metabolic control) in the adolescent. This is a very interesting result. Family environment is important in the complex mechanism of adaptation to diabetes self-care having also an impact on metabolic control (Grey & Berry, 2004). In a study about behavioral therapy with families of adolescents with diabetes, when the relationship between parents and adolescents with diabetes improved, parents' coping with their adolescents' diabetes got better producing also better outcomes, such as good metabolic control in the adolescent (Wysocki et al., 2000).

Adolescent's emotional representation of diabetes (as a threatening disease) predicted higher levels of glycated haemoglobin (poor metabolic control). In a study about health beliefs in adolescents with type 1 diabetes, negative illness perception, like illness severity and susceptibility were predictors of poor metabolic control. On the other hand, lower family's comprehension (illness coherence) of diabetes predicted bad metabolic control in the adolescent. This result emphasizes the importance of parents' understanding of the impact of diabetes on their child suggesting that those parents who understand less the disease may exercise less parental supervision and provide less family support regarding diabetes's management and, as a consequence, metabolic control decreases.

In terms of quality of life, higher school support predicted higher quality of life. This result is in accordance with the literature. Peers relationships are paramount on the psychological well-being of adolescents with diabetes (Helgeson et al., 2009). In fact, relationships with peers can positively or negatively (e.g. conflict experiences) influence quality of life of adolescents with type 1 diabetes. Adolescents who have more positive attitudes with their school experience tended to experience lower problems and worries with diabetes's management (Lehmkuhl & Nabors, 2007).

Lower quality of life was predicted by higher perceptions of diabetes consequences and higher perceptions of emotional representation (more threatening). This result is in accordance with the literature. In fact, using the same illness perceptions questionnaire, with adults with type 2 diabetes, lower quality of life was found to be related to stronger beliefs of diabetes consequences and negative emotional representations (Edgar et al., 2003). Also, in another study, illness beliefs predicted quality of life i.e. consequences and emotional representations of diabetes were found to predict low quality of life in adolescents (Paddison et al., 2008).

6. Conclusion

In this study, the importance of family factors (family support and parental coping) become evident on diabetes outcomes. As a result, it is important to include parents on intervention programs regarding diabetes in adolescence, School support is also an important factor and future studies should address how peers, teachers and school environment may help or hinder adherence, metabolic control and quality of life. According to results, psychological interventions should be included in the treatment protocol of adolescents receiving medical treatment.

Adolescents and parents' illness representations were predictors of adherence, metabolic control and quality of life, showing the importance of these constructs on diabetes outcomes and should, therefore, be included in intervention programs. Future studies should address how contradictory illness representations between parents and adolescents impact diabetes outcomes particularly if the adolescent perceives parents as intrusive trying to force their diabetes' representations on them.

It would be also interesting to assess family functioning from the adolescent point of view, besides parents' perspective (the only one addressed in the present study) and find out whether parents and adolescents' different perspectives, regarding family functioning, may impact diabetes outcomes.

7. References

Almeida, J. & Pereira, M. G. (no prelo). *Escala Comportamental de Suporte Social Familiar para Adolescentes com Diabetes* (DFBS).

Almeida, J. & Pereira, M.G. (2008). Questionário de Avaliação da Qualidade de Vida para Adolescentes com Diabetes: Estudo de validação do DQOL. *Análise Psicológica, 2* (26), 295-307.

American Diabetes Association (2003). Test of Glycemia in Diabetes. Clinical Pratice Recommendations. *Diabetes Care,* 26 (1), 106-108.

Amillategui, B. , Calle, J. R. , Alvarez, M. A. Cardiel, M. A., & Barrio, R. (2007). Identifying the special needs of children with Type 1 diabetes in the school setting. An overview of parents' perceptions. *Diabetic Medicine,* 24(10), 1073-1079.

Amoros, M., Sanchez, J., & Carrillo, F. (2003). Adherencia al tratamiento. In Quiles, Sebastian & Carrillo (Eds.), *Manual de Psicología de la Salud con Niños, Adolescentes y Familia,* (pp. 73-94). Ediciones Pirâmide: Madrid.

Anderson, B. J., Auslander, W. F., Jung, K. C., Miller, J. P., & Santiago, J. V. (1990). Assessing family sharing of diabetes responsibilities. *Journal of Pediatric Psychology,* 15, 477-492.

Anderson, B., Brackett, J, Finkelstein, D., & Laffel, L. (1997). Parental Involvement in Diabetes Management Tasks: Relations to Blood Glucose Monitoring and Metabolic Control in Adolescents with Insulin-Dependent Diabetes-Mellitus. *The Journal of Pediatrics,* 130 (2), 257-265.

Anderson, B.J., & Laffel, L.M.B. (1997). Behavioral and psychology research with school aged children with type 1 diabetes. *Diabetes Spectrum,* 10 (4), 277-284.

Anderson, B.J., Miller, P., Auslander, W.F., & Santiago, J.V. (1981). Family Characteristics of Diabetic Adolescents: Relationship to Metabolic Control. *Diabetes Care,* 4, 586-594.

Barros, L. (2003). *Psicologia Pediátrica: perspectiva desenvolvimentista.* 2ªEdição. Climepsi Editores: Lisboa.

Bearman, K. J., & La Greca, A. M. (2002). Assessing friend support of adolescents' diabetes care: the diabetes social support questionnaire-friends version. *Journal of Pediatric Psychology,* 27(5), 417-428.

Beveridge, R.M., Berg, C.A., Wiebe, D.J., & Palmer, D.L. (2006). Mother and Adolescent representations of illness ownership and stressful events surrounding diabetes. *Journal of Pediatrics Psychology*, 31, 818-827.

Bishop, G. (1994). Interacting with the health care system. In Bishop (Ed.), *Health Psychology: Integrating mind and body* (pp. 220-227). Needham-Heights: Allyn and Bacon.

Brito, T.B., & Sadala, M.L.A. (2009). Diabetes mellitus juvenil: a experiência de familiares de adolescentes e pré-adolescentes. *Ciência & Saúde Coletiva*, 14 (3), 947-960.

Broadbent, E., Petrie, K. J., Main, J., & Weinman, J. (2006). The Brief Illness Perception Questionnaire. *Journal of Psychosomatic Research*, 60 631- 637.

Burroughs, T.E., Harris, M.A., Pontious, S.L., & Santiago, J.V. (1997). Research on social support in adolescents with IDDM: A critical review. *Diabetes Educator*, 23, 438-448.

Butler, D.A., Zuehlke, J.B., Tovar, A., Volkening, L.K., Anderson, B.J., & Laffel, L.M.B. (2008). The impact of modifiable family factors on glycemic control among youth with type 1 diabetes. *Pediatric Diabetes*, 9 (Part II), 373-381.

Cameron, F. J., Skinner, T. C., De Heaufort, C. E., Hoey, H., Swift, P. G. F., Aanstoot, H. et al., (2008). Are family factors universally related to metabolic outcomes in adolescents with type 1 Diabetes? *Diabetes Medicine*, 25 (4), 463-468.

Carroll M.F & Shade D.S. (2001). Ten pivotal questions about diabetic ketoacidosis. *Postgraduate Medicine*, 110, 89 –95.

Close H, Davies AG, Price DA, Goodyer IM. (1986). Emotional difficulties in diabetes mellitus. *Archives of Diseases Childhood*. 61(4), 337–340 .

Correia, A.C.R. (2010). *Coping e Auto-Eficácia em Pais de Crianças e Adolescentes com Diabetes tipo 1*. Tese de Mestrado em Psicologia Clínica e da Saúde não publicada. Faculdade de Ciências Humanas e Sociais. Porto. Portugal.

Delamater, A. M. (2009). Psychological care of children and adolescents with diabetes. *Pediatric Diabetes*, 10 (Suppl. 12), 175-184.

Diabetes Control and Complications Trial Research Group (DCCT) (1994). Effect of intensive diabetes treatment on the development and progression of long term complications in adolescents with insulin-dependent diabetes mellitus. *Journal of Pediatrics*, 12, 177-188.

Dickenson, L.M., Ye, X., Sack, J., & Hueston, W.(2003). General quality of life in youth with diabetes: Relationship to patient management and Diabetes – Specific Family and Conflict. *Diabetes Care*, 26, 3067-3073.

Duarte, R. (2002). *Epidemiologia da Diabetes*. In R. Duarte, J. Caldeira, J. Parreira, L. Sagreira, A. Odette & P. Lisboa (Eds). *Diabetologia Clínica*, Lidel - Edições Técnicas Lda. Lisboa.

Duke, D. C., Geffken, G. R., Lewin, A. B., Williams, L. B., Storch, E. A., & Silverstein, J. H. (2008). Glycemic Control in Youth with Type 1 Diabetes: Family Predictors and Mediators. *Journal of Pediatric Psychology*, 33 (7), 719-727.

Edgar, R. A. & Skinner, T. C. (2003). Illness Representation and Coping as Predictors of Emotional Well-being in Adolescents with Type 1 Diabetes. *Journal of Pediatric Psychology*, 28 (7), 485-493.

Eiser, C. 1990). *Chronic Childhood Disease*. New York: Cambridge University Press.

Elkind, D. (1984). *All grown up and no place to go: Teenagers in crisis*. Reading, MA: Add is on-Wesley.

Ellerton, M. L.; Stewart, M. J., Ritchie, J. A., & Hirth, A. M. (1996). Social support in children with a chronic condition. *Canadian Journal of Nursing Research*, 28 (4), 15-36.

Ellis, D. A., Podolski, C. L., Frey, M., Naar-King, S., Wang, B., & Moltz, K. (2007). The Role of Parental Monitoring in Adolescent Health Outcomes: Impact on Regimen Adherence in Youth with Type 1 Diabetes. *Journal of Pediatric Psychology*, 32(8), 907-917.

Epstein, N., Baldwin, L. & Bishop, D. (1983). The McMaster Family Assessment Device. *Journal of Marital and Family Therapy*, 9, 171-180.

Erikson, E. H. (1968) .*Identity, Youth and Crisis*. New York: Norton

Fagulha, A., Santos, I., & Grupo de Estudo da Diabetes (2004). Controlo glicémico e tratamento da Diabetes tipo 1 da Criança e Adolescente em Portugal. *Acta Médica Portuguesa*, 17, 173-179.

Figueiras, M.J. & Alves, N. C.(2007). Lay perceptions of serious illnesses: An adapted version of the Revised Illness Perception Questionnaire (IPQ-R) for healthy people. *Psychology and Health*, 22 (2), 143-158.

Fisher, E.B., Delamater, A.M., Bertelson, A.D., & Kirkley, B.G. (1982). Psychological factors in diabetes and its treatment. *Journal of Consulting and Clinical Psychology*, 50(6), 993-1003.

Fukunishi, I., Akimoto, M., Horikawa, N., Shirasaka, K., & Yamazaki, T. (1998). Stress and Social Support in glucose tolerance abnormality. *Journal of Psychosomatic Research*, 45 (4), 362-269.

Glasgow, R. E., Ruggiero, L., Eakin, E. G., Dryfoos, J., & Chobanian, L. (1997). Quality of life and associated characteristics in a large national sample of adults with diabetes. *Diabetes Care*, 20 (4), 562-567.

Gonder-Frederick, L., Cox, D. J., & Ritterband, L. M. (2002). Diabetes and behavioral medicine: The second decade. *Journal of Consulting and Clinical Psychology*, 70(3), 611-625

Grey, M. & Berry, D. (2004). Coping Skills Training and Problem Solving in Diabetes. *Current Diabetes Reports*, 4, 126-131.

Grey, M., Boland, E., Yu, C., Sullivan-Bollyai, A., & Tamborlane, W.V. (1998). Personal and Family Factors Associated with Quality of Life in Adolescents with Diabetes. *Diabetes Care*, 212 (6), 909-914.

Griva, K., Myers, L. B., & Newman, S. (2000). Illness perceptions and self-efficacy beliefs in adolescents and young adults with insulin dependent diabetes mellitus. *Psychology and Health*, 15, 733–750.

Guttmann-Bauman, I., Flaherty, B. P., Strugger, M. & McEvoy, R. C. (1998). Metabolic Control and Quality-of-Life Self-Assessment in Adolescents With IDDM. *Diabetes Care*, 21 (6), 915-918.

Hanas, R. (2007). *Diabetes Tipo 1 em Crianças, Adolescentes e Jovens Adultos*. Abbott Diabetes Care. Lidel - Edições técnicas Lda: Lisboa.

Hanson, C. L., Cigrang, J. A., Harris, M. A., Carle, D. L., Relyea, G., & Burghen, G. A. (1989). Coping styles in youths with insulin-dependent diabetes mellitus. *Journal of Consulting and Clinical Psychology*, 57, 644–651.

Hanson, C.L. (2001). Quality of life in families of youths with chronic conditions. In H.M. Koot & J.L. Wallander (Eds.), *Quality of life in child and adolescent illness: Concepts, methods and findings* (pp. 182-209). New York: Brunner-Routledge.

Haynes, A., Bower, C., Bulsara, M. K., Finn, J., Jones, T. W. and Davis, E. A. (2007), Perinatal risk factors for childhood Type 1 diabetes in Western Australia—a population-based study (1980–2002). *Diabetic Medicine*, 24, 564–570.

Helgeson, V. S., Lopez, L. C., & Kamarck, T. (2009). Peer Relationships and Diabetes: Retrospective and Ecological Momentary Assessment Approaches. *Health Psychology*. 28(3), 273-282.

Helgeson, V. S., Siminerio, L., Escobar, O. & Becker, D. (2009). Predictors of Metabolic Control among Adolescents with Diabetes: A 4-Year Longitudinal Study. *Journal of Pediatric Psychology*, 34(3), 254–270.

Hirschberg, S.L. (2001). *The Self-regulation of health behaviour in children with insulin dependent diabetes mellitus.* Dissertation presented to the Faculty of Pacific Graduate School of Psychology. Palo Alto, California.

Hoey, H., Aanstoot, H. J., Chiarelli, F., Daneman, D., Danne, T., Dorchy, H. et al., (2001). Good Metabolic Control is Associated with Better Quality of Life in 2101 Adolescents with Type 1 Diabetes. *Diabetes Care*, 24 (11), 1923-1928.

Holmbeck, G. N., Colder, C., Shapera, W., Westhoven, V., Kenealy, L., & Updegrove, A. (2000). Working with adolescents: Guides from developmental psychology. In P. C. Kendall (Ed.), *Child and adolescent therapy: Cognitive behavioral procedures* (2nd ed.; pp. 334–385). New York: Guilford Press.

Ingersoll, G. & Marrero, D. (1991). A modified Quality of Life Measure for Youths: Psycometrics Properties. *The Diabetes Educator*, 17 (2), 114-118.

Jacobson A. M., Hauser, S. T., Wolfsdorf, J. I., Houlihan, J., Milley, J. E. & Watt, E. (1987). Psychological Predictors of Compliance in Children with Recent Onset of Diabetes Mellitus. *Journal of Pediatrics*, 805-811.

Kakleas, K., Kandyla, B., Karayianni, C., & Karavanaki, K. (2009). Psychosocial problems in adolescents with Type 1 diabetes mellitus. *Diabetes & Metabolism*. University of Athens.

Kovacs, M., & Feinberg, T. (1982). Coping with juvenile onset diabetes mellitus. In A. Baum & J. Singer (Eds), *Handbook of Psychology and Health*, 2,165-212. Erlbaum: Hillsdale, NJ.

Kovacs, M., Kass, R. E., Schnell, T. M., Goldston, D., & Marsh, J. (1989). Family functioning and metabolic control of school-aged children with IDDM. *Diabetes Care, 12,* 409-414.

Kristeller, J. l., & Rodin, J. (1984). A Three-stage model of treatment continuity: compliance, adherence and maintenance. In A. Baum, S. Taylor & J. Singer (Eds.), *Handbook of Psychology and Health.* (Vol. IV, pp. 85-112). New Jersey: Lawrence Erlbaum Associates.

La Greca, A. M. (1992). *Brief Manual for the Self Care Inventory.* University of Miami.USA.

La Greca, A. M. (1992). Peer Influences in Pediatric Chronic Illness: An Update. *Journal of Pediatric Psychology;* 17 (6), 775-784.

La Greca, A. M., & Bearman, K. J. (2002). The Diabetes Social Support Questionnaire-Family Version: Evaluating Adolescents' Diabetes-Specific Support From Family Members. *Journal of Pediatric Psycholog,* 27 (8), 665-676.

La Greca, A. M., & Thompson, K.M (1998). Family and friend Support for Adolescents with Diabetes. *Análise Psicológica,* 1 (XVI), 101-113.

La Greca, A. M., Auslander, W. F., Greco, P., Spetter, D., Fisher, E. B., Jr., & Santiago, J. V. (1995). I get by with a little help from my family and friends: Adolescents' support for diabetes care. *Journal of Pediatric Psychology, 20,* 449–476.

Laffel, L., Connell, A., Vangsness, L., Goebel-Fabri, A., Mansfield, A., & Anderson, B. (2003). General Quality of life in Youth with type 1 Diabetes. Relationship to patient management and diabetes-specific family conflict. *Diabetes Care,* 26, (11), 3067- 3073.

Lehmkuhl, H., & Nabors, L. (2007). Children with Diabetes: Satisfaction with School Support, Illness Perceptions and HbA1C Levels. *Journal of Developmental and Physical Disabilities,* 20, 101-114.

Leite (2005). Programa de promoção da adesão terapêutica em crianças diabéticas. In M. Guerra & L. Lima, (Eds.), *Intervenção Psicológica em Grupos em Contextos de Saúde.* Climepsi Editores: Lisboa.

Leventhal, H., Diefenbach, M.A., & Leventhal, E. A. (1992). Illness Cognition: Using common sense to understand treatment adherence and affect cognition interactions. *Cognitive Therapy and Research,* 16, 143-163.

Leventhal, H., Meyer, D., & Nerenz, D. (1980). The common-sense representation of illness danger. In S. Rachman (Ed.), *Contributions to Medical Psychology* (Vol. 2, pp. 7–30). New York: Pergamon Press.

Leventhal, H., Nerenz, D. R., & Steele, D. J. (1984). Illness representation and coping with health threats. In A. Baum, S. E. Taylor, & J. E. Singer (Eds.), *Handbook of Psychology and Health* (pp. 219 –252). Hillsdale, NJ: Lawrence Erlbaum Associates.

Lewin, A. B., Heidgerken, A. D., Geffken, G. R., Williams, L. B., Storch, E. A., Gelfand, K. M. & al., (2006). The Relation Between Family Factors and Metabolic Control: The Role of Diabetes Adherence. *Journal of Pediatric Psychology,* 31 (2), 174-183.

Lewin, A. B., La Greca, A. M., Geffken, G. R., Williams, L. B., Duke, D. C., Storch, E. A. & et al., (2009). Validity and Reliability of an Adolescent and Parent Rating Scale of Type 1 Diabetes Adherence Behaviors: The Self-Care Inventory (SCI). *Journal of Pediatric Psychology,* 34(9), 999-1007.

Macrodimitris S.D., & Endler N.S. (2001). Coping, control, and adjustment in Type 2 diabetes. Health Psychology, 20(3), 208-16.

Malik, J. A., & Koot, H. M. (2009). Explaining the Adjustment of Adolescents With Type 1 Diabetes. Role of diabetes-specific and psychosocial factors. *Diabetes Care,* 32, 774-779.

Manne, S.L., Jacobson, P.B.,Gorfinkle,K., Gerstein, F., & Redd, W.H. (1993).Treatment adherence diffilculties among children with cancer: the role of parenting style. *Journal of Pediatric Psychology,* 18 (1), 47-62.

McCubbin, H. I., McCubbin, M. A., Patterson, J. M., Cauble, A.E., Wilson, L. R., & Warwick, W. (1983). CHIP – Coping Health Inventory for Parents: An Assessment of Parental Coping Patterns in the Care of the Chronically Ill Child. *Journal of Marriage and Family,* 359-370.

McKelvey, J., Waller, D. A., North, A. J., Marks, J. F., Schreiner, B., Travis, L. B., & Murphy, J.N. Reliability and Validity of the Diabetes Family Behavior Scale (DFBS). *The Diabetes Educator,* 19, 125-132.

McNabb, W. L. (1997). Adherence in diabetes: can we define it an can we measure it? *Diabetes Care,* 20 (2), 215-218.

Miller, K. B., & La Greca, A. M. (2005). Adjustment to chronic illness in girls. In D. J. Bell, S. L. Foster, & E. J. Mash (Eds.), *Handbook of behavioral and emotional problems in girls* (pp. 489–522). New York: Kluwer Academic/Plenum Press Publishers.

Miller-Johnson, Emery, R, Marvin, R., Clarke, W., Loevinger, R., & Martin, M. (1994). Parent-Child Relationships And The Management Of Insulin-Dependent Diabetes Mellitus. *Journal of Consulting and Clinical Psychology*, 62 (3), 603-610.

Mortensen, H., Hougaard, P., & Hvidore Study Group (1997). Comparison of metabolic control in a cross-sectional study of 2873 children and adolescentts with IDDM from 18 countries. *Diabetes Care*, 20, 714-720.

Mortensen, H.B., Robertson, K.J., Aanstoot, H.J. Danne, T., Holl, R.H., Hougaard, P., et al., (1998). Insulin management and metabolic control of Type 1 diabetes mellitus in childhood and adolescence in 18 countries. Diabetic Medicine, 15, 752–759,

Moss-Morris, R., Weinman J., Petrie, K.J. Horn, R., Cameron, L. & Buick, D. (2002). The Revised Illness Perception Questionnaire (IPQ-R). Psychology and Health ,17 (1), 1-16.

Northam, E, Anderson, P, Adler, R., & Warne, M. (1996). Psychosocial and Family Functioning In Children with Insulin-Dependent Diabetes at Diagnosis and One Year Later. *Journal of Pediatric Psychology*, 21, 699-717.

Novato, T.S. (2009). *Factores preditivos de Qualidade de Vida Relacionada à Saúde em Adolescentes com Diabetes Mellitus tipo 1*. Tese não publicada de Pós-Graduação em Enfermagem na Saúde do Adulto. Brasil.

Nunes, M.D.R. & Dupas, G. (2004). Entregando-se à vivência da doença do filho: a experiência da mãe da criança/adolescente diabético. *Texto e Contexto de Enfermagem*, 13 (1), 83-91.

Olsen, B., Berg, C. A. and Wiebe, D. J. (2005). Dissimilarity in mother and adolescent illness representations of type 1 diabetes and negative emotional adjustment. *Psychology and Health*, 23 (1), 113-129.

Organización Mundial de la Salud (1965).Problemas de salud de la adolescência. Série de Informes técnicos, Geneva: OMS, 308,29p.

Paddison, C.A.M., Alpass, F.M., & Stephens, C.V. (2008). Psychological variables account for variation in metabolic control and quality of life among people with type 2 diabetes in New Zealand. *International Journal of Behavioural Medicine* 15: 180–186, 2008.

Papalia, D., Olds, S., & Feldman, R. (2001). *O Mundo da criança*. McGraw-Hill: Lisboa.

Patino, A. M., Sanchez, J., Eidson, M., & Delamater, A. M. (2005). Health Beliefs and Regimen Adherence in Minority Adolescents with Type 1 Diabetes. *Journal of Pediatric Psychology*, 30 (6), 503-512.

Pereira, M. G., & Almeida, J. P. (2001). CHIP – *Coping Health Inventory for Parents: An Assessment of Parental Coping Patterns in the Care of the Chronically Ill Child*. Research Version of University of Minho.Braga.Portugal.

Pereira, M.G., Berg-Cross, L., Almeida, P., & Machado, C. J. (2008). Impact of Family Environment and Support and Adherence, Metabolic Control, and Quality Life in Adolescents with Diabetes. *International Journal of Behavioral Medicine*, 15, 187-193.

Petrie, K. J., Weinman, J., Sharpe, N., & Buckley, J. (1996). Role of patients' view of their illness in predicting return to work and functioning after myocardial infarction: Longitudinal study. *British Medical Journal*, 312, 1191–1194..

Ray, C., Epstein N., Keitner, G., Miller, I., & Bishop, D. (2005). Evaluation and Treating Families: The McMaster Approach. *Routledge Taylor & Francis Group*. New York.

Rocha. L. (2010). *Variáveis familiares, adesão, controlo metabólico e qualidade de vida na diabetes tipo 1:* Um estudo com adolescentes e familiares Unpublished dissertation. University of Minho. Braga. Portugal.

Santos, R. J. (2001). *Adolescentes com Diabetes Mellitus Tipo 1: Seu cotidiano e enfrentamento da doença.* Dissertação apresentada ao Programa de Pós-Graduação em Psicologia da Universidade Federal do Espírito Santo. Brasil.

Sarafino, E. P. (1990). *Health psychology: Biopsychosocial Interactions.* New York: John Wiley & Sons.

Searle, A., Norman, P., Thompson, R., & Vedhara, R. (2007). Illness representations among patients with type 2 diabetes and their partners: Relationships with self-management behaviours. *Journal of Psychosomatic Research*, 63, 175-184.

Seiffe-Krenke, I.(1998). Psychological Adjustment of Adolescents with Diabetes: Functional or Dysfunctional for Metabolic Control? *Journal of Pediatric Psychology*, 23 (5), 313-322.

Silva, I. (2003). *Qualidade de vida e variáveis psicológicas associadas a sequelas de diabetes e sua evolução ao longo do tempo.* Tese de Doutoramento não publicada, Faculdade de Psicologia e de Ciências da Educação, Universidade do Porto.Portugal.

Silva, I., Pais Ribeiro, J., Cardoso, H., & Ramos, H. (2002). Questionário de Auto-cuidados na Diabetes – contributo para a criação de um instrumento de avaliação da adesão ao tratamento. *Psiquiatria Clínica*, 23 (3), 227-237.

Skinner T. C., Hampson S. E., & Fife-Schaw, C. (2002). Personality, personal model beliefs, and self-care in adolescents and young adults with Type 1 diabetes. *Health Psychology*, 21, 61–70.

Skinner, T. C., & Hampson, S. E. (2001). Personal models of diabetes in relation to self-care, well-being, and glycemic control: A prospective study in adolescence. *Diabetes Care*, 24, 828–833.

Skinner, T. C., John, M., & Hampson, S. E. (2000). Social support and personal models of diabetes as predictors of self-care and well-being: A longitudinal study of adolescents with diabetes. *Journal of Pediatric Psychology*, 25(4), 257–267.

Snoek F.J., Pouwer F., Welch G.W., & Polonsky WH.(2000). Diabetes-related emotional distress in Dutch and U.S. diabetic patients: cross-cultural validity of the problem areas in diabetes scale. *Diabetes Care*, 23(9), 1305-9.

Sperling, A. M. (1996). Diabetes Mellitus. In W. Nelson, R. Behrman, & A.Arvin (Ed.). *Nelson Textbook of Pediatrics*, 15ª Edição, WB Sanders & Company: Philadelphia.

Stern, M. & Zevon, M.A (1990). Stress, Coping and Family Environment: the Adolescent's Response to Naturally Occurring Stressors. *Journal of Adolescent Research*, 5, 290-305.

Thomas, A. M., Peterson, L., & Goldstein, D. (1997). Problem solving and diabetes regimen adherence by children and adolescents with IDDM in social pressure situations: A reflection of normal development. *Journal of Pediatric Psychology*, 22, 541–561.

Trindade, I. (2000). Abordagem Psicológica do doente crónico em centros de saúde. In I.Trindade, & J. Teixeira (Eds), Psicologia nos cuidados de saúde primários (pp. 47-53). Climepsi Editores: Lisboa.

Warren, L. & Hixenbaugh, P. (1998). Adherence and Diabetes. In L.B. Myers, & K. Midence (Eds), *Adherence to treatment in medical conditions* (pp.423-453). Harwood Academic Publishers: Netherlands

Watkins K.W., Klem L, Connell C.M., Hickey, T., Fitzgerald. J.T., Ingersoll-Dayton B. (2000) Effect of adults self-regulation of diabetes on quality of life. *Diabetes Care* 2000; 23, 1511-1515.

Wysocki et al. (2000). Randomized, Controlled Trial of Behavior Therapy for Families of Adolescents with Insulin-Dependent Diabetes Mellitus. *Journal of Pediatric Psychology*, 25 (1), 23-33.

Wysocki, T (1993). Associations Among Teen-Parent Relationships, Metabolic Control, and Adjustment to Diabetes in Adolescents. *Journal of Pediatric Psychology*, 18 (4), 441-452.

Wysocki, T., & Greco, P. (2006). Social support and diabetes management in childhood and adolescence: Influence of parents and friends. *Current Diabetes Reports, 6,* 117-122.

Wysocki, T., Greco, P., Harris, M. A., Bubb, J., & White, N. H. (2001). Behavior therapy for families of adolescents with IDDM: Maintenance of treatment effects. *Diabetes Care, 24, 441-446.*

Zanetti, M.L. & Mendes, I.A.C. (2001). Análise das actividades relacionadas às actividades diárias de crianças e adolescentes com diabetes mellitus tipo1: depoimento de mães. *Revista Latino-Americana de Enfermagem,* 9 (6), 25-30.

7

Inadequate Coping Attitudes, Disordered Eating Behaviours and Eating Disorders in Type 1 Diabetic Patients

Ricardo V. García-Mayor and Alejandra Larrañaga
Eating Disorders Section, Endocrinology, Diabetes,
Nutrition and Metabolism Department,
University Hospital of Vigo
Spain

1. Introduction

Diabetes mellitus has been found to be the sixth leading cause of death for those living in the United States affecting the young and old at an alarming rate (National Center for Health Statistics, 2011). Type 1 diabetes typically has an early onset in life, but can occur at any age. It primarily develops when the body's own immune system attacks and destroys pancreatic beta cells, which produce the hormone insulin that regulates blood glucose levels. This type of diabetes accounts for 5 to 10 % of all diagnosed cases. Type 2 diabetes affects mainly adult subjects, its prevalence around the world has increased in relationship with the increase of the prevalence of overweight and obesity, attributed to lifestyle changes such as sedentary habits and overeating. Consequently, diabetes is one of the most challenging and burdensome chronic diseases of the 21st century, and it is a growing threat to the world's public health (King et al, 1995; King et al, 1998). Diabetes mellitus, especially type 1 form represent a very hard experience that requires subsequent psychological adaptation. Unfortunately, this often does not occur and it is followed by frustration and the non-acceptance of the disease. Problems with coping are one of the important consequences of the disease and the cause of uncountable problems in the future.

The management of type1 diabetes and its associated health-risk factors are often complex and require considerable patient education and frequent medical monitoring (Koopmanschap, 2002). The participation of the patients is basic in order to obtain a correct degree of metabolic control; however, this carries as a consequence considerable amount of stress. People on insulin must learn how to regulate their blood sugars by monitoring blood glucose levels daily while carefully attending to their food intake and an exercise regimen. Careful blood glucose monitoring is necessary to prevent wide variations in blood sugars that affect both short term and long term health and functioning. Hypoglycaemia reactions are a concern in the short run not only because they are frightening and disruptive, but also because, when severe, they can lead to unconsciousness, coma and death (Cox & Gonder-Frederick, 1992). The constant stress of maintaining tight glycaemia control can result in two types of psychological distress (a) subclinical emotional distress, and (b) diagnosable psychological disorders (Rubin & Payrot, 2001). Additionally, psychiatric conditions can occur independently without being a consequence of diabetes. It has been shown that individuals with diabetes have a disproportionately higher rate of psychiatric disorders (Bogner et al, 2007; Llorente & Urrutia, 2006), with affective and anxiety disorders being more commonly diagnosed than in the general population (De Mont-Marin et al, 1995). This is evidenced by research showing high rates of psychiatric disorders, particularly depression and anxiety, for example, Fettahoglu et al., (Fettahoglu et al, 2007) found over 40% increased risk in having any type of psychiatric disorder in patients with diabetes, and Gülseren et al. (Gülseren et al, 2001) found that depression and anxiety account for 45% of psychiatric disorders in patients with diabetes. These results show the negative impact that diabetes can have on an individual's psychosocial adjustment, and the need for research to determine the most appropriate and common coping strategies to deal with the stress of illness.

Other psychological problems of these patients are Eating Disorders (ED). The classical ED are anorexia nervosa (AN) and bulimia nervosa (BN), but recently another entity was recognized, the so called eating disorders not otherwise specified (EDNOS), which are incomplete forms of classical ED that are diagnosed when patients did not fulfill the classical ED diagnostic criteria. Type 1 diabetic patients have a high risk of suffering from ED due to these patients have to select the food they eat carefully in an early period of their development and because both entities, type 1 diabetes and ED, often affect adolescents and young adults. Furthermore, type 1 diabetic patients suffer from other eating behavior anomalies, which mainly appear in girls, that consist in splitting insulin doses or restricting food intake in order to reduce their body weight, but with the high price of the metabolic disturbance and subsequent chronic vascular complications if such behavior persists over time.

In this chapter we will review these psychological anomalies suffered by type 1 diabetic patients, especially problems with coping attitudes, disordered eating behaviors (DEB) and eating disorders (ED), and also discuss some aspects of their forms of presentation, management and prevention.

2. Search strategy for identification and selection of studies

We identified relevant studies published in English by searching MEDLINE from January 1990 to December 2010. We included randomised and quasi-randomised controlled studies, clinical series, reviews and systematic reviews on type 1 diabetic patients with inadequate coping attitudes, disordered eating behaviors and eating disorders, in which children, adolescents and young adults with type 1 diabetes were properly defined. As study strategy, relevant questions about type 1 diabetes and eating disorders were previously determined: coping with diabetes, epidemiology, clinical forms of eating disorders and specific behavioral anomalies in type 1 diabetic patients, metabolic consequences and vascular complications, management and prevention.

3. Inadequate coping attitudes in type 1 diabetic patients

People suffering from any type of chronic disease, need to make minor or major lifestyle adjustments. Diabetes, in particular, can eventually take its toll on the emotional, psychological, and physical well being of any person. These adjustments can lead to either successful adherence to medical regimens and control of the disease, or among other things, ineffective or maladaptive coping. The literature reveals that successfully adjusting to a chronic illness yields the following outcomes: successful performance of adaptive tests, absence of psychological disorders, low experience of negative affect, improved functional status, and appraisals of well-being in varying life domains (Stanton et al, 2001). Coping can generally be defined as cognitive and/or behavioral attempts to manage and tolerate situations that are appraised as stressful to an individual. No single coping strategy or dimension can be considered maladaptive. The quality of the coping strategy and process is evaluated according to its impact on the outcome of interest. From the previous conceptual definition, Folkman and Lazarus (Folkman & Lazaruz, 1980; Folkman & Lazaruz, 1985; Folkman & Lazaruz, 1988) distinguished two primary dimensions of coping (or categories): emotion-focused (composed of individual coping strategies such as seeking emotional support) and problem-focused (composed of individual coping strategies such as making a plan of action). These coping categories described efforts to either alleviate the personal emotional stress induced by the stressor or alter the source of stress in the environment. Use of problem-focused coping has been found to be associated with better metabolic control, emotional status, and better adjustment overall in patients with diabetes (Lundman & Norberg, 1993); use of emotion-focused coping has been found to be associated with poor adjustment and adherence to health regimens in chronically ill samples (Bombardier et al, 1990).

Diabetic patients initially experience high levels of depression and anxiety (Lustman et al, 1997; Tuncay, 2008). Anderson et al. (Anderson et al, 2001) found that adults with diabetes have twice the odds of comorbid depression. It was also found that this prevalence was much higher in women than in men. Within their sample, one in every three individuals had a level of depression that impaired their ability to function on a daily basis which in turn affected quality of life, regimen adherence, and blood glucose control. Regarding to coping strategies, it has been shown that problem-focused coping was positively associated with glycaemia control and negatively associated with anxiety and depression (Maes et al, 1996). Smari and Valtysdottir (Smari & Valtysdottir, 1997) also found that problem-focused coping was associated with lower blood glucose levels — indicative of better adjustment. On the contrary, individuals who engaged in more emotion-focused types of coping experienced more anxiety, depression, and higher levels of glycaemia. It is obvious that any deviation from a normal routine or health status serves as a continual source of stress that leads to the individuals' inability to care for themselves (White et al, 1992). Therefore, management of this stress via coping strategies is crucial for psychological and physical health.

An author found that treating depression through therapy is effective for individuals with diabetes so they may regain confidence and abilities to control the disease, leading to improved quality of life and social and physiological functioning (Eisenberg, 1992). The treatment includes the development of coping skills through training programs (Grey & Berry, 2004) as well as patient empowerment (Anderson et al, 1995). DeRidder and Schreurs (DeRidder & Schreurs, 2001) observed that diabetic patients in particular are inclined to use coping strategies that are aimed at reducing the negative emotions surrounding the disease and its maintenance. If this suggestion was found to be empirically true across diabetes studies and patients, it may portend a particularly problematic issue since these strategies were generally viewed as less adaptive. It is apparent that stress permeates the management of diabetes and thus use of effective coping skills is imperative not only in illness management but general stress management as well. At present, there is no systematic quantitative review of the stress and coping literature in diabetes that links coping strategies to indices of adjustment. Thus, a summary statement of the adaptive versus maladaptive strategies identified for these coping-adjustment relations cannot be made with any degree of confidence.

4. Epidemiology of disordered eating behavior and eating disorders in type 1 diabetic patients

Disordered eating behavior (DEB) is common in young women living in westernized countries, where thinness is valued and dietary restraint is pursued (Attie & Brook-Gunn, 1989). Prevalence studies in North America indicate that full syndrome bulimia nervosa may be found in 1-3% of adolescents and young adult women and subthreshold disorders are even more common (American Psychiatric Association, 1994; Fairburn & Beglin, 1990; Jones et al, 2001). The rates of these disorders are lower but rising in less-westernized countries such as Asia and Africa as Western attitudes towards weight and shape become more pervasive (Hoek, 1993; Lee, 1993; Lee & Lee 1996). Differences in the prevalence of eating disorders varies according to different ethnic groups (Abrams et al, 1993; Kumanyika, 1993), however, a study found that ethnic differences in eating disorder symptoms disappeared when body mass index (BMI) was controlled (Arriaza & Mann, 2001). At present, there is no information on the effect of culture and race on eating disorders in people with diabetes.

The risk of eating disturbances has been postulated to be higher in type 1 diabetic patients than in the general population due to multiple interacting factors related to diabetes and its treatment (Colton et al, 1999; Rodin & Daneman, 1992). Diabetes management imposes some degree of perceived dietary restraint, particularly patients who eat according to a predetermined meal plan, rather than in response to internal cues for hunger and satiety. Such neglect of internal cues may contribute to dietary dysregulation in susceptible individuals (Polivy & Herman, 1985). The relationship between higher weight and DEB presents a management dilemma for clinicians, since both dietary restraint and higher weight are clear risk factors for the development of ED and their negative health consequences.

Although until recently it has been unclear whether there is a specific association of eating disorders with diabetes, some studies have suggested an increased incidence of eating disorders in young women with diabetes (Birk & Spencer, 1987; Engstrom et al, 1999; Hudson et al, Lloyd et al, 1987; 1985; Rodin et al, 1985; Rodin et al, 1986/1987; Rodin et al, 1991; Rosmark et al, 1986; Stancin et al, 1989; Steel et al, 1987; Vila, et al, 1993; Vila et al, 1995) whereas others did not find such an increase (Bryden et al, 1999; Fairburn et al, 1991; Friedman et al, 1995; Mannucci et al, 1995; Marcus et al, 1992; Meltzer et al, 2001; Peveler et al, 1992; Powers et al, 1990; Robertson & Rosenvinge, 1990; Striegel-Moore et al, 1992; Wing et al, 1986). However, the conclusions of these studies are limited by the small sample sizes of females in the age of the highest risk for eating disturbances, the absence of control groups, their low statistical power, and/or by the lack of structured diagnostic interviews for the assessment of eating disorders.

A study examined the association between ED and type 1 diabetic girls, aged 12-19, for at least 1 year. Subjects with diabetes were 2.4 times more likely than non diabetic controls to have a clinical ED and 1.9 times more likely to have a subthreshold ED (Affenito & Adams, 2001). In another investigation, the prevalence of ED in a population-based cohort of female adolescents with type 1 diabetes was compared with that found in aged-matched controls. DEB was found in 16.9% of adolescents with diabetes compared with 2.2% of the controls (Hoek, 1993). A longitudinal study of 87 patients with diabetes aged at baseline 11-25 years, in whom eating habits and attitudes were assessed by a semistructured research diagnostic interview, showed that 14.9%, at baseline, and 26%, at the end of the follow-up period, had evidence of bingeing or purging while insulin misuse for weight control was reported by 35.6% of the patients (Peveler et al, 2005). A recent study from France (Ryan et al, 2008) concluded that abnormal eating behavior is present in French diabetic patients at higher levels than among the general population.

Thus, nowadays, there is clear evidence that EB and DEB are more prevalent in type 1 diabetic women than in the general population.

5. Clinical forms of eating disorders in type 1 diabetics

The three diagnostic forms of ED are AN, BN and EDNOS. Common to all three is a core problem in which the self-evaluation is unduly influenced by body weight or shape. This can be characterized by an extreme pursuit of thinness, in the case of AN, or recurrent episodes of binge eating and compensatory caloric purging behaviors, in the case of BN. EDNOS encompasses those ED that are clinically significant enough to compromise the patient health and the quality of life, but do not meet formal diagnostic criteria for AN or BN (American Psychiatric Association, 1994).

Eating disorders that meet Diagnostic and Statistical Manual of Mental Disorders four edition (DSM-IV) diagnostic criteria, mostly bulimia nervosa and EDNOS, are more than twice as common in girls with diabetes compared to their non-diabetic peers, furthermore, subthreshold eating disorders were also almost twice as common in girls with diabetes compared to controls (American Psychiatric Association, 1994). In line with these studies, it was found that the ED associated with bingeing and purging are the most common types of ED among girls with diabetes as they are in girls in the general population (American Psychiatric Association, 1994; Fairburn & Beglin, 1990; Jones et al, 2001). Restricting ED are much less common conditions (Jones et al, 2000), thus a specific association between anorexia nervosa and type 1 diabetes has not been demonstrated (Rodin et al, 2002).

In a longitudinal study by Colton et al, (Colton et al, 2007), at 5 years, 49% of a cohort of girls with type 1 diabetes reported current disordered eating behavior (DEB), 43.9% active dietary restraint, 6.1% binge-eating episodes, 3.1% self-induced vomiting, 3.1% insulin omission and 25.5% excessive exercise for weight control. Furthermore, 13.3% met criteria for an ED: three girls had bulimia nervosa, three had an eating disorder not otherwise specified and seven had a subthreshold ED.

Using the DSM-III-R or the DSM-IV for interview-based diagnosis, the prevalence of AN varies between 0.0-1.8% for diabetic patients, whereas 0.0-0.6% for controls. The prevalence of BN was 0.0-5.8% and 0.0-2.0%, respectively (Engström et al, 1999; Fairburn et al, 1991; Jones et al, 2000; Mannucci et al, 1995; Peveler et al, 1992; Robertson et al, 1990; Striegel-Moore et al, 1992; Vila et al 1995). In a study that aimed to determine the prevalence of ED in young adolescents, 98 type 1 diabetic patients and 575 age-matched controls were studied. The authors found neither AN nor BN case among diabetics and controls. However, the prevalence of EDNOS was significantly higher in adolescent diabetics than in controls both in boys (1.7% vs. 0.9% respectively) and girls (5.3% vs. 1.6% respectively). In addition, subthreshold ED were more common in male diabetic adolescents than in non-diabetic peers (García-Reyna et al, 2004). In a meta-analysis by Mannucci et al (Mannucci et al, 2005), they found that the prevalence of AN in type 1 diabetes was not significantly different from that in controls, being 0.27 vs. 0.06 %, respectively, while the prevalence of BN was 1.23 vs. 0.69 %, respectively, $p < 0.05$, in line with previous studies (Affenito et al, 1997; Jones et al, 2000; Vila et al, 1995).

The cited data indicate that young type 1 diabetic patients have a higher prevalence of BN, EDNOS and subthreshold ED than their non-diabetic peers. Data are summarized in Table 1.

Clinical forms	Globally	Girls	Boys
AN	0.0-1.8 %	0.27 %	-
BN	0.0-5.8 %	1.23-13.3 %	-
EDNOS	7 %	5.3 %	1.7 %
DEB	16.9 %	14.9-49.4 %	-
Insulin misuse	-	3.1-35.6 %	-

Table 1. Estimated prevalence of ED and DEB in type 1 diabetic patients.

6. Specific behavioral anomalies in type 1 diabetics

It is well-known the association of chronic illness, such as type 1 diabetes, asthma, attention deficit disorder, physical disabilities and seizure disorders, with DEB (Neumark-Sztainer et al, 1995; Neumark-Sztainer et al, 1998). Adolescents with chronic illness present higher body dissatisfaction engaged in more high risk weight loss practices (Neumark-Sztainer et al, 1995). These data were confirmed by other studies (Neumark-Sztainer et al, 1998).

While adjusting to the changes of puberty, the adolescence is a period of rapid physical and psychological growth and development. During this time to control weight and to overcome body dissatisfaction, some adolescents commonly diet or exercise. Other may present more severe misbehaviors such as bingeing and purging, the use of laxatives or the adherence to an overly strict exercise regimen.

Before diagnosis and treatment, individuals with type 1 diabetes are likely to lose a large amount of weight. However, once the treatment begins the weight usually returns. By controlling diabetes with insulin injections many diabetics face a constant struggle with their weight (Collazo Clavell, 2010). As insulin encourages fat storage, many people with type 1 diabetes have discovered the relationship between reducing the amount of insulin they take and their corresponding weight loss (Mathur & Conrad, 2008; Mathur & Conrad, 2008). It is well-known that adolescents with type 1 diabetes tend to exhibit increased difficulty in maintaining optimal weight and also are more inclined to be concerned about their weight than their non-diabetic counterparts (Bryden et al, 1999).

Since weight management during this state of development can be especially difficult for those with type 1 diabetes, some diabetics may restrict or omit insulin, a condition known as diabulimia, as a form of weight control (Baginsky, 2009; Hasken et al, 2010; Ruth-Sahd et al, 2009). This is not a medically recognized condition yet, but describes the situation of a considerable number of type 1 diabetic patients.

Insulin restriction becomes a more significant problem in older adolescents, perhaps as parental supervision of insulin administration decreases. It becomes more common a potential worsening in severity and frequency throughout early adulthood. Once the pattern of frequent and habitual insulin restriction became entrenched, the cycle of negative feelings about body image, shape and weight; chronically elevated blood sugars; depression, anxiety and shame; and poor diabetes self-care can be complex and difficult to treat.

In a study that looked at 143 adolescents with type 1 diabetes who completed the Assessing Health and Eating among Adolescents with Diabetes survey; unhealthy weight control practice was observed in 37.9 % of females and 15.9% of males. Among the females, 10.3% reported skipping insulin and 7.4 % reported taking less insulin to control their weight (Neumark-Sztainer et al, 2002). Only one male reported doing either of these behaviors. In another 4 years follow-up study of 91 girls with diabetes aged 12 to 18, dieting was reported by 38% of the sample, binge eating by 45%, insulin omission by 14 % and self-induced vomiting by 8% at baseline, these behaviors were even more common at follow-up, when most of the girls were in the age of the highest risk for ED. At this time, more than half of the sample reported dieting for weight loss and binge eating, and one-third reported deliberate insulin omission to prevent weight gain (Rydall et al, 1997).

In general terms, it is estimated that between 30% and 40% of adolescents and young adults with diabetes skip or reduce insulin after meals to lose weight (Hasken 2010).

7. Metabolic consequences and vascular complications of disordered eating behaviors and eating disorders in type 1 diabetics

There is a spectrum of severity of disturbance of eating habits and attitudes, and subthreshold eating problems, seen as relatively mild in non diabetic patients, can give rise to clinically important disturbances of self-care and glycaemia control in diabetics. In general terms, glycosilated hemoglobin was higher in patients with diabetes who had ED compared with those with diabetes without ED (Affenito & Adams, 2001). A study by Rydall et al (Rydall et al, 1997), found that the mean HbA1c was significantly higher among girls with clinical DEB compared to those moderately disordered of eating habits or with no disordered behavior. Another 3-year longitudinal study by Figueroa Sobrero et al (Figueroa Sobrero et al, 2010) revealed that the presence and persistence of disordered eating behavior is associated with worse prognosis in type 1 diabetic children and adolescents.

The lack of proper insulin treatment in type 1 diabetics may lead to many harmful physical effects. Reducing insulin to lose weight increases the risk of dehydration, break down of muscle tissue, high risk of developed infections and fatigue. If this behavior continues, it may also result in kidney failure, eye disease leading to blindness, vascular disease and even death.

In particular, patients who misuse insulin to control body weight (Crow et al, 1998; Rodin et al, 1989), are thought to be at increased risk for microvascular complications (Rydall et al, 1997; Steel et al, 1987), but the extent of the risk has not been well characterized, as most studies have been cross-sectional. Clinical outcome in terms of physical and psychological health are not known with certainty. One longitudinal study of patients with diabetes and DEB over 9 years, found a low rate of microvascular complications (Pollock et al, 1995). On the contrary, another study, taking place over 4 years, found that insulin-dependent girls with DEB had an increased risk for retinopathy (Rydall et al, 1997). A more recent longitudinal study observed that diabetic patients aged 11 to 25 years with DEB or insulin misuse had a significant risk for the development of two or more serious complications, such as repeated episodes of diabetic ketoacidosis, increased rate of hospital admission and mortality (Peveler et al, 2005).

Therefore, ED in type 1 diabetics have clearly shown to be associated with impaired metabolic control (Jones et al, 2000; Vila et al, 1993; Friedman S et al, 1995; Affenito et al 1997; Affenito et al 1998; Rydall et al, 1997), more frequent episodes of ketoacidosis (Polonsky et al, 1994), and an earlier than expected onset of diabetes-related microvascular complications, particularly, retinopathy (Affenito et al, 1997; Colas et al, 1991; Rydall et al, 1997; Steel et al, 1987; Ward et al, 1995). In this sense, disordered eating status was more predictive of diabetic retinopathy than was the duration of diabetes, which is a well-established risk factor for microvascular complications (Diabetes Control and Complications Trial Research Group, 1993). Furthermore, ED in type 1 diabetic patients is associated with high mortality (Walker et al, 2002).

Regarding to mortality, an 11-year follow-up study reports that insulin restriction conveyed more than a three-fold increased risk of mortality in type 1 diabetic patients after controlling for age, body mass index and HbA1c values. Age of death was younger among insulin restrictors, with a mean age of death of 45 years, as compared to 58 years among those reporting appropriate insulin use (Goebel-Fabbri et al, 2007).

Insulin restriction becomes a more significant problem in older adolescents and in early adulthood. Once the pattern of frequent and habitual insulin restriction becomes entrenched, its consequent poor diabetes self-care can be complex and difficult to treat. Figure 1.

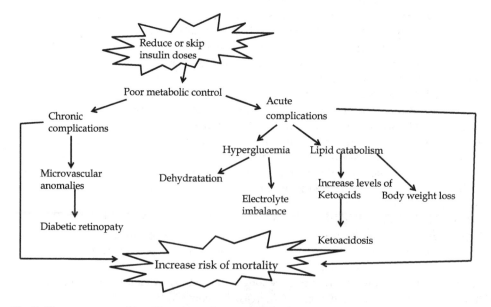

Fig. 1. Consequences of insulin misuse in type1 diabetic patients.

8. Management of inadequate coping attitudes in type 1 diabetic patients

Several major trial carried out in the past decades, have demonstrated that intensive diabetes management for type 1, as well as type 2 diabetes, can delay or prevent the onset and progression of many complications of the disease, especially microvascular complications (DCCT, 1993; UKPDS, 1998). Such studies also have demonstrated that achieving excellent glycaemia control requires complex self-management behaviors to be learned and maintained.

Traditionally, diabetes education has focused on increasing knowledge about diabetes and its care and increasing skills to perform self-care behaviors, such as blood glucose monitoring. However, it is clear that although knowledge and skills are important prerequisites to diabetes self-management, additional training in the application of this knowledge and skills in day-to-day living are necessary for longer-term maintenance and improved outcomes. Cognitive-behavioral interventions such as coping skills training focus primarily on improving behavioral skills are necessary to achieve better glycaemia and psychosocial outcomes in patients with diabetes and in their relative members (Grey & Berry, 2004).

8.1 Social problem solving

Social problem solving assists individuals when they are faced with peer or family pressures or any decision in which they are confronted with a dilemma. Social problem solving is a process by which an individual learns to think through the steps of having a problem and reaching a decision about how to handle the problem. The process assists individuals to look at all possible outcomes of situations and the possible consequences of their decisions (Duangdao & Roesch, 2008).

8.2 Conflict resolution

The basis of conflict resolution is the acquisition of skills necessary to resolve conflict in a positive manner that results in positive outcomes for all parties involved in the conflict (Deustsch & Brickman, 1994). The first step in this training is development of the understanding that in any conflict both parties can win and that every conflict should be approached in this manner. The individual is helped to focus on clear communication and problem-solving skills. Once the conflict is identified, all possible outcomes and the consequences to these outcomes are explored. Role-playing can then be set up to try out the communication of the decision. Role-play is used as both forms of practice and feedback on communication skills.

8.3 Communication skills training

This kind of training aims to help individuals express themselves in ways that are clear, appropriate, and constructive. Two main skills are identified under communication skills training: social skills training and assertiveness training. Models for social skills training include those by Carteledge & Milburn (Carteledge & Milburn, 1980) and Goldstein *et al.* (Goldstein et al, 1980). These models strive to teach individuals how to work with others in a way that will result in positive outcomes for all. Assertiveness training permits one to communicate in ways that are direct, honest, and appropriate. Working groups allow members to observe the behavior of others as well as practice and obtain feedback on how effectively they communicate with the other members of the group.

8.4 Coping skills training

Coping skills training has been utilized by Grey and Barry (Grey & Berry, 2004) in individuals with diabetes, particularly, in the area of problem solving. The framework is derived from Bandura's conceptualization of self-efficacy, where the individuals act as the catalyst for positive changes in their lives (Bandura, 1986). When a person can practice and rehearse a new behavior, such as learning how to cope successfully with a problem situation, self-efficacy or self-concept can be enhanced. Further, by enhancing self-efficacy, problems with psychosocial well-being may be decreased. When an individual cannot cope effectively with a problem situation, confidence is decreased for dealing with the next problem, and less successful coping patterns are employed (Marlatt & Gordon, 1985).

This kind of training was originally developed for work with youth to prevent drug and alcohol use, training in the use of coping skills can teach personal and social behaviors that can assist individuals in dealing with potential stressors they encounter in their daily lives and the stress reactions that may result from these situations (Forman et al, 1993). In children and youth, such interventions have been demonstrated to reduce substance abuse (Forman et al, 1993), improve social adjustment (Bierman & Furman, 1984), prevent smoking (DelGreco et al, 1986) and reduce responses to stressors (Elias et al, 1986). In adults, coping skills training has been used to address drug and alcohol use and weight reduction.

8.5 Cognitive-behavioural modification

The cognitive-behavioural modification process comprises three steps. The first is working with the individual to reflect on how they think and then respond to situations. The individual's thoughts are then examined to consider if the thoughts are based on fact or assumption. Once the thoughts are examined the next step is to solve the social problem. The last step consists in teaching the individual to use his or her thoughts to help follow through on the decision made in the previous step. The group members can list their negative thoughts and then the member and the group can formulate alternate positive thoughts to counter the negative thoughts.

8.6 Coping skills training with children and adolescents

The use of coping skills training for youth with diabetes was based on the hypothesis that improving coping skills would improve the ability of youth to cope with the problems faced on a day-to-day basis in managing diabetes. Initially, a number of studies were conducted in five to 10 years old school-children and preadolescents using coping skills training (Gross et al, 1982; Gross et al, 1983; Johnson et al, 1982). The results of these studies suggested that coping skills training increased appropriate verbal assertiveness and performance in social situation, but not glycaemia control. An experimental pilot study by Boardway et al (Boardway et al, 1993) also supported the potential of this intervention to assist adolescents to manage diabetes, the authors observed that diabetes-specific stress was found to decrease significantly after stress management training, but glycaemia control, coping styles, self-efficacy, and adherence to regimen remained unchanged.

Some controlled studies (Davidson et al, 1997; Grey et al, 1998; Grey et al, 2000) were conducted to determine whether coping skills training would improve glycaemia and psychosocial outcomes in adolescents with type 1 diabetes mellitus implementing intensive diabetes management. They showed that, at 3 months, adolescents who received coping skills training had lower hemoglobin A1c levels and less distress about coping with their diabetes than adolescents receiving intensive management alone. Furthermore, adolescents who received coping skills training found it easier to cope with their diabetes and experienced less negative impact from diabetes on their quality of life than those who did not receive the training. The authors also demonstrated that the effects on glycaemia control and quality of life associated with coping skills training combined with intensive diabetes management can be sustained over 1 year (Grey et al, 2000).

Hains et al, (Hains et al, 2001) examined the impact of a cognitive behavioral intervention for distressed adolescents with type 1 diabetes mellitus. They studied six youths who had increased levels of anxiety, diabetes stress, or anger who received eight individual sessions using cognitive restructuring with problem solving through a conceptualization phase, skill acquisition phase, and application phase. Four patients demonstrated improvement on anxiety, anger expression, or diabetes stress, compared with baseline.

The results of the aforementioned studies suggest that in children and adolescents with type 1 diabetes, coping skills training increases the repertoire of skills that youth have to self-manage diabetes. Thus, they can improve their metabolic control and their quality of life.

8.7 Coping skills training with parents and children or adolescents

Family environment has been found to play an important role in the adaptation of children with type 1 diabetes (McDougal, 2002). It has been shown that family interventions decrease parent-child conflicts about diabetes and improve metabolic control (Grey et al, 2003; Wysocki et al, 2000; Wysocki et al, 2001). One study that includes 119 families of adolescents with type 1 diabetes mellitus, assessed the effectiveness of an experimental group receiving Behavioral-Family Systems Therapy compared to both education and support groups in reducing parent-adolescent conflict in diabetes management. The Behavioral-Family Systems Therapy intervention targeted parent-adolescent conflict by focusing on family problem solving, communication skills training, cognitive restructuring, and aspects of functional and structural family therapy over 10 sessions. The results revealed that the experimental group showed significant improvement in parent-adolescent relationships, decreased diabetes-specific family conflicts, and increased treatment adherence when compared with education and support groups. At 6-month follow-up, parent-adolescent relationships remained significantly improved for the experimental group as compared to the control group. At 12 months, diabetes-specific family conflict was significantly improved compared to the control group. The experimental group showed improved treatment adherence compared with the control and education groups that both showed deteriorated adherence (Wysocki et al, 2000; Wysocki et al, 2001).

When parental involvement decreases, which is frequent in early adolescence, the metabolic control tends to deteriorate. Anderson et al. (Anderson et al, 1995) studied an office-based intervention to maintain parent adolescent teamwork in diabetes management. The study variables included parental involvement in diabetes care, family conflict, and subsequent metabolic control. Eighty-five patients aged 10 to 15 years were randomly assigned to one of three groups, which included teamwork, attention control, or standard control for 24 months. The teamwork families reported less conflict at 12 months. More adolescents in the teamwork group when compared to the comparison groups improved their HbA1c levels from the 12- to 24-month period. The results suggested the value of parent-adolescent partnership in diabetes management.

The results of the mentioned studies of coping skills training and problem-solving interventions in children, and adolescents with diabetes, as well as parents of children with diabetes, have demonstrated that these interventions are effective in assisting people to improve diabetes self management and to achieve better diabetes outcomes (Grey & Berry, 2004).

9. The management of eating behavioral anomalies in type 1 diabetics

No treatment outcome studies to date have examined treatment efficacy for DEB and ED in type1 diabetics, for this reason, many of the recommendations have not yet been empirically evaluated. ED have been shown to convey their own significant medical risk and also appear to persist and worsen over time. Treatment aimed at promoting family co-management of diabetes treatment tasks and decreasing diabetes-related family conflict have already been shown to promote improved diabetes outcomes in children and teens with type 1 diabetes (Nansel et al, 2008).

Despite the fact that little research has been done to determine the best treatment approaches for the problem of type 1 diabetic patients with ED or DEB, a multidisciplinary care team is considered the standard to treat these people. Such a team should include an endocrinologist/diabetologist, a nurse educator, a nutritionist with ED and/or diabetes training and a psychologist or social worker to provide weekly therapy. Depending on the severity of related psychiatric symptoms, such as depression and anxiety, a psychiatrist for psychopharmacologic evaluation and treatment should also be consulted. Team members must be allowed to frequently an openly communicate with each other to maintain congruent treatment approaches, messages and goals. Patients may require a medical or psychiatric inpatients hospitalization until they are medically stable and emotionally ready to engage in treatment as outpatients. Early in the treatment, monthly appointments with a team endocrinologist or nurse educator may be necessary to maintain medical stability, and monthly appointments with the nutritionists are also recommended. Laboratory tests, especially HbA1c and electrolytes, and weight checks should occur routinely at medical appointments. Unfortunately, such specialty services are rarely available to individuals with diabetes.

As a result, detection of insulin restriction may be unlikely until after the problem has become habitual and entrenched. Goebel-Fabbri et al (Goebel-Fabbri 2008) suggest that insulin restriction can be captured by a single screening item "I take less insulin than I should". The use of this question in routine clinical practice has the potential to identify at-risk subjects and, consequently, to make possible an early intervention. However, further studies are needed to assess the clinical utility of adopting such a question as a screening tool to identify insulin restrictors.

The overall goal of the treatment of patients with type 1 diabetes and DEB and ED is to return the patients to a state of premorbid physical and mental health. Treatment begins with emphasis on nutritional rehabilitation, weight restoration and adequate diabetes control (Anzai et al, 2002; Krakoff, 1991).

Psychotherapy should begin immediately for the patient and family, but it is not effective for the patient when is in a starvation mode (Walsh et al, 2000).

9.1 Diabetes treatment

The diabetes team has the important responsibility of monitoring insulin regimens and providing education about diabetes management and potential complications to patients and families (Krakoff, 1991). There are no studies looking at treatment of ED/DEB in youth with type 1 diabetes. The traditional approaches to poor blood glucose control involving a stricter and more intensive monitoring of the diabetic management may increase the risk for disordered eating (Colton et al, 1999). For this reason, it is recommended a less rigid approach in the insulin regimen and nutrition therapy to improve DEB. Lowering the amount of time spent on diabetes management during the day may help to lessen stress associated with the diabetes, which may in turn help alleviate DEB. Krokoff (Krokoff, 1991) suggested that self-destructive insulin manipulation within the context of an ED may also be an indirect call for help, signaling the need for more parental/adult intervention in patient's physical and mental health.

Trento et al, (Trento et al, 2009) suggest that offering a carbohydrate counting program within a group care management approach may help patients with type 1 diabetes acquire better self-efficacy and restructure their cognitive and lifestyle potential.

Technological advances can also be used to address specific treatment issues seen in these patients. For example, the first challenge that most patients face is weight gain associated with insulin restart. Patients need to be taught to indentify insulin edema, which may make them feel fat, bloated and uncomfortable, as temporary water retention that is different from the development of fatty tissue. Special tools designed to measure water-related weight versus lean muscle mass versus fat mass could help patients tolerate the temporary weight gain related to edema (Goebel-Fabbri 2008). Additionally, newer insulin analogs show evidence of improving weight profiles which could be of help (Goebel-Fabbri 2008; Russell-Jones & Khan, 2007).

9.2 Nutritional management

The dietician must balance the difficult tasks of providing diabetes education, ED education, writing meal plans and defining weight goals for patients and families (Anzai et al, 2002; Krakoff, 1991). The challenge presents when trying to balance the goal of slow weight gain and /or maintenance with diabetes meal planning. As the patient continues to increase calorie intake, insulin doses will need to be adjusted to match the amount of food eaten avoiding hyperglycemia. It is recommend a realistic goal of good blood glucose control instead of optimal blood glucose levels as the body readjusts to refeeding and the patient begins to benefit from psychotherapy. Multiple daily injections regimens that use insulin to carbohydrate ratios provide greater flexibility with meal times and amounts of food but do require increased blood glucose monitoring and insulin injections. Such intense diabetes management may increase the potential for disordered eating as the child or adolescent must think constantly about the effects of food, insulin and exercise on his or her blood glucose levels. This may not be an ideal approach to diabetes meal planning during the treatment and recovery from the ED. As the individual's physical and psychological health improves, the incorporation of more flexible meal-planning strategies may be useful. Care professionals, including nutrition therapists and diabetes educators, should be sensitive to weight-related changes and concerns in youth with type 1 diabetes. It is important for all health care professionals to be aware that weight loss may be related to glycaemia control.

9.3 Psychological therapy

Psychotherapy individual, group, and family therapy are the most common ways to treat ED. There are no studies showing the best psychotherapy modality for patients with type 1 diabetes and ED or DEB. Some authors propose individual therapy to help patients to recover from ED and diabetes mismanagement (Krokoff, 1991). Adolescents with type 1 diabetes often struggle with emotional issues related to having the illness and use an ED as a maladaptive coping mechanism. Individual therapy can help patients to develop more healthy coping strategies. Often families of patients with diabetes and ED have not adequately coped with the feelings of grief related to having a chronic illness in the family and thus they have not adequately supported the patient with diabetes. Dysfuntional family dynamics can exacerbate difficulties of adjusting to the illness and of resolving issues of grief and loss associated with the diagnosis. Family therapy is recommended to help the family in developing more functional ways of relating and in addressing issues of grief and loss that may be contributing to ED symptoms.

Psychoeducation is a useful method to aid the patient to develop skills that will help him or her to cope with a chronic disease. Therefore, it can be helpful in type 1 diabetic patients who have difficulties accepting the disease.

Psycho-pharmaceutical agents may be useful to treat comorbid mental health problems (Rosen, 2003). Table 2.

One uncontrolled study of cognitive behavior therapy (Peveler & Fairburn, 1992) and several case reports of other treatment approaches for ED associated with type1 diabetes have been reported (Nielsen et al, 1987; Peveler & Fairburn, 1989; Ramirez et al, 1990). Further research is needed to demonstrate whether more intensive, prolonged or alternative interventions may have a more significant impact on metabolic control and other diabetes-related outcomes.

Components	Recommendations
Diabetes therapy	Avoid intensive insulin regimens Avoid intensive glucose monitoring Use insulin analog with better weight gain profile Measure body weight with bioimpedance devices Involve family member in metabolic control
Nutrition	Less rigid diet recommendations Avoid excessive attention to the foods Meal planning based on family customs
Psychotherapy	Family therapy Psychoeducation Individual or group psychotherapy promote self-esteem Individual psychotherapy to promote adequate coping
Pharmacotherapy	Drugs to treat comorbidities associated with ED or DEB: depression, anxiety, etc.

Table 2. Components for the treatment of type 1 diabetic patients with ED or DEB.

10. Prevention

Since most type 1 diabetic patients do not admit to having an ED, this condition is commonly detected first by health care professionals (Walsh et al, 2000). The diabetes team may be the first to discover an ED and can play a crucial role in recommending proper treatment to the patient and family. It is unlikely that diabetes management will improve until appropriate treatment begins for the concurrent ED.

The results of studies on coping skills training and problem-solving interventions in children, adolescents, and adults with diabetes, as well as parents of children with diabetes, have demonstrated that these interventions are effective assisting people to improve diabetes self-management and to achieve better diabetes outcomes.

In childhood, the data suggest that interventions should include both children or adolescents and their parents within the first years after the diagnosis to improve self-management through learning problem-solving skills. Health care providers need to pay particular attention to adolescents with poorer glycaemia control and quality of life when they intensify their treatment, because they are less likely to reach treatment goals and may require additional support. Serious problems with self-management usually emerge during early adolescence and are difficult to correct [41,42]. The family management of diabetes should include a cooperative relationship between the patient, his or her family, and the diabetes health care provider team. The complexities of diabetes care demand a multifaceted approach that includes a strong foundation of diabetes education, medical supervision, reinforcement of positive self-care behaviors, and behavioral interventions that include problem solving and coping skills training. It is imperative to use problem solving strategies with psychological support that meet the developmental stage and level of adjustment for all family members involved in diabetes care.

Clinic-based group interventions for young women with diabetes and DEB may be the most practical and nonstigmatizing approach to prevention and early intervention for this problem. Rigid approaches to the dietary management of diabetes can contribute to the development of DEB. Rigid dieting has been shown to be a risk factor for ED in nonobese, nondiabetic women (Stewart et al, 2002). In type 1 diabetic patients feelings of deprivation associated with the perceived requirement for dietary restraint may trigger episodes of binge eating and subsequent insulin omission to prevent weight gain. Further, the weight gain associated with intensive diabetes management may amplify body dissatisfaction and the drive for thinness in susceptible girls (Daneman et al, 1998; Daneman & Rodin, 1999). For these reasons less intensive regimens are recommended in the initial stage of diabetes treatment, especially in young women.

It is recommended that the health care professional who treat young women with type 1 diabetes maintain a high index of suspicion for the presence of an eating disturbance, particularly among those patients with persistent poor metabolic control, repeated episodes of ketoacidosis and/or weight and shape concerns.

Screening for disordered eating behaviors in type 1 diabetics would be the best approach to get an early detection of behavioral abnormalities in these patients, however, a validated screening tool is not available yet (Dion Kelly et al, 2005). Clinicians working with adolescent and young adult women diabetes should be cognizant of patterns that might indicate the presence of DEB in their patients. They can include extreme concerns about weight and body shape, unusual patterns of intense exercise, sometimes accompanied or followed by frequent hypoglycemia, unusually low-calorie meal plans, unexplained elevations in HbA1c values, repeated problems with diabetic ketoacidosis and amenorrhea (Olmsted et al, 2008). Recently, Markowitz et al. (Markowitz et al, 2010) proposed a 16-items diabetes-specific self-reported measure of disordered eating for brief screening tool for disordered eating in diabetes. Table 3.

Individual or group intervention aimed to increase self-esteem, appearance and body acceptance, and family-based interventions with the objective of developing flexible approaches to food and meal planning may help to avoid the development of DEBs in type 1 diabetic patients.

CLUES
Adolescents or young women with type 1 diabetes
Patients with high concern on body weight or shape
Patients with not adequate coping with diabetes
Poor metabolic control including frequent episodes of ketoacidosis
Type 1 diabetic patients with amenorhea

Table 3. Clues to early diagnose ED or DEB in type 1 diabetics

11. Conclusions

Diabetes self-management is crucial to prevent early morbidity. Although more experimental research is needed, especially in minority populations and the non-adolescent age range, the addition of coping skills training and problem solving interventions to the clinical care of patients with diabetes appears warranted. Such interventions can be incorporated into routine diabetes education programs or the content included in regular diabetes care visits. Interventions using coping skills training and problem solving for children, adolescents, and adults with diabetes and their families should be individualized to their lifestyle, respect individual differences and routines, incorporate social support, and be reinforced and followed over time. Behavioral theory should be used in the design of future approaches.

Today is well-known that disordered eating behaviors and subthreshold disordered eating disorders are more prevalent in girls with type 1 diabetes than their peers without diabetes. DEB persists over time and its rates and symptoms severity increase with age. In type 1 diabetic women, the predominant ED are BN and EDNOS. Furthermore, these patients also develop specific DEB such as diet restriction, and insulin misuse in order to lose weight, with the consequent impairment of their metabolic control which is followed by acute diabetic complications such as diabetic ketoacidosis, dehydration or electrolyte anomalies, and chronic microvascular complications, mainly diabetic retinopathy, that even increase the risk of mortality.

Full established DEB and ED are difficult to manage. The management of these conditions requires a multidisciplinary team formed by an endocrinologist/diabetologist, nurse educator, nutritionist, psychologist and, frequently, a psychiatrist who should be consulted to evaluate and treat with psycho pharmaceutical products the possible psychiatric comorbidities of these patients. Unfortunately, the mentioned team is often not available for patients.

The best psychological methods to treat these anomalies are not determined yet. According to personal experience, patients tend to be treated individually or in group and, frequently, it is needed familiar therapy. Results of the treatment of these entities from experienced health professionals are waiting.

The key for the management of type 1 diabetic patients with ED or DEB is the early diagnosis and treatment. Unfortunately, validated questionnaires to screen type 1 diabetic population are not available so far. Therefore it is important that the staff of the diabetes team who treats these patients should know the relationship between poor diabetes metabolic control and intentional misuse of insulin, or the recommended diet to control weight gain. They also should know that strict diet and intensive insulin regimens are risk factors for the development of DEB or ED. Therefore, it would be important to be alert to detect excessive concern about body weight, shape or body dissatisfaction in these patients.

Eating disorders in type 1 diabetic patients represent some of the most complex patient problems to treat both medically and psychologically. Given the extent of the problem and the severe medical risk associated with it, more clinical and technological research aimed to improve its treatment is critical to the future health of this at-risk population.

12. References

Abrams, KK., Allen, L., & Gray, JJ. (1993). Disordered eating attitudes and behaviors, psychological adjustment, and ethnic identity: a comparison of black and white female college students. *Int J Eating Disord*, Vol.14, No. 1, (July 1993), pp. 49-57.

Affenito, SG., & Adams, CH. (2001). Are eating disorders more prevalent in females with type 1 diabetes mellitus when the impact of insulin omission is considered? *Nutr Rev*, Vol. 59, No. 6, (June 2001), pp. 179-182.

Affenito, SG., Backstrand, JR., Welch, GW., Lammi-Keefe, CJ., Rodriguez, NR., & Adams, CH. (1997). Subclinical and clinical eating disorders in IDDM negatively affect metabolic control. *Diabetes Care*, Vol. 20, pp. 182-184.

Affenito, SG., Rodriguez, NR., Backstrand, JR., Welch, GW., & Adams, CH. (1998) Insulin misuse by women with type 1 diabetes mellitus complicated by eating disorders does not favorably change body weight, body composition, or body fat distribution. *J AmDiet Assoc*, Vol.98, pp. 686-688.

American Psychiatric Association. Diagnostic and statistical manual of mental disorders. 4th ed. Washington (DC): American Psychiatric Association, 1994.

Anderson, RM., Funnel, MM., Butler, PM., Arnold, MS., Fitzgerald, JT., & Feste, CC. (1995). Patient empowerment. Results of a randomized controlled trial. *Diabetes Care*, Vol. 18, pp. 943-949.

Anzai, N., Lindsay-Dudley, K., & Bidwell, RJ. (2002). Impatient and partial hospital treatment for adolescent eating disorders. *Child Adolesc Psychiatr Clin North Am* , Vol. 11, pp. 279-309.

Arriaza, CA., & Mann, T. (2001). Ethnic differences in eating disorder symptoms among college students: the confounding role of body mass index. *J Am Coll Health*, vol. 49, pp. 309-315.

Attie, I., & Brooks-Gunn, J. (1989). Development of eating problems in adolescent girls: a longitudinal study. *Dev Psychol*, vol. 25, pp. 70-79.

Baginsky, P. (2009).A battle to overcome "Diabulimia". *Am Fam Physician*, vol. 79, pp. 263.

Bandura A. (1986). Social Foundations of Thought and Action: A SocialCognitive Theory. Prentice Hall. Englewood Cliffs, NJ.

Bierman, KL., & Furman, W. (1984). The effects of social skills training andpeer involvement on social adjustment of preadolescents. *Child Development*, Vol. 55, pp. 155–162.

Birk, R., & Spencer, ML. (1987).The prevalence of anorexia nervosa, bulimia and induced glycosuria in IDDM females. *Diabetes Educ*, vol. 15, pp. 336-341.

Boardway, RH., Delameter, AM., Tomakowsky, J., & Gutai, JP. (1993). management training for adolescents with diabetes. *Journal of Pediatric Psychology*, Vol. 18, pp. 183–195.

Bogner, HR., Morales, KH., Post, EP., & Bruce, ML. (2007). Diabetes, depression, and death. *Diabetes Care*, vol. 30, pp. 3005-3010.

Bombardier. CH., D'Amico, C., & Jordan, JS. (1990). The relationship of apprisal and coping to chronic illness adjustment. *Behavioral and Research Therapy*, Vol. 28, pp. 297-304.

Bryden, KS., Neil, A., Mayou, RA., Peveler, RC., Fairburn, CG., & Dunger, DB. (1999). Eating habits, body weight and insulin misuse: a longitudinal study of teenagers and young adults with type 1 diabetes. *Diabetes Care*, vol. 22, pp. 1956-1960.

Bryden, KS., Neil, A., Peveler, RC., Fairburn, CG., & Dundger, DB. (1999). Eating habits, body weight, and insulin misused. A longitudinal study of teenagers and young adults with type 1 diabetes. *Diabetes Care*, vol. 22, pp. 1956-1960.

Carteledge, MG., & Milburn, JF.(1980). eds: *Teaching Skills to Children: Innovative Approaches*. Pergamon, Elmsford, NY.

Colas, C., Mathieu, P., & Tehobroutsky, G. (1991). Eating disorders and retinal lesions in type 1 (insulin-dependent) diabetic women (letter). *Diabetología*, vol.34, pp.288.

Colton, PA., Olmsted, MP., Daneman, D., Rydall, AC., & Rodin, GM. (2007). Five-year prevalence and persistence of disturbed eating behavior and eating disorders in girls with type 1 diabetes. *Diabetes Care*, vol. 30 pp. 2861-2862.

Colton, PA., Rodin, GM., Olmsted, MP., & Daneman, D. (1999). Eating disturbances in young women with type 1 diabetes mellitus: mechanisms and consequences. *Psychiatr Ann*, vol. 40, pp. 193-201.

Cox, DJ., & Gonder-Frederick, L. (1992). Major developments in behavioural diabetes research. *J Consult Clin Psychol*, vol. 60, pp. 628-638.

Crow, SJ., Keel, PK., & Kendall, D. (1998). Eating disorders and insulin-dependent diabetes mellitus. *Psychosomatics*, vol. 39, pp. 233-243.

Daneman, D., Olmsted, M., Rydall, A., Maharaj, S., & Rodin, G. (1998). Eating disorders in young women with type 1 diabetes: prevalence problems and prevention. *Horm Res*, vol. 50, pp. 79-86.

Daneman, D., & Rodin, G. (1999). Eag disorders in young women with type 1 diabetes: a cause for concern? *Acta Paediatr*, vol. 88, pp. 117-119.

Davidson, M., Boland, EA., & Grey, M. (1997). Teaching teens to cope: coping skills training for adolescents with diabetes mellitus. *Journal Social Pediatric Nursery*, Vol. 2, pp.65-72.

DelGreco, L., Breitbach, L., Rumer, S, McCarthy, RH., & Suissa, S. (1986). Four-year results of a youth smoking prevention program using assertiveness training. *Adolescence*, Vol. 21, pp. 631–640.

De Mont-Marin, F., Hardy, P., Lepine, JP., Halfon, P., & Feline, A. (1995). Six-month and lifetime prevalences of psychiatric disorders in patients with diabetes mellitus. *European Psych*, vol.10, pp. 245-249.

DeRidder, D., & Schreus, K. (2001). Developing interventions for chronically ill patients: is coping a helpful concept?. *Clinical Psychology Review*, Vol. 2, pp. 205-240.

Deutsch, M., & Brickman, E. (1994). Conflict resolution. *Pediatric Review*, Vol. 15, pp. 16–22.

Diabetes Control and Complications Trial Research Group (DCCT) (1993). The effect of intensive treatment of diabetes on the development and progression of long-term complications in insulin-dependent diabetes mellitus. *N Engl J Med*, vol. 329, pp. 977-986.

Dion Kelly, S., Howe, CJ., Hendler, JP.,& Lipman, TH. (2005). Disordered eating behaviors in youth with type 1 diabetes. *The Diabetes Educator*, Vol. 31, pp. 572-583.

Duangdao, KM., & Roesch, SC. (2008). Coping with diabetes in adulthood: a meta-anlysis. *Journal of Behavior Medicine*, Vol. 31, pp. 291-300.

Eisenberg, L. (1991). Treating depression and anxiety in primary care. Closing the gap between knowledge and practice. *New England Journal of Medicine*, Vol. 326, pp. 1080-1084.

Engstrom, I., Kroon, M., Advirdsson, CG., Segnestam, K., Snellman, K., & Aman, J. (1999). Eating disorders in adolescent girls with insulin-dependent diabetes mellitus: a population- based case-control study. *Acta Paediatr*, vol. 88, pp. 117-119.

Fainburn, CG., & Beglin, SJ.(1990). Studies of the epidemiology of bulimia nervosa. *Am J Psychiatry*, vol. 147, pp. 401-408.

Fairburn, CG., Peveler, RC. (1991). Davies, B., Mann, JL., & Mayou, RA. Eating disorders in young adults with insulin dependent diabetes mellitus: a controlled study. *Br Med J*, vol. 303, pp. 17-20.

Fettahoglu, EC., Koparan, C., Özatalay, E., & Turkkahraman, D. (2007). The psychological difficulties in children and adolescents with insuline dependent diabetes mellitus. *Psych in Türkiye*, vol. 9, pp. 32-36.

Figueroa-Sobrero, A., Evangelista, P., Mazza, C., Basso, P., López, SM., Scaiola, E., Honfi, M., Ferraro, M., Eandi, ML., & Walz, F. (2010).Three-year follow up of metabolic control in adolescents with type 1 diabetes with and without eating disorders. *Arch Argent Pediatr*, vol. 108, pp. 130-135.

Folkman, S., & Lazarus, RS. (1980). An analysis of coping in a middle-aged community sample. *Journal of Health and Social Behavior*, Vol. 21, pp. 219-239.

Folkman, S., & Lazarus, RS. (1985). If it changes it must be a process: Study of emotion and coping during three stages of a college examination. *Journal of Personality and Social Psychology*, Vol. 48, pp. 150–170.

Folkman, S., & Lazarus, RS. (1988). Manual for the ways of coping questionnaire. Consulting Psychologist Press. Palo Alto (CA).

Forman, SG. (1993). Coping Skills Training for Children and Adolescents. Jossey-Bass. San Francisco, CA.

Friedman, S., Vila, G., Timsit, J., Boitard, C., & Mouren-Simeoni, MC. (1995). Troubles des conduits alimentaires et equilibre metabolique dans une population de jeunes adultes diabetiques insulino-dependants. *Ann Med-Psychol*, vol. 153, pp. 282-285.

García-Reyna, NI., Gussinyer, S., Raich, RM., Gussinyer, M., Tomás, J., & Carrascosa, A. (2004). Trastornos de la conducta alimentaria en adolescentes jóvenes con diabetes mellitas tipo 1. *Med Clin (Barc)*, vol. 122, pp. 690-692.

Goebel-Fabbri, AE., Franko, DL., Pearson, K., Anderson, BJ., & Weinger, K. (2008). Insulin restriction and associated morbidity and mortality in women with type 1 diabetes. *Diabetes Care*, vol. 31, pp. 415-419.

Goebel-Fabbri, AE. (2008). Diabetes and eating disorders. *J Diabetes Sci Technol*,vol. 2, pp. 530-532.

Goldstein, AP., Sprafkin, RP., Gershaw, NJ., & Klein, P. (1980). Skillstreaming the Adolescent: A Structured Learning Approach to Teaching Prosocial Skills. Research Press. Champaign.

Goldston, DB., Kovacs, M., Obrosky, DS., & Iyenger, S. (1995). A longitudinal study of life events and metabolic control among youths with insulin-dependent diabetes mellitus. *Health Psychology*, Vol. 14, pp. 409-414.

Grey, M., Boland, EA., Davidson, M., Yu, C., Sullivan-Bolyai, S., & Tamborlane, WV. (1998). Short-term effects of coping skills training as an adjunct to intensive therapy in adolescents. *Diabetes Care*, Vol. 21, pp. 902–908.

Grey, M., Boland, EA., Davidson, M., Yu, C., & Tamborlane, WV. (2000). Coping skills training for youth with diabetes mellitus has long-lasting effects on metabolic control and quality of life. *Journal of Pediatrics*, Vol.137, pp. 107–113.

Grey, M., & Berry, D. (2004). Coping skills training and problem solving in diabetes. *Current Diabetes Reports*, Vol. 4, pp. 126-131.

Gross, AM., Johnson, WC., Wildman, H., Mullett, N. (1982). Coping skills training with insulin-dependent pre-adolescent diabetics. *Child Behavior Therapy*, Vol. 3, pp. 141–153.

Gross, AM., Heiman, L., Shapiro, R., & Schultz, RM. (1983). Children with diabetes: social skills training and hemoglobin A1c levels. *Behavior Modification*, Vol. 7, pp. 151–165.

Gülseren, L., Hekimsoy, Z., Gülseren, S., Bodur, Z., & Kültür, S. (2001). Depression-anxiety, quality of life and disability in patients with diabetes mellitus. *Turkish J Psych*, Vol. 12, pp. 89-98.

Hains, AA., Davies, WH., Parton, E., & Silverman, AH. (2001). Brief report: a cognitive behavioral intervention for distressed adolescents with type I diabetes. *Journal of Pediatric Psychology*, Vol. 26, pp. 61–66.

Hasken, J., Kresl, L., Nydegger, T., & Temme, M. Diabulimia and the role of school health personnel (2010). *Journal of School Health*, Vol. 80, pp. 465-469.

Hoek, HW. (1993). Review of the epidemiological studies of eating disorders. *Int Rev Psychiatry*, vol. 5, pp. 61-74.

Hudson, JL., Wentworth, SM., Hudson, MS., & Pope, HG. (1985). Prevalence of anorexia nervosa and bulimia among young diabetic women. *J Clin Psychiatry*, vol. 46, pp. 88-93.

Johnson, SB., Pollack, R., Silverstein, J., Rosenbloom AL., Spillar R., McCallum M., & Harkavy J. (1982). Cognitive and behavioral knowledge about insulin-dependent diabetes among children and parents. *Pediatrics*, Vol. 69, pp. 708-713.

Jones, JM., Bennett, S., Olmsted, MP., Lawson, ML., & Rodin, G. (2001). Disodered eating attitudes and behaviours in teenaged girls: an Ontario school-based study. *Can Med Assoc J*, vol. 165, pp. 547-552.

Jones, JM., Lawson, ML., Daneman, D., Olmsted, MP., & Rodin, G.(2000). Eating disorders in adolescent females with and without type 1 diabetes: cross sectional study. *Br Med J*,vol. 320, pp. 1563-1566.

King, H., Aubert, RE., & Herman, WH. (1998). Global burden of diabetes, 1995–2025 – Prevalence, numerical estimates, and projections. *Diabetes Care*, vol. 21, pp. 1414-1431.

King, H., Gruber, W., & Lander, T. (1995). Implementing National Diabetes Programmes.Report of a WHO Meeting Geneva: World Health Organization Division of Non-communicable Diseases.

Koopmanschap, M. (2002). Coping with Type II diabetes: the patient's perspective. *Diabetologia*, vol.45, pp. S18-S22.

Kovacs, M., Goldston D., Obrosky, DS., & Iyenger, S. (1992). Prevalence and predictors of pervasive noncompliance with medical treatment among youths with insulin-dependent diabetes mellitus. *Journal of American Academy Childs and Adolescent Psychiatry*, Vol. 31, pp. 1112-1119.

Krakoff, DB. (1991). Eating disorders as a special problem for persons with insulin-dependent diabetes mellitus. Nurs *Clin North Am*, vol. 26, pp. 707-714.

Kumanyika, SK., Wilson, JF., & Guilford-Davenport, M. (1993). Weight-related attitudes and behaviors of black women. *J Am Diet Assoc*, vol. 93, pp. 416-422.

Lee, S. (1993). How abnormal is the desire for slimness? A survey of eating attitudes and behaviour among Chinese undergraduates in Hong Kong. *Psychol Med*, vol. 23, pp. 437-451.

Lee, AM., & Lee, S. (1996). Disordered eating and its psychosocial correlates among Chinese adolescent females in Hong Kong. *Int J Eating Disord*, vol. 20, pp. 177-183.

Lundman, B., & Norberg, A. (1993). Coping strategies in people with insulin-dependent diabetes mellitus. *Diabetic Education*, Vol. 19, pp.198-204.

Lustman, PJ., Clouse, RE., Griffith, LS., & Carney, RM. (1997). Screening for depression in diabetes using the Beck Depression Inventory. *Psychosomatic Medicine*, Vol. 59, pp. 24-31.

Llorente, MD., & Urrutia, V. (2006). Diabetes, psychiatric disorders, and the metabolic effects of antipsychotic medications. *Clin Diabetes*, vol. 24, pp. 18-26.

Lloyd, GG., Steel, JM., & Young, RJ. (1987). Eating disorders and psychiatric morbidity in patients with diabetes mellitus. *Psychother Psychosom*, vol. 48, pp. 189-195.

Maes, S., Leventhal, H., & DeRidder, D. (1996). Coping with chronic diseases. Handbook of coping. Wiley. New York.

Mannucci, E., Ricca, V., Mezzani, B., Di Bernardo, M., Piani, F., Vannini, R., Cabras, PL., & Rotella, CM. (1995). Eating attitudes and behavior in IDDM patients: a case controlled study. *Diabetes Care*, vol.18, pp. 1503-1504.

Mannucci, E., Rotella, F., Ricca, V., Moretti, S., Placidi, GF., & Rotella, CM. (2005). Eating disorders in patients with type 1 diabetes: A meta-analysis. *J Endocrinol Invest*, vol. 28, pp. 417-419.

Marcus, MD., Wing, RR., Jawad, A.,& Orchard, TJ. (1992). Eating disorders symptomatology in a registry-based sample of women with insulin-dependent diabetes mellitus. *Int J Eatting Disord*, vol.12, pp. 425-430.

Markowitz, JT., Butler, DA., Volkening, LK., Anitisdel, JE., Anderson, B., & Laffel, LMB. (2010). Brief screening tool for disordered eating in diabetes. *Diabetes Care*, Vol. 33, pp. 495-500.

Marlatt, GA., & Gordon, JR. (1985). Relapse Prevention: Maintenance Strategies in Addictive Behavior Change. The Guilford Press. New York, NY.

McDougal, J. (2002). Promoting normalization in families with preschool children with type 1 diabetes. *Journal of Specialty Pediatric Nursering*, Vol. 7, pp. 113–120.

Meltzer, LJ., Bennett Johnson, S., Prine, JM., Banks, RA., Desrosiers, PM., & Silverstein, JH. (2001). Disordered eating, body mass and glycaemia control in adolescents with type 1 diabetes. *Diabetes Care*, vol. 24, pp.678-682.

Nansel, TR., Anderson, BJ., Laffel, LM., Simons-Morton, BG., Weissberg-Benchell, J., Wysocki, T., Iannotti, RJ., Holmbeck ,GN., Hood, KK., & Lochrie, AS. (2009). A multisite trial of a clinic-integrated intervention for promoting family management of pediatric type 1 diabetes: feasibility and design. *Pediatr Diabetes*, vol. 10, pp.105-115.

National Centre for Health Statistics. 2011. USA Government.

Neumark-Sztainer, D., Patterson, J., Mellin, A., Ackard, DM., Utter, J., Story, M., & Sockalosky, J. (2002). Weight control practices and disordered eating behaviors among adolescent females and males with type 1 diabetes: associations with sociodemographics, weight concerns, familial factors, and metabolic outcomes. *Diabetes Care*, vol.25, pp.1289-1296.

Neumark-Sztainer, D., Story, M., Falkner, NH., Beuhring, T., & Resnick, M. (1998). Disordered eating among adolescents with chronic illness and disability. *Arch Pediatr Adolesc Med*, vol. 152, pp.871-878.

Neumark-Sztainer, D., Story, M., Resnick, M., Garwick, A., & Blum, R. (1995). Body dissatisfaction and unhealthy weight-control practices among adolescents with and without chronic illness: a population-based study. *Arch Pediatr Adolesc Med*, vol. 149, pp.1330-1335.

Nielsen, S., Borner, H., & Kabal, M. (1987). Anorexia nervosa/ bulimia in diabetes mellitus: a review and presentation of 5 cases. *Acta Psychiatr Scand*, vol.75, pp.464-473.

Olmsted, MP., Coton, PA., Daneman, D., Rydall, AC., & Rodin, GM. (2008). Prediction of the onset of disturbed eating behavior in adolescent girls with type 1 diabetes. *Diabetes Care*, Vol. 31, pp. 1978-1982.

Peveler, RC., Bryden, KS., Neil, HAW., Fairburn, CG., Mayou, RA., Dunger, DB., & Turner, HM. (2005). The relationship of disordered eating habits and attitudes to clinical outcomes in young adult females with type 1 diabetes. *Diabetes Care*, vol. 28, pp.84-88.

Peveler, RC., & Fairburn, CG. (1999). Anorexia nervosa in association with diabetes mellitus: a cognitive-behavioural approach to treatment. *Behav Res Ther*, vol.27, pp.95-99.

Peveler, RC., & Fairburn, CG. (1992). The treatment of bulimia nervosa in patients with diabetes mellitus. *Int J Eating Disord*, vol.11, pp.45-53.

Peveler, RC., Fairburn, CG., Boller, I., & Dunger, DB. (1992). Eating disorders in adolescents with IDDM: a controlled study. *Diabetes Care*, vol. 15, pp.1356-1360.

Polivy, J., & Herman, CP. (1985). Dieting and binging: a casual analysis. *Am Psychol*, vol. 40, pp.193-201.

Polonsky, WH., Anderson, BJ., Lohrer, PA., Aponte, JE., Jacobson, AM., & Cole, CF. (1994). Insulin omission in women with IDDM. *Diabetes Care*, vol.17, pp.1178-1185.

Pollock, M., Kovacs, M., & Charron-Prochownik, D. (Eating disorders and maladaptive dietary/insulin management among youths with childhood-onset insulin-dependent diabetes mellitus

Powers, PS., Malone, JL., Coovert, DL., & Schulman, RG. (1990). Insulin-dependent diabetes mellitus and eating disorders: a prevalence study. *Compr Psychiatry*, vol.31, pp.205-210.

Robertson, P., & Rosenvinge, JH. (1990). Insulin-dependent diabetes mellitus: a risk factor in anorexia nervosa or bulimia nervosa? An empirical study of 116 women. *J Psychosom Res*, vol. 34, pp.535-541.

Ramirez, LC., Rosenstock, J., Strowig, S., Cercone, S., & Raskin P. (1990). Effective treatment of bulimia with fluoxetine, a serotonin reuptake inhibitor in patient with type 1 diabetes mellitus. *Am J Med*, vol. 88, pp. 540-541.

Rodin, G., Craven, J., Littlefield, C., Goldbloom, D., & Daneman, D. (1989). Insulin misuse through omission or reduction of dose. Psychosomatics, vol.30, pp.465-466.

Rodin, G., Craven, J., Littlefield, C., Murray, M., & Daneman, D. (1991). Eating disorders and intentional insulin undertreatment in adolescent females with diabetes. *Psychosomatics*, vol.32, pp.171-176.

Rodin, G., & Daneman, D. (1992). Eating disorders and IDDM: a problematic association. *Diabetes Care*, vol.15, pp.1402-1412.

Rodin, GM., Daneman, D., Johnson, LE., Kenshole, A., & Garfinkel, P. (1985). Anorexia nervosa and bulimia in female adolescents with insulin dependent diabetes mellitus: a systematic study. *J Psychiatr Res*, vol. 19, pp.381-384.

Rodin, GM., Johnson, LE., Garfinkel, P., Daneman, D., & Kenshole, A. (1986/1987). Eating disorders in female adolescents with insulin dependent diabetes mellitus. *Int J Psychiatry Med*, vol.16, pp. 49-57.

Rodin, GM., Olmsted, MP., Rydall, AC., Maharaj, SI., Colton, PA., Jones, JM., Biancucci, LA., & Daneman, D. (2002). Eating disorders in young women with type 1 diabetes mellitus. *J Psychosom Res*, vol. 53, pp.943-949.

Rosen, DS. (2003). Eating disorders in children and young adolescents: etiology, classification, clinical features and treatment. *Adolesc Med*, vol.14, pp. 49-59.

Rosmark, B., Berne, C., Holmgrem, S., Lago, C., Renholm, G., & Sohlberg, S. (1986). Eating disorders in patients with insulin-dependent diabetes mellitus. *J Clin Psychiatry*, vol. 47, pp.547-550.

Rubin. RR., & Payrot, M. (2001). Psychological Issues and Treatments for People with Diabetes. *Journal of Clinical Psychology*, vol. 57, pp.457-462.

Russell-Jones, D., & Khan, R. (2007). Insulin-assosociated weight gain in diabetes-causes, effects and coping strategies. *Diabetes Obesity & Metabolism*, Vol. 9, pp. 799-812.

Ruth-Sahd, LA., Schneider, M., & Haagen, B. (2009). Diabulimia: what it is and how to recognize it in critical care. *Dimens Crit Care Nurs*, vol. 28, pp. 147-153.

Ryan, M., Gallanagh, J., Livingstone, MB., Gaillard, C., & Ritz P. (2008). The prevalence of abnormal eating behaviour in a representative sample of the French diabetic population. *Diabetes & Metabolism*, vol. 34, pp.581-586.

Rydall, AC., Rodin, GM., Olmsted, MP., Devenyi, RG., & Daneman, D. (1997). Disordered eating behavior and microvascular complications in young women with insulin-dependent diabetes mellitus. *N Engl J Med*, vol.336, pp.1849-1854.

Smari, J., & Valtysdottir, H. (1997). Dispositional coping, psychological distress, and disease-control in diabetes. *Personality and Individual Differences*, Vol. 22, pp. 151–156.

Stancin, T., Link, DL., & Reuter, JM. (1989). Binge eating and purging in young women with IDDM. *Diabetes Care*, vol. 12, pp.601-603.

Stanton, AL., Collins, CA., & Sworowski, LA. (2001). Adjustment to chronic illness: Theory and research. In: *Handbook of health psychology*, Baum A, Revenon TA & Singer JS, pp. 387-403, Mahway NK, Erlbaum.

Steel, JM., Young, RJ., Lloyd, GG., & Clarke, BF. (1987). Clinically apparent eating disorders in young diabetic women: associations with painful neuropathy and other complications. *Br Med J*, vol. 294, pp.859-862.

Stewart, TM., Williamson, DA., & White, MA. (2002). Rigid vs. flexible dieting: association with eating disorder symptoms in nonobese women. *Appetite*, vol. 38, pp. 39-40.

Striegel-Moore, RH., Nicholson, TJ., & Tamborlane, WV. (1992). Prevalence of eating disorder symptoms in preadolescent and adolescent girls with IDDM. *Diabetes Care*, vol. 15, pp.1361-1368.

Trento, M., Borgo, E., Kucich, C., Passera, P., Trinetta, A., Charrier, L., Cavallo, F., & Porta, M. (2009). Quality of life , coping ability, and metabolic control in patients with type 1 diabetes managed by group care and a carbohydrate counting program. *Diabetes Care*, Vol. 32, pp. e134.

Tuncay, T., Musabak, I., Engin Gok, D., & Kutlu, M. (2008). The relationship between anxiety, coping strategies and characteristics of patients with diabetes. *Health and Quality of Life Outcomes*, Vol. 6, pp. 79-88.

UKPDS Group (1998). Intensive blood-glucose control with sulphonylureas or insulin compared with conventional treatment and risk of complications in patients with type 2 diabetes. *Lancet*, Vol. 352, pp. 837–843.

Vila, G., Nollet-Clemencon, C., Vera, L., Crosnier, H., Robert, JJ., & Mouren-Simeoni, MC. (1993). Etude des troubles des conduits alimentaires dans une population d`adolescents souffrant de diabete insulino-dependant. *Can J Psychiatry*, vol.38, pp. 606-610.

Vila, G., Robert, JJ., Nollet-Clemencon, C., Vera, L., Crosnier, H., Rault, G., Jos, J., & Mouren-Simeoni, MC. (1995). Eating and emotional disorders in adolescent obese girls with insulin-dependent diabetes mellitus. *Eur Child Adolesc Psychiatry*, vol. 4, pp. 270-279.

Walker, JD., Young, RJ., Little, J., & Steel, JM. (2002). Mortality in concurrent type 1 diabetes and anorexia nervosa. *Diabetes Care*, Vol. 25, pp. 1664-1665.

Walsh, JME., Wheat, ME., & Freund, K. (2000). Detection, evaluation and treatment of eating disorders: the role of the primary care physician. *J Gen Intern Med*, vol.15, pp.577-590.

Ward, A., Troop, N., Cachia, M., Watkins, P., & Treasure, J. (1995). Doubly disabled: diabetes in combination with an eating disorder. *Postgrad Med J*, vol. 71, pp.546-550.

Wing, RR., Nowalk, MP., Marcus, MD., Koeske, R., & Finegold, D. (1986). Subclinical eating disorders and glycaemia control in adolescents with type 1 diabetes. *Diabetes Care*, vol. 9, pp.162-167.

White, NE., Richter, JM., & Fry, C. (1992). Coping, social support and adaptation to chronic illness. *Western Journal of Nursing Research*, Vol. 14, pp. 211–224.

Wysocki, T., Greco, P., Harris, MA., Bubb, J., & White, NH. (2001). Behavior therapy for families of adolescents with diabetes: maintenance of treatment effects. *Diabetes Care*, Vol. 24, pp. 441–446.

Wysocki, T., Harris, MA., Greco, P., Bubb, J., Danda, CE., Harvey, LM., McDonell, K., Taylor, A., & White, NH. (2000). Randomized controlled trial of behavior therapy for families of adolescents with insulin-dependent diabetes mellitus. *Journal of Pediatric Psychology*, Vol. 25, pp. 23–33.

8

Contributing Factors to Poor Adherence and Glycemic Control in Pediatric Type 1 Diabetes: Facilitating a Move Toward Telehealth

Joseph P. H. McNamara[1], Adam M. Reid[2], Alana R. Freedland[3],
Sarah E. Righi[1] and Gary R. Geffken[1]
[1]*University of Florida, Department of Psychiatry*
[2]*University of Florida, Department of Clinical and Health Psychology*
[3]*University of Florida, Department of Counselor Education*
USA

1. Introduction

The study of family's with children with T1D and their regimens has led to a burgeoning literature by psychologist's with an interest in the relationship between adherence and glycemic control. Research in pediatric or child health psychology may be described as focusing on studying behavioral health, or psychological factors including learning, development, psychopathology, and culture as they interact with biological and physiological factors involved with illness, and in many cases, chronic illnesses. T1D is a chronic illness where an increasingly complex medical regimen for the child's illness interacts with the child's family, their school, their peers, and their culture. T1D is a chronic illness where the research of child health psychologists and other health care professionals can be seen as providing a prototype or model of other chronic illness of childhood that have a lower prevalence, and hence have a literature that is comparatively less developed than that of T1D.

2. The challenges of type 1 diabetes

Type 1 Diabetes (T1D) is a complex and challenging disease for children and adolescents due to the necessary integration of daily medical tasks (e.g., blood glucose monitoring) and lifestyle modifications. Evidence suggests that a substantial percentage of children are non-adherent to these demands.[1,2] Although some of those who are non-adherent experience few negative consequences, a large number of non-adherent children are at risk for significant medical complications including diabetic ketoacidosis (DKA), neuropathy, nephropathy, retinopathy, and cardiovascular disease.[3] Despite improvements in fluid and insulin therapy, fatality rates are still estimated at 1 to 2% of youth who experience a DKA episode. Non-adherence can also negatively impact clinical decisions made by health care providers such as prescribing incorrect insulin doses. Further, poor adherence results in increased morbidity and mortality, as well as problematic medication use and excessive use of health care services.[4,5] Numerous factors have a significant impact on adherence and glycemic control.

3. Family and psychological factors influencing adherence and glycemic control

Research suggests that family factors have a large impact on adherence and glycemic control in populations with pediatric T1D. Young children's management of T1D is highly dependent on family factors due to their high reliance on parental care. Parenting style is an important variable to examine when measuring adherence and glycemic control. Davis and colleagues[6] found parental warmth was associated with better adherence among preschool through elementary aged children with T1D. Parental restrictiveness was associated with low glycemic control. Establishing good self-care habits at an early age is critical in the maintenance of T1D since young children diagnosed with T1D are more likely to experience longer disease duration.[7] Healthy habits, such as engagement in physical activity, are crucial for the management of T1D. Mackey and Streisand[8] found parental support of exercise activity to be related to higher rates of physical activity in youth with T1D. Support included encouragement and parent participation in the exercise activity. Healthy eating behaviors are also essential to the management of T1D. In a qualitative study examining the effects of family meals on youth with T1D, the authors found that family meals were important to the participants.[9] The participants found it easier to maintain healthy eating habits when they shared meals with their families. In contrast parental conflict, characterized by criticism of exercise activity, was negatively associated to rates of physical activity. This study implicates the importance of including family-focused strategies in nutritional interventions.

While diet and exercise are important for the management of T1D, new technologies such as continuous subcutaneous insulin infusion (CSII) or the insulin pump have made their way into diabetic management. Evidence supports use of the insulin pump to improve quality of life and patients using the pump exhibit higher levels of glycemic control compared to patients on daily injections.[10] While the pump allows patients to achieve improved glycemic control, maintaining these results is difficult and often deteriorates over time.[11] According to Wiebe and colleagues,[12] low parental involvement was associated with lower pump duration. Parent involvement was lowest among older adolescents. The authors concluded that older adolescents' desire for independence might have affected parental involvement. Therefore it is important for clinicians to promote shared responsibility for pump management. Assessment of parental support prior to implementation of the insulin pump can provide clinicians with valuable information pertaining to the appropriateness of its use. The Diabetes Family Behavior Checklist (DFBC) is a common instrument used for the assessment of parental support for pediatric T1D.[13] Lewin and colleagues[14] found the measure to display high internal consistency and moderate to high convergent validity with other instruments measuring family behaviors related to diabetes, adherence, and glycemic control. The authors concluded that using both parent and child forms of the DFBC as well as administering these forms separately were important for the validity of the assessments.

In addition to parental support, authoritative parenting, classified by parental demand and responsiveness, has been associated with higher metabolic control and self-care in adolescents with T1D.[15] Authoritative mothering displayed the closest relationship to improved glycemic control and self-care. This could be explained by the mothers' higher involvement in care than the fathers in the study. Both maternal permissiveness and authoritarian parenting styles were associated with poorer diet adherence.[15] Similar to these findings, Lloyd and colleagues[16] found maternal empathy to be positively correlated

Contributing Factors to Poor Adherence and Glycemic Control in Pediatric Type 1 Diabetes: Facilitating a Move Toward Telehealth

143

with adherence and glycemic control in a sample of T1D adolescents. It is common for mothers to be more involved in the care giving process than their male counterparts, which can often lead to high levels of stress among mothers with children with T1D. In a study by Lewin, Storch, Silverstein, Baumeister, Strawser, and Geffken[17] illness-related stressors linked with a mother's caretaking role were highly correlated to a mother's stress and state anxiety. Parenting stress was positively correlated to child behavior problems. Similarly, Hilliard, Monaghan, Cogen, and Streisand[18] found that general anxiety and parenting stress were associated with parents' perceptions of their children's problematic behavior in children with T1D.

In addition to the management of T1D and behavioral problems, parenting stress has been related to initial diagnosis of the disorder. Streisand and colleagues[19] found that parents exhibited the highest levels of anxiety and depressive symptoms at the time of their child's diagnosis. These results implicate the importance of providing additional support and education to parents of newly diagnosed children as well as assessing for anxious and depressive symptoms. Parents are also at risk for developing chronic sorrow pertaining to the diagnosis of pediatric T1D. Results of a study examining chronic sorrow showed that parents exhibited a grief reaction upon initial diagnosis and continued to experience intermittent emotional distress.[20] The mothers in the study sample were more comfortable talking about their grief than fathers, however, both mothers and fathers displayed evidence of chronic sorrow. With growing evidence supporting the positive association between parenting stress and other issues related to T1D, recent interventions have been created to focus specifically on these issues among parents of children with the disorder. In a study by Monaghan, Hilliard, Cogen, and Streisand,[21] the authors assessed the efficacy and practicality of a telephone-based intervention designed for parents of children with T1D. The intervention aimed to improve parental quality of life by decreasing parenting stress, increasing social support and improving the management of pediatric T1D. The subjects scored lower on parenting stress and higher on social supportpost-intervention. This evidence suggests the utility of interventions with families coping with T1D. The Pediatric Inventory for Parents has been proven to be an effective instrument for measuring parenting stress in mothers of children with T1D.[14] The instrument displayed internal consistency reliability and validity for this population.

Current research suggests that family conflict may also have a negative impact on the management of pediatric T1D. In a study examining youth and adolescents with T1D, perception of family conflict was the highest predictor of medical adherence.[22] Perception of family cohesion predicted improved adherence. Parent-child conflict has also been linked to poor adherence as well as poor metabolic control in children with T1D.[23] Similarly, Williams, Laffel, and Hood[24] found a positive relationship between psychological distress and diabetes-specific conflict in pediatric T1D. The results of these studies indicate the importance of family cohesion for better management of pediatric T1D. According to the findings of Harris, Freeman, and Beers[25] Behavioral Family Systems Therapy (BFST) produced an improvement in mother-adolescent conflict related to diabetes specific issues as well as an improvement in general parent-adolescent conflict.

Given the impact of family cohesion on diabetes management, it is no surprise that spousal support is also an important factor in the examination of adherence and glycemic control in children with T1D. Marital conflict has been shown to influence the link between mother-adolescent relationships and adherence. Lewandowski and Drotar[26] found that higher levels of perceived spousal support were associated with lower mother-adolescent conflict and higher medical adherence of adolescents with T1D. Single-parent households have been associated with lower adherence.[27] In a study on family dynamics in adolescents with T1D, the authors found that divorced, separated and single-parent families appeared to pose the highest risk to poor glycemic control among this population.[28] The study also showed that parent-child agreement on blood glucose monitoring responsibility was related to more frequent monitoring. The results from this study provide support for interventions aimed at facilitating the transition from parental responsibility to adolescent responsibility of metabolic management. Clinicians should be aware of these implications when assessing for diabetes management. The Diabetes Family Conflict Scale is a clinical tool that is used to measure negative emotions surrounding blood glucose monitoring, quality of life and perceived parental burden caused by the management of diabetes.[29] This measure is the most commonly used assessment for measuring diabetes-related family conflict. Hood, Butler, Anderson, and Laffel[30] revised the scale to include updated technology and language pertaining to diabetes management. The revised scale has high construct validity, predictive validity and internal consistency.

Similar to the aforementioned family factors, several child behavioral patterns also contribute to poor adherence and glycemic control. How a child behaves is one of the most important predictors of a multitude of important outcomes, including academic success,[31] social acceptance,[32] and development of psychological problems.[33] Two of these psychological problems are externalizing and internalizing behaviors, which are two of the biggest broad spectrum behavioral classification terms used in psychological literature since its popularization with the work of Achenbach.[34] Externalizing problems, problems that are manifested in outward behavior and reflect a child's negative reactions to his or her environment, and internalizing problems, behaviors in which youth direct feelings and emotions inward, are predictive of numerous behavioral outcomes, especially adherence and glycemic control within the pediatric diabetes literature.[35][36]

Externalizing symptoms have been found to relate to a poorer prognosis for youth with diabetes.[37] This likely can be explained by the poor adherence and glycemic control in these youth with diabetes.[38][39][40] Children with externalizing problems, such as oppositional or aggressive behaviors, likely fail to listen to their parents when told to take their insulin injection or maintain an appropriate diet regimen, as evidenced by Duke & colleagues[41] who conducted a study on 120 youth with diabetes and found that adherence mediated the relationship between externalizing behaviors and low HbA$_{1c}$ levels. Attention deficit-hyperactivity disorder, a common externalizing disorder, has received little attention in the pediatric diabetes literature. One case study of two children with co-morbid ADHD and diabetes found that standard behavioral treatment for ADHD significantly reduce problems with adherence to the diabetes treatment regimen.[41][42] Emerging research investigating improvements in adherence and glycemic control as the result of treatments tailored solely toward addressing co-morbid internalizing disorders, such as depression or generalized anxiety disorder, reveal similar results.[42][43] Keeping in mind the clear inhibiting role of externalizing and internalizing problems (highlighted below) on adherence, and the importance of adherence in glycemic regulation, future treatment plans for youth with T1D should incorporate concurrent psychological therapy.

Parent reported internalizing disorders are believed to be present in approximately 28% of individuals with diabetes[44][45] and, similar to externalizing disorders, co-morbid presenting internalizing disorders have been associated with a worse prognosis in youth with T1D.[46] As suggested by empirical findings both cross sectionally and longitudinally,[47][36][35][46] one reason for this worse prognosis likely stems from poorer adherence and glycemic control as a result of the internalizing symptoms. For example, a youth with depression may struggle to adhere to the recommendations of their primary care physician due to a lack of motivation, feelings of helplessness, and decreased energy. Indeed, research has shown that depressed individuals do often engage in less self-care and health promoting activities.[48] It has been proposed that a bidirectional relationship may exist between depression and glycemic control, implying that lower glycemic control may lead to increased dysphoria while dysphoria may in turn lead to worse adherence which causes poorer glycemic management.[49]

These children who struggle to adhere to their doctor's recommendations and manage their diabetes properly will continue to experience the multiple health-related issues associated with diabetes, as well as put themselves at risk for more serious health problems as they get older, such as coronary heart disease.[50] Clearly, externalizing and internalizing disorders can have a crippling effect on adherence and glycemic control in diabetic youth, yet, the standard approach to treatment fails to address these internalizing and externalizing problems. A new approach which could circumvent some of the barriers to treatment caused by these internalizing and externalizing symptoms, such as poor self-care, lack of motivation, and avoidance behaviors would likely improve the poor prognosis of these youth with type 1 diabetes. An example of addressing these treatment barriers would be incorporating motivational interviewing, a therapeutic approach aimed at increasing motivation and self-esteem, that has been found to improve glycemic control in youth with diabetes.[51]

The role of depression in causing poorer adherence and glycemic control can be explained further when examining the role of peer victimization in this relationship. Peer victimization, as used in the psychological literature, can be overt forms (such as physical and verbal assault) and/or relational forms (social ostracism),[52] and both kinds of peer victimization are higher in several clinical pediatric populations, such as in youth with learning disorders,[53] obesity,[54] endocrine disorders,[55] inflammatory bowel disease,[56] etc. While little research has been conducted on peer victimization in a population of youth with diabetes, some recent studies have replicated the previous results with other chronic health conditions, finding that youth with diabetes have higher rates of relational peer victimization than their peers without diabetes.[57] Further, the importance of investigating the impact of victimization in diabetes is highlighted by Storch & colleagues[57] further findings that, within the sample of youth with diabetes, children who had higher rates of peer victimization were more likely to be depressed, lonely, and socially anxious. As discussed earlier, research in the past few years has began to identify depression as a driving mechanism of the link between peer victimization and poor adherence and glycemic control. Research by Storch & colleagues[58] found that depression partially mediated the relationship between peer victimization and diabetes self-management, or simply put that peer victimized, youth with diabetes manage their diabetes worse as they endorse higher levels of depression. Specifically related to their self-management, this study found that the more the youth were victimized by their peers, the worse HbA1c, adherence to glucose testing, and dietary management. While these findings are certainly preliminary, they do have important clinical implications. Forth most, clinicians treating pediatric diabetes need to be aware that they are working with an at risk population for peer victimization. Assessment procedures for peer victimization should be implemented in order to develop a better understanding of a probable cause for any presenting depression related issues with the child or adolescent.

Higher cognitive functions that underlie problem solving abilities, specifically executive functioning, has been found to be more developed in youth who are better at forseeing long term consequences.[59] Thus it is no surprise that higher executive functioning is associated with adherence to the diabetes regimen.[60] In other words, children who are better at measuring the risks of not monitoring there glucose intake, carrying around snacks or other recommendations of their doctor are more likely to adhere to their diabetes regimen. Recent research has identified that children with higher executive functioning are better at problem solving, planning, organization, and working memory and that all of these derivatives of executive functioning have been associated with adherence, which in turn was associated with higher glycemic control.[61][62] It is important for clinicians to be aware of youth's deficits in executive functioning and understand the value in discussing problem solving techniques with the children, which likely could improve overall diabetes management.[63] Future research in pediatric diabetes should investigate possible paradigms that could improve aspects of a child's problem solving abilities related to diabetes in a clinically feasible manner.

Other research has suggested that executive functioning may relate less to adherence in younger youth with diabetes,[63] but this may result from the increased involvement from parents in younger children, which improves glycemic control,[64][65] and therefore future research should investigate the relationship between parental executive functioning and younger children's glycemic control. Parents do play an obviously beneficial role in how a youth manages their diabetes, such as monitoring their adherence to treatment recommendations,[66] however, parents can also negatively impact their child's prognosis as the result of parental accommodation. Parental accommodation relates to parents giving in to their youth's resistance to beneficial treatment recommendations or treatment procedures in order to lower their child's anxiety, increase mood, or just as a result of the parent's poor insight into the necessity of the procedure.

Parental accommodation has received little attention in the diabetes literature, but is well researched in other pediatric populations, specifically related to the treatment of anxiety disorders.[67] This literature discusses how parents can create a barrier to the treatment of pediatric anxiety disorders by facilitating avoidance of anxiety provoking stimuli, such as a spider or germs, so that their child does not become anxious, even though this serves to reinforce the maladaptive anxiety. Research on parental accommodation is beginning to identify a similar predicament in pediatric diabetes populations. Simply put, parents are the frontline caregivers for their youth with diabetes.[68] They generally are responsible for preparing insulin injections or controlling the blood glucose levels consumed in their youth's diet. All too often however, parents are poorly educated on their child's diabetes regimen, which leads to poor HbA$_{1C}$ levels,[69] or the youth may be resistant to their parents enforcement of the treatment recommendations. If the latter is the case, parents who accommodate to their youths resistance (e.g. allowing youth to not adhere to their diet, not routinely check their urine for ketones, etc.) and utilize permissive parenting styles are more likely to have youth with worse glycemic control than parents who are more strict and encourage mature decision making in relation to diabetes management (authoritative parenting style).[70] Thus, emerging research on diabetes underlines the importance of educating parents on the management of their child's diabetes and suggests that certain parenting approaches, specifically ones which allow for youth to take charge of their diabetes management but also sets strict boundaries about what is expected (such as mandatory daily checking of glucose levels, maintaining dietary restrictions, etc.) results in better adherence and improved glycemic control in youth with type 1 diabetes. Additionally, a child's adherence to their diabetes regimen is a product of the tools they use to monitor glucose and administer insulin.

4. New technology influencing adherence and glycemic control

Many aspects of medical care are undergoing a technological revolution; diabetes management is no exception. The advent of portable insulin pumps has had positive implications for youth with T1D mellitus in that this new technology simplifies diabetes management and allow for a more flexible lifestyle. Insulin pumps allow users to follow a less strict diet than non-pump users. Moreover, insulin pumps administer insulin more accurately than by hand thereby rendering individual insulin injections unnecessary and decreasing the incidence of severe hypoglycemia[71][72]

Compared to those administering multiple daily injections (MDI), youth using a continuous subcutaneous insulin infusion (CSII), more simply known as an insulin pump, have significantly lower A1C levels[73][73] and reduced daily insulin requirements.[74] Compared to MDI regimens, children using CSII experienced a significant reduction in their glycosylated hemoglobin level.[74] In addition to the positive effects of using a CSII, pumps are safe and well tolerated even among young children.[75][76]

The sensor-augmented insulin pump (SAP), a sophisticated tool, is an advancement in CSII technology that facilities the administration of insulin and monitors blood glucose. These insulin pumps represent a new era of diabetes management that simplifies the daily treatment regimens youth and their parents must follow. For instance, among youth using either a conventional insulin pump or SAP for a duration of six months to 3 years, SAP users' glycosylated hemoglobin level improved significantly more than that of conventional insulin pump users'.[77] In a study by Hirsch and colleagues,[78] SAP users had significantly decreased hypoglycemia and improved A1C levels as compared with conventional insulin pump users. As diabetes management becomes easier due to technological developments in insulin pump design, children and adolescents will become more likely to adhere to their diabetes regimens.

Technological devices in diabetes management are not the only promising tools for youth with Type 1 Diabetes. Carbohydrate counting is a simple and effective strategy that helps youth and their parents decide how much insulin to administer and can lead to an improvement in glycemic control. In a study by Mehta, Quinn, Volening, and Laffel[79] with children aged 4 through 12 found a relationship between parents who precisely counted the amount of carbohydrates consumed each day and lower A1C levels. Furthermore researchers found that it is feasible for children and their caregivers to accurately estimate the amount carbohydrates in food. In a study with 2530 children and children with diabetes, 73 percent were within 10-15 grams of the actual carbohydrate amount.[80] However, a study by Bishop and colleagues[81] found that in their sample of 48 adolescents aged 12 to 18, most youth could not accurately count carbohydrates. However they found that children who did successfully count carbohydrates had significantly lower A1C levels. As evidenced by the aforementioned studies, knowing how to accurately count carbohydrates is strongly associated with adherence to diabetes treatment.

Assessment of diabetes related knowledge is a means of understanding a patient's level of illness-specific knowledge as a necessary prerequisite of a youth's adherence to their diabetes regimen. The Diabetes Awareness and Reasoning Test (DART) is composed of 122 questions that effectively measures general diabetes knowledge, nutrition, diabetes care at school, hyperglycemia/hypoglycemia, insulin pump, problem solving, blood glucose testing, and sick days diabetes care. The DART was given to both children and their caregivers and A1C levels of each child were provided. It was shown that the children's insulin pump sub-score and children's parents total DART score significantly predicted A1C levels in that higher test scores predicted lower A1C levels.[82] The PedCarbQuiz is another questionnaire that was completed by adolescents or their caregivers and measures carbohydrate and insulin-dosing knowledge. Similar to the results of the study by Heidgerken and colleagues,[82] higher scores achieved by adolescent and their caregivers on the PedCarbQuiz[83] significantly correlated with lower A1C levels. The relationship between diabetes knowledge and A1C levels underlines the importance of diabetes management education in treatment adherence. New interventions are being developed to help enhance adherence and glycemic control.

5. Role of new interventions

Woolston and colleagues[84] stated the principles for new interventions should be family-focused with services provided in the home to enhance effectiveness. The team providing these services should be multidisciplinary in nature, in order to identify concerns from different perspectives that might benefit the family. This type of intervention should help the child and family achieve self-sufficiency and ultimately no longer require the in-home services.

An innovative approach to home-based intervention is through telehealth. Telehealth interventions permit diabetes educators and mental health providers trained in behavioral treatment of diabetes adherence to assist their patients in their home environment without contending with logistical challenges of scheduling face-to-face contact.[85][86] Telemedicine provides an immediate and efficient way for health care providers and their patients to communicate. This improved communication increases the timeliness of feedback, which makes treatment more efficient and responsive.[87]

In a review of how telehealth could be integrated into mental health care, Stamm[88] noted that one of the great strengths of telehealth is that it can overcome significant barriers to treatment, including economics and geography. These barriers are often identified in mental health, as patients report that they cannot keep their appointments because they cannot afford transportation, or because they do not have the flexibility in their job to leave work to attend sessions. Additionally, telehealth allows providers to increase their availability over a wider geographical area, since patients will no longer have to travel long distances to receive appropriate services.[89]

Two of the ways in which telehealth can be used has been used with patients with diabetes are home telemonitoring and telephone support.[90] Home telemonitoring can be further divided based on a timing distinction: real-time interaction or delayed.[92] Phone calls and videoconferencing fall into this category. Delayed telemonitoring involves data or information that is accessed by a provider after the patient initially sends the information. Telephone support is provided by the clinician but does not necessarily require electronic transmission of patient data.[92]

Video teleconferencing has been examined as a means of maintaining face-to-face contact between provider and patient. Stamm[89] noted that advances in technology are fueling improvements in the utility of these services. A review of the literature provided support for telehealth services in increasing the likelihood of therapy attendance with no loss in treatment benefits. Preliminary data suggests that this approach may be effective in increasing adherence to medical regimens, and can be used as a tool to support ongoing therapy. Piette and colleagues[91] designed an intervention where adult patients with diabetes received biweekly telephone calls from diabetes educators to discuss diabetes care. The educators were allowed to individualize the information provided to the specific needs of each patient. They found that their intervention improved glycemic control, and reduced diabetes-related symptoms.[90] Additionally, they found that this intervention reduced patient-reported depressive symptoms, improved self-efficacy with regard to diabetes care, and reduced the number of days spent in bed. These patients also reported greater satisfaction with the level of health care provided.[91]

Polisena and colleagues[92] metaanalysis on telehealth for diabetes found that telehealth had a positive impact on both the utilization of health services as well as glycemic control. In the 26 studies they examined, they consistently found significant benefits of home telemonitoring on glycemic control, reduced hospital visits, and shorter hospital stays. The results on telephone support in the metaanalysis by Polisena and colleagues[92] were less clear although some studies found increased patient satisfaction and reported improved quality of life. A possible reason for the inconsistent findings within the telephone support was the significant variability in the strategies used.[92]

A possible strategy to address this problem in youth with T1D would be implementing Behavioral Family Systems Therapy (BFST) through telehealth. BSFT has shown to improve family relationships and communication in families with children who have diabetes.[92][93] In addition, Wysocki and colleagues[95] found that BSFT led to improved treatment adherence and metabolic control.

BSFT includes numerous strategies to improve adherence.[95][96] More specifically, BSFT has 4 treatment strategies including problem solving, communication skills training, structural family therapy for role clarification, and cognitive restructuring. The first strategy is a structured approach to problem solving. As adolescence can be a period of increased conflict between parents and teens, the use conflict resolution skills to reduce family tension can be very therapeutic. The steps in the problem solving technique are: a) define the problem, b) set a goal, c) brainstorm ways to accomplish the chosen goal, d) evaluate the ideas, e) implement the plan, and f) revise the goal.[95][96]

The second strategy in BFST is communication skills training that focuses on improving communication between parents and adolescents around diabetes related tasks and adherence. Often parents and adolescents engage in negative communication patterns, particularly during times of conflict or when negotiating adherence strategies. The communication skills training component is designed to remediate negative communication patterns within the family. This can be an idiosyncratic component, which allows the therapist to tailor interventions to the specific needs of the families. The steps in communication skills are: a) feedback, b) instruction, c) modeling, and d) behavioral rehearsal.[95][96]

The third strategy in BSFT that is useful in improving adherence and glycemic control in families with youth with T1D is the use of structural family therapy to focus on defining roles within the family. Individuals may have ideas about the roles of each family member that have not been shared with other family members. Role confusion within the family can contribute to increased communication problems and conflict. Role clarification and explicit role negotiation within the family, as explicated in structural family therapy, can be used to reduce problems in the family that adversely impact adherence and glycemic control.[95][96]

The fourth strategy in BFST that can be used therapeutically to improve adherence and glycemic control in families with youth with T1D is cognitive restructuring. Cognitive restructing can used to address cognitive distortions and irrational thinking that can impair problem solving ability within the family. Cognitive distortion can contribute to the maintenance of maladaptive communication patterns and conflict between parents and adolescents, and thereby adversely impacting regimen adherence. Helping parents and adolescents to restructure or "soften" their strong unproductive belief patterns can facilitate more effective communication.[95][96]

Several studies conducted within the research program of Geffken and colleagues provide evidence for the effectiveness of telehealth family psychotherapy for youth with T1D. A case study[94] and case series[95] demonstrated decreased HbA1c in participants as well as improved family dynamics surrounding the diabetes regimen. An open trial of 27 adolescents[96] demonstrated a 0.7% reduction in HbA1c and no diabetes related hospitalizations in an at-risk sample of youth. Additionally, results from a controlled trial show improved metabolic control and family interactions.[97][98] Specifically, relative to those in the wait-list, families in immediate treatment had an average decrease in HbA1c of 1.32% and fewer disagreements around the diabetes regimen between parents and children ($p<.05$). Participants also showed improved adherence to their regimen at end of treatment ($p<.05$). After a one-month follow-up period, however, many participants did not maintain their treatment gains. Over one third had an increase of 0.6% or greater in HbA1c, suggesting that additional sessions would likely aid in maintaining treatment gains. Of the remaining youth, approximately one third maintained gains, while the remaining youth were unable to be reached for follow-up assessments. Although not systematically assessed, our non-study related interactions with these youth (i.e., consultations during their scheduled endocrinology visits) suggest that the overwhelming majority of these youth experienced partial or full relapses. Taken together, these studies demonstrate that intensive telehealth family psychological treatment using a BSFT model improves adherence to the medical regimen, glycemic control, and family dynamics.

According to Azar and Gabbay[87], telemedicine interventions have a wide range of variability. Some systems are more basic and focus phone, email or short message services to faciliatate communication between patients and their providers. In contrast other systems use complex web interfaces that can include home meter information as well as logs for diet and activitiy levels.[99] For example, Carelink, an insulin-pump monitoring system accessed online, significantly improved glycemic control equally among children in both rural and urban areas even though children in rural areas visited clinics less frequently. The Carelink system allowed children and their parents to upload and access information about their glucose levels, amount of insulin required each day, and informed patients of where their blood sugar levels were in comparison to their goal daily sugar level. If dose adjustments were necessary, the diabetes care provider emailed or called their patient to alert them of the change.[100]

6. Conclusions

This review of the literature demonstrates a wide variety of psychological variables may mediate the relationship between regimen adherence and glycemic control in the families of youth with T1D. These psychological variables range from parental warmth and support to coerciveness and conflict in the parent-child relationship. It was also demonstrated that a wide variety of childhood behavioral patterns such as internalizing and externalizing, behavioral self-regulation and executive functioning, and peer-victimization may have similar relationships with regimen adherence and glycemic control in youth with T1D. The role of diabetes knowledge and the importance of it's measurement are suggested. Finally the development of new technology in diabetes care and management have been reviewed. The value of newer telehealth technologies are highlighted towards the latter sections of the review. The review demonstrates that Telehealth, used via the telephone or internet, is a cost-effective, convenient way for patients and their healthcare providers to manage and communicate about their diabetes regimen. The work by Geffken and colleagues demonstrates that telehealth can particularly useful for service delivery with families with youth with T1D. Telehealth allows treatment for families with youth with T1D with considerable barriers to their diabetes management such as those who require complex treatments and more frequent consultation with their diabetes care provider than distance or funding will allow. This review provides evidence on the value and critical inclusion of behavioral health services and research for the treatment of families youth with T1D.

7. References

[1] M.A. Rapoff, & M.U. Barnard, "Compliance with pediatric medical regimens", *Patient compliance in medical practice and clinical trials.* New York: Raven Press, 73-98. 1991.

[2] M. Kovacs, D. Goldston, S. Obrosky, & S. Iyengar, "Prevalence and predictors of pervasive noncompliance with medical treatment among youths with insulin-dependent diabetes mellitus" *Journal of the American Academy of Child and Adolescent Psychiatry,* Vol. 31, pp. 1112-1119. 1992.

[3] Diabetes Control and Complications Research Group, "The effect of intensive treatment of diabetes on the development and progression of long-term complications in insulin-dependent diabetes mellitus", *New England Journal of Medicine,* Vol. 329, pp.977-986.1993.

[4] K.L. Lemanek, J. Kamps, & N.B. Chung, "Empirically supported treatments in pediatric psychology: Regimen adherence", *Journal of Pediatric Psychology,* Vol. 26, pp. 253-275. 2001.

[5] A.L.Quittner, D.L. Espelage, C. Ievers-Landis, & D. Drotar, "Measuring adherence to medical treatment in childhood chronic illness: Considering multiple methods and sources of information", *Journal of Clinical Psychology in Medical Settings,* Vol. 7, pp. 41-54. 2002.

[6] C. L. Davis, A. M. Delamater, K. H. Shaw, A.M. La Greca, M. S. Eidson, J. Perez-Rodriguez, & R. Nemery, "Parenting styles, regimen adherence, and glycemic control in 4- to 10-year-old children with diabetes", *Journal of Pediatric Psychology,* Vol. 26(2), pp. 123-129. 2001.

[7] Diabetes Control and Complications Trial Research Group, "Effect of intensive diabetes treatment on the development and progression of long-term complications in adolescents with insulin-dependent diabetes mellitus: Diabetes control and complications trial", *The Journal of Pediatrics,* Vol. 125(2), pp. 177-188. 1994.

[8] E. R. Mackey, & R. Streisand, "Brief report: The relationship of parental support and conflictto physical activity in preadolescents with type 1 diabetes", *Journal of Pediatric Psychology,*Vol. 33(10), pp. 1137-1141. 2008.

[9] A. J. Rovner, S. N. Mehta, D. L. Haynie, E. M. Robinson, H. J. Pound, D. A.Butler et al., "Perceived benefits, barriers, and strategies of family meals among children with type 1 diabetes mellitus and their parents: Focus-group findings", *Journal of the American Dietetic Association*, Vol. 110(9), pp. 1302-1306. 2010.

[10] J. R. Wood, E. C. Moreland, L. K. Volkening, B. M. Svoren, D. A. Butler, & L. M. B. Laffel, "Durability of insulin pump use in pediatric patients with type 1 diabetes", *Diabetes Care*, Vol. 29(11), pp. 2355-2360. 2006.

[11] I. Rabbone, A. Bobbio, K. Berger, M. Trada, C. Sacchetti, & F. Cerutti, "Age-related differences in metabolic response to continuous subcutaneous insulin infusion in pre-pubertal and pubertal children with type 1 diabetes mellitus", *Journal of Endocrinological Investigation*, Vol. 30(6), pp. 477-483. 2007.

[12] D. J. Wiebe, A. Croom, K. T. Fortenberry, J. Butner, J. Butler, M. T. Swinyard, et al., "Parental involvement buffers associations between pump duration and metabolic control among adolescents with type 1 diabetes", *Journal of Pediatric Psychology*, Vol. 35(10), pp.1152-1160. 2010.

[13] L. C. Schafer, K. D. McCaul, & R. E. Glasgow, "Supportive and nonsupportive family behaviors: Relationships to adherence and metabolic control in persons with type I diabetes", *Diabetes Care*, Vol. 9(2), pp. 179-185. 1986.

[14] A. B. Lewin, E. A. Storch, J. H. Silverstein, A. L. Baumeister, M. S. Strawser, & G. R. Geffken, "Validation of the pediatric inventory for parents in mothers of children with type 1 diabetes: An examination of parenting stress, anxiety, and childhood psychopathology", *Families, Systems, & Health*, Vol., 23(1), pp. 56-65. 2005.

[15] M. S., Greene, B., Mandleco, S. O. Roper, E. S. Marshall, & T. Dyches, "Metabolic control, self-care behaviors, and parenting in adolescents with type 1 diabetes: A correlational study", *The Diabetes Educator*, Vol. 36(2), pp. 326-336. (2010).

[16] S. M. Lloyd, M. Cantell, D. Pacaud, S. Crawford, & D. Dewey, "Brief report: Hope, perceived maternal empathy, medical regimen adherence, and glycemic control in adolescents with type 1 diabetes", *Journal of Pediatric Psychology*, Vol.34(9), pp. 1025-1029. 2009.

[17] A. B. Lewin, G. R. Geffken, A. D. Heidgerken, D. Duke, W. Novoa, L. B. Williams, & E.A. Storch, "The diabetes family behavior checklist: A psychometric evaluation", *Journal of Clinical Psychology in Medical Settings*, Vol. 12(4), pp. 315-322. 2005.

[18] M. E. Hilliard, M. Monaghan, F. R. Cogen, & R. Streisand, "Parent stress and child behaviour among young children with type 1 diabetes", *Child: Care, Health & Development*, Vol. 37(2), pp. 224-232. 2011.

[19] R. Streisand, E. R. Mackey, B. M. Elliot, L. Mednick, I. M. Slaughter, J. Turek, & A. Austin, "Parental anxiety and depression associated with caring for a child newly diagnosed with type 1 diabetes: Opportunities for education and counseling", *Patient Education & Counseling*, Vol. 73(2), pp. 333-338. 2008.

[20] S. Bowes, L. Lowes, J. Warner, & J. W. Gregory, "Chronic sorrow in parents of children with type 1 diabetes", *Journal of Advanced Nursing*,Vol. 65(5), 992-1000. 2009.

[21] M. Monaghan, M. E. Hilliard, F. R. Cogen, & R. Streisand, "Supporting parents of very young children with type 1 diabetes: Results from a pilot study", *Patient Education & Counseling*, Vol. 82(2), pp. 271-274. 2011.

[22] S. T. Hauser, A. M. Jacobson, P. Lavori, J. I. Wolfsdorf, R. D. Herskowitz, J. E. Milley, et al., "Adherence among children and adolescents with insulin-dependent diabetes

mellitus over a four-year longitudinal follow-up: II. immediate and long-term linkages with the family milieu", *Journal of Pediatric Psychology*, Vol. 15(4), pp. 527-542. 1990.

[23] S. Miller-Johnson, R. E. Emery, R. S. Marvin, W. Clarke, R. Lovinger, & M. Martin, "Parent-child relationships and the management of insulin-dependent diabetes mellitus", *Journal of Consulting and Clinical Psychology*, (1994). Vol. 62(3), pp. 603-610. 1994.

[24] L. B. Williams, L. M. B. Laffel, & K. K. Hood," Diabetes-specific family conflict and psychological distress in paediatric type 1 diabetes", *Diabetic Medicine*, Vol. 26(9), pp. 908-914. 2009.

[25] M. A. Harris, K. A. Freeman, & M. Beers, "Family therapy for adolescents with poorly controlled diabetes: Initial test of clinical significance", *Journal of Pediatric Psychology*, Vol. 34(10), pp. 1097-1107. 2009.

[26] A. Lewandowski, & D. Drotar, "The relationship between parent-reported social support and adherence to medical treatment in families of adolescents with type 1 diabetes", *Journal of Pediatric Psychology*, Vol. 32(4), pp. 427-436. 2007.

[27] K. M. Grabill, G. R. Geffken, D. Duke, A. Lewin, L. Williams, E. Storch, & J. Silverstein, "Family functioning and adherence in youth with type 1 diabetes: A latent growth model of glycemic control", *Children's Health Care*, Vol. 39(4), 279-295. 2010.

[28] F. J. Cameron, T. C. Skinner, C. E. de Beaufort, H. Hoey, P. G. F. Swift, H. Aanstoot, et al., "Are family factors universally related to metabolic outcomes in adolescents with Type 1 diabetes?", *Diabetic Medicine*, Vol. 25(4), pp. 463-468. 2008.

[29] D. Rubin Young-Hyman, & M. Peyrot "Parent-child responsibility and conflict in diabetes care", *Diabetes*, Vol.38:28. 1989.

[30] K. K. Hood, D. A. Butler, B. J. Anderson, & L. Laffel, "Updated and revised diabetes family conflict scale", *Diabetes Care*, Vol. 30(7), pp.1764-1769. 2007.

[31] D. Arnold, "Co-occurrence of externalizing behavior problems and emergent academic difficulties in young high-risk boys: A preliminary evaluation of patterns and mechanisms," *Journal of Applied Developmental Psychology*, Vol. 18, pp. 317-330, 1997.

[32] D. Schwartz, K.A. Dodge, G.S. Pettit, J.E. Bates, & The Conduct Problems Prevention Research Group, "Friendship as a moderating factor in the pathway between early harsh home environment and later victimization in the peer group," *Developmental Psychology*, Vol. 36, pp. 646-662, 1999.

[33] C.R. Petty, J.F. Rosenbaum, D.R. Hirshfeld-Becker, A. Henin, S. Hubley, S., LaCasse, et al., "The Child Behavior Checklist broad-band scales predict subsequent psychopathology: a 5-year follow-up," *Journal of Anxiety Disorders*, Vol. 22, pp. 532-539, 2008.

[34] T.M. Achenbach, "Integrative guide for the 1991 CBCL/4-18,YSR, and TRF profiles," Burlington: University of Vermont, Department of Psychiatry, 1991.

[35] D. M. Cohen, M. A., Lumley, S. Naar-King, T. Partridge, & N. Cakan, "Child behavior problems and family functioning as predictors of adherence and glycemic control in economically disadvantaged children with type 1 diabetes: A prospective study," *Journal of Pediatric Psychology*, Vol. 29, pp. 171-284, 2008.

[36] L. Greening, L. Stoppelbein, C. Konishi, S.S. Jordan, & G. Moll, "Child routines and youths' adherence to treatment for type 1 diabetes," Vol. 32, pp. 437-447, 2007.

[37] M. Kovacs, D. Charron-Prochownik, & D. S. Obrosky, " A longitudinal study of biomedical and psychosocial predictors of multiple hospitalizations among young people with insulin-dependent diabetes mellitus," *Diabetic Medicine*, Vol. 12, pp. 142-148, 1995.

[38] C.M. McDonnell, E.A. Northam, S.M. Donath, G.A. Werther, & F.J. Cameron, "Hyperglycemia and externalizing behavior in children with type 1 diabetes," *Diabetes Care, 30*, pp. 2211–2215, 2007.

[39] S. Naar-King, A. Idalski, D. Ellis, M. Frey, T. Templin, P.B. Cunningham, et al."Gender differences in adherence and metabolic control in urban youth with poorly controlled type 1 diabetes: The mediating role of mental health symptom," *Journal of Pediatric Psychology*, 31, pp. 793-802, 2005.

[40] D.K. Duke, G.R. Geffken, A.B. Lewin, L.B. Williams, E.A. Storch, & J.H. Silverstein, "Glycemic control in youth with type 1 diabetes: Family predictors and mediators," *Journal of Pediatric Psychology*, Vol. 33, 719-727, 2008.

[41] K. Gelfand, G. Geffken, A. Lewin, A. Heidgerken, M. Grove, T. Malasanos, et al, "An initial evaluation of the design of pediatric psychology consultation service with children with diabetes," *Journal of Child Health Care*, Vol. 8, pp.113-123, 2004.

[42] L. M. Sancheza, A.M. Chronisa & S.J. Hunter, "Improving Compliance With Diabetes Management in Young Adolescents With Attention-Deficit/Hyperactivity Disorder Using Behavior Therapy," *Cognitive and Behavioral Practice*, Vol. 13, pp. 134-145, 2006.

[43] S.M. Markowitz, J.S. Gonzalez, J.L. Wilkinson, & S.A. Safren, "A Review of Treating Depression in Diabetes: Emerging Findings," *Psychosomatics*, Vol. 15, pp. 1-18, 2011.

[44] R.M. Ghandour, M.D. Kogan, S.J. Blumberg, & D.F. Perry, "Prevalence and correlates of internalizing mental health symptoms among CSHCN," *Pediatrics*, Vol. 125, pp. e269-e277, 2010.

[45] P.J. Lustman & R. E. Clouse, "Depression in diabetic patients: the relationship between mood and glycemic control," *Journal of Diabetes Complications*, Vol. 19, pp. 113–122, 2005.

[46] M.M. Garrison, W.J. Katon, & L.P. Richardson. "The impact of psychiatric comorbidities on readmissions for diabetes in youth." *Diabetes Care*, Vol. 28, pp. 2150-2154, 2005.

[47] V. S. Helgeson, K. A. Reynolds, L. Siminerio, O. Escobar, & D. Becker, "Parent and adolescent distribution of responsibility for self-care: Links to health outcome." Journal of Pediatric Psychology, Vol. 33, pp. 497-508, 2008.

[48] A.M. La Greca & J.S. Skyler, "Psychological issues in IDDM; A multivariate framework," in *Stress, Coping, and Disease*, Erlbaum, 1991, pp. 169-109.

[49] P. J. Lustman, R.J. Anderson, K.E. Freedland, M. de Groot, R.M. Caney, & R.E. Clouse, "Depression and poor glycemic control: a meta-analytic review of the literature. *Diabetes Care*, Vol. 23, pp. 934-942, 2000.

[50] S. He, H. Cao, C.G.M. Magnusson, M. Eriksson-Berg, M. Mehrnaz, K. Schenck-Gustafsson, & M. Blombäck, "Are increased levels of von Willebrand factor in chronic coronary heart disease caused by decrease in von Willebrand factor cleaving protease activity? A study by immunoassay with antibody against intact bond," *Thrombosis Research*, Vol. 103, pp. 241–248, 2001.

[51] Channon, S. J., Huws-Thomas, M. V., Rollnick, S., Hood, K., Cannings-John, R. L., Rogers, C. et al., "A multicenter randomized controlled trial of motivational interviewing in teenagers with diabetes." *Diabetes Care*, Vol. 30, 1390–1395, 2007.

[52] N. R. Crick, & M. A. Bigbee, "Relational and overt forms of peer victimization: A multiinformant approach," *Journal of Consulting and Clinical Psychology*, Vol. 66, 337–347, 1998.

[53] A. Baumeister, E.A. Storch, & G.R. Geffken, "Peer victimization in children with learning disabilities," *Child and Adolescent Social Work Journal*, Vol. 25, pp.11-23, 2008.

[54] C.S. Lim, P.A. Graziano, D.M. Janicke, W.N. Gray, L.M. Ingerski, & J.H. Silverstein,"Peer Victimization and Depressive Symptoms in Obese Youth: The Role of Perceived Social Support Children's Health Care," *Children's Heath Care*, Vol. 40, pp. 1-15, 2011.

[55] E.A. Storch, A. Lewin, J.H. Silverstein, A.D. Heidgerken, M.S. Strawser, A. Baumeister, et al., "Social-psychological correlates of peer victimization in children with endocrine disorders," *The Journal of Pediatrics*, Vol. 145, pp. 784-789, 2004.

[56] D.M. Janicke, W.N. Gray, N.A. Kahhan, K.W. Follansbee Junger, K.K. Marciel, et al., "Brief Report: The Association Between Peer Victimization, Prosocial Support, and Treatment Adherence in Children and Adolescents with Inflammatory Bowel Disease," *Journal of Pediatric Psychology*, Vol. 34, pp. 769-773, 2009.

[57] E.A. Storch, A. Lewin, J. Silverstein, A. Heidgerken, M. Strawser, A. Baumeister, et al., "Peer victimization, and psychosocial adjustment in children with type 1 diabetes," *Clinical Pediatrics*, Vol. 43, pp. 467-471, 2004

[58] E.A. Storch, A. Heidgerken, G.R. Geffken, A. Lewin, V. Ohleyer, M. Freddo, et al., "Bullying, regimen self-management, and metabolic control in youth with type 1Diabetes," *Journal of Pediatrics*, Vol. 148, pp. 784-787, 2006.

[59] A. Bechara, A.R. Damasio, H. Damasio, & S.W. Anderson, "Insensitivity to future consequences following damage to human prefrontal cortex," *Cognition*, Vol. 50, pp. 7-15, 1994.

[60] D.M. Bagner, L.B. Williams, G.R. Geffken, J.H. Silverstein, & E.A. Storch, "Type 1 diabetes in youth: The relationship between adherence and executive functioning," *Children's Healthcare*, Vol. 36, pp.169-179, 2007.

[61] K. McNally, J. Rohan, J. Pendley, A. Delamater, & D. Drotar, "Executive functioning, treatment adherence, and glycemic control in children with Type 1 Diabetes," *Diabetes Care*, Vol. 33, pp. 1159–1162, 2010.

[62] L.B. Williams, "Executive functioning, parenting stress, and family factors as predictors of diabetes management in pediatric patients with type 1 diabetes using intensive insulin regimens," *University of Florida, 2008*.

[63] T. Wysocki, R. Iannotti, J. Weissberg-Benchell, K. Hood, L. Laffel, B.J. Anderson, et al., "Diabetes problem solving by youths with type 1 diabetes and their caregivers: Measurement, validation and longitudinal associations with glycemic control," *Journal of Pediatric Psychology*, Vol. 33, pp. 875-884, 2008.

[64] O. Hsin, A.M. La Greca, J.M. Valenzuela, C.T. Moine, & A.M. Delamater, "Adherence and glycemic control among Hispanic youth with type 1 diabetes: role of family involvement and acculturation," *Journal of Pediatric Psycholology*, Vol. 26, 2009.

[65] M. Grey, E. Boland, C. Yu, S. Sullivan-Bolyai, & W. Tamborlane, "Personal and family factors associated with quality of life in adolescents with diabetes." *Diabetes Care*, Vol. 21, pp. 909-914, 1998.

[66] D.A. Ellis, C.L. Podolski, M. Frey, S. Naar-King, B. Wang, & K. Moltz, "The role of parental monitoring in adolescent health outcomes: Impact on regimen adherence in youth with type 1 diabetes." *Journal of Pediatric Psychology*, Vol. 32, pp. 907-917, 2007.

[67] C. Suveg, T.L. Roblek, J. Robin, A. Krain, S. Schendbrand, & G.S. Ginsburg, "Parental involvement when conducting cognitive-behavioral therapy for children with anxiety disorders," *Journal of Cognitive Psychotherapy*, Vol. 20, pp. 287–301, 2006.

[68] M., Kovacs, T. L. Feinberg, S. Paulauskas, R. Finkelstein, M. Pollack, & M. Crouse-Novak, "Initial psychological responses of parents to the diagnosis of insulin-dependent diabetes mellitus in their children," *Diabetes Care*, Vol. 8. pp. 568–575, 1985.

[69] H. Tahirovic & A. Toromanovic, "Glycemic control in diabetic children: role of mother's knowledge and socioeconomic status," *European Journal of Pediatrics*, Vol. 169, pp. 961-964, 2010.

[70] M.S. Greene, B. Mandleco, S.O. Roper, E.S. Marshall & T. Dyches, "Metabolic control, self-care behaviors, and parenting in adolescents with type 1 diabetes: a correlational study," *Diabetes Education*, Vol. 36, pp. 326–336, 2010.

[71] American Diabetes Association, *Living with diabetes: Advantages of using an insulin Pump*, 2010.

[72] J. C. Pickup, & A. J. Sutton, "Severe hypoglycaemia and hypocaemic control in type 1 diabetes: Meta-analysis of multiple daily insulin injections compared with continuous subcutaneous insulin infusion", *Diabetic Medicine*, Vol. 25(7), pp. 765-774. 2008.

[73] C. A. Paris, G. Imperatore, G. Klingensmith, D. Petitti, B. Rodriguez, A. M. Anderson, et al., "Predictors of insulin regimens and impact on outcomes in youth with type 1 diabetes: The search for diabetes in youth study", *Journal of Pediatrics*, Vol. 155(2), pp. 183-189. 2009.

[74] E. Pankowska, M. Blazik, P. Dziechciarz, A. Szypowska, & H. Szajewska, "Continuous subcutaneous insulin infusion vs. multiple daily injections in children with type 1 diabetes: A systematic review and meta-analysis of randomized control trials", *Pediatric Diabetes*, Vol. 10(1), pp. 52-58. (2008).

[75] L. A. Fox, L. M. Buckloh, S. D. Smith, T. Wysocki, & N. Mauras, "A randomized controlled trial of insulin pump therapy in young children with type 1 diabetes", *Diabetes Care*, Vol. 28(6), pp. 1277-1281. 2005.

[76] J. N. Churchill, R. L. Ruppe, & A. Smaldone, "Use of continuous insulin infusion pumps in young children with type 1 diabetes: A systematic review", *Journal of Pediatric Health Care*, Vol. 23(3), pp.173-179. 2008.

[77] A. E. Scaramuzza, D. Iafusco, I. Rabbone, R. Bonfanti, F. Lombardo, R. Schiaffini, et al., "Use of integrated real-time continuous glucose monitoring/insulin pump system in children and adolescents with type 1 diabetes: A 3-year follow-up study", *Diabetes Technology & Therapeutics*, Vol. 13(2), pp. 99-103. 2011.

[78] I. B. Hirsch, J. Abelseth, B. W. Bode, J. S. Fischer, F. R. Kaufman, J.Mastrototaro, et al., "Sensor-augmented insulin pump therapy: Results of the first randomized treat-to-target study", *Diabetes Technology & Therapeutics*, Vol. 10(5), pp. 377-383. 2008.

[79] S. N. Mehta, N. Quinn, L. K. Volkening, & M. B. Laffel, "Impact of carbohydrate counting on glycemic control in children with type 1 diabetes", *Diabetes Care*, Vol. 32(6), 1014-1016. 2009.

[80] C. E. Smart, K. Ross, J. A. Edge, B. R. King, P. McElduff, & C. E. Collins, "Can children with type 1 diabetes and their caregivers estimate the carbohydrate content of meals and snacks?", *Diabetic Medicine*, (2010). (2010). Vol. 27(3), pp. 348-353. 2010.

[81] F. K. Bishop, D. M. Maahs, G. Spiegel, D. Owen, G. J. Klingensmith, A. Bortsov, et al., "The carbohydrate counting in adolescents with type 1 diabetes (CCAT) study", *Diabetes Spectrum*, Vol. 22(1), pp. 56-62. 2009.

[82] A. D. Heidgerken, L. Merlo, L. B. Williams, A. B. Lewin, K. Gelfand, T. Malasanos, et al., "Diabetes awareness and reasoning test: A preliminary analysis of development and psychometrics", *Children's Health Care*, Vol. 36(2), pp. 117-136. 2007.

[83] M. B. Koontz, L. Cuttler, M. R. Palmert, M. O'Riordan, E. A. Borawski, J. McConnell, & E. O. Kern, "Development of validation of a questionnaire to assess carbohydrate and insulin-dosing knowledge in youth with type 1 diabetes", *Diabetes Care*, Vol. 33(3), pp. 457-462. 2010.

[84] J.L. Woolston, S.J. Berkowitz, M.C. Schaefer, & , J.A. Adnopoz, "Intensive, integrated, in-home psychiatric services: The catalyst to enhancing outpatient intervention", *Child and Adolescent Psychiatric Clinics of North America*, Vol. 7, 615-633. 1998.

[85] E. A. Balas, F. Jaffrey, G. J. Kuperman, S. A. Boren, G. D. Brown, F. Pinciroli, & J. A. Mitchell, "Electronic communication with patients: Evaluation of distance medicine technology", *Journal of the American Medical Association*, Vol. 278, pp. 152-159. 1997.

[86] D. C. Klonoff, "Diabetes and telemedicine: Is the technology sound, effective, cost effective,and practical?", *Diabetes Care,*Vol. 26, pp. 1626-1628. 2003.

[87] M. Azar, & R. Gabbay, "Web-based management of diabetes through glucose uploads: Has the time come for telemedicine?" *Diabetes Research and Clinical Practice, Vol. 83*, pp. 9-17. 2009.

[88] B. H. Stamm, "Integrating telehealth into mental health care", *In T. L. Jackson (Ed.), Innovations in clinical practice: A source book*, Vol. 18. pp. 385-400.2000.

[89] N. Holt, & M.A. Crawford, "Medical information service via telephone: The pioneer of physician consultation services", *Annals of the New York Academy of Science*, Vol. 670. pp. 155-162. 1992.

[90] J. Polisena, K. Tran, K. Cimon, B. Hutton, S. McGill, & K. Palmer, "Home telehealth for diabetes management: A systematic review and meta-analysis", *Diabetes, Obesity & Metabolism*, Vol. 11(10). pp. 913-930. 2009.

[91] J.D. Piette,M. Weinberger M, S. J. McPhee, C.A. Mah, F.B. Kraemer, L.M., Crapo, "Do automated calls with nurse follow-up improve self-care and glycemic control among vulnerable patients with diabetes?" *Am J Med*, Vol. 108, pp. 20-27. 2000.

[92] T. Wysocki, M. A. Harris, L. M. Buckloh, D. Mertlich, A. S. Lochrie, A. Taylor, et al., "Effects of behavioral family systems therapy for diabetes on adolescents' family relationships, treatment adherence, and metabolic control", *Journal of Pediatric Psychology*, Vol. 31, pp. 928-938. 2006.

[93] T. Wysocki, M. A. Harris, P. Greco, J. Bubb, C.E. Danda, L.M. Harvey, et al., "Randomized, controlled trial of behavior therapy for families of adolescents with insulin-dependent diabetes mellitus", *Journal of Pediatric* Psychology, Vol. 25, pp. 23–33. 2000.

[94] J.W. Adkins, E.A. Storch, A.B. Lewin, L. Williams, J.H. Silverstein, T. Malasanos, et al., "Home-based behavioral health intervention: Use of a telehealth model to address poor adherence to type-I diabetes medical regimens", *Journal of Telehealth and Telemedicine*, Vol. 12, pp. 370-372. 2006.

[95] K. Gelfand, G. Geffken, M. Halsey-Lyda, A. Muir, & T. Malasanos, "Intensive telehealth management of five at risk adolescents with diabetes", *Journal of Telehealth and Telecare,*Vol. 9, pp. 117-121. 2003.

[96] A. Heidgerken, E.A. Storch, L. Williams, A. Lewin, J.H. Silverstein, J. Adkins, et al., "Telehealth intervention for adolescents with type 1 diabetes", *Journal of Pediatrics,* Vol. 148, pp. 707-708. 2006.

[97] H.D. Lehmkuhl, E.A. Storch, C. Cammarata, K. Meyer, O. Rahman, J. Silverstein, et al., "Telehealth Behavior Therapy for the Management of Type I Diabetes in Adolescent", *Journal of Diabetes and Science Technology,* Vol. 4(1), pp. 199-208. 2010.

[98] E.A. Storch, G. Geffken, J. Adkins, D. Duke, K. Kiker, T. Malasanos, & J. Silverstein,"Wait-list controlled trial of telehealth behavior therapy: Preliminary results", *Scientific Proceedings of Therapeutic Patient Education,* Vol. 68. 2006.

[99] R. Bellazzi, M. Arcelloni, G. Bensa, H. Blankenfeld, E. Brugués, E. Carson,. . . M. Stefanelli, "Design, methods, and evaluation directions of a multi-access service for the management of diabetes mellitus patients", *Diabetes Technology & Therapeutics,* Vol. 5(4), pp. 621-629. 2003.

[100] E. A. Corriveau, P. J. Durso, E. D. Kaufman, B. J. Skipper, L. A. Laskaratos, & K. B. Heintzman, "Effect of carelink, an internet-based insulin pump monitoring system, on glycemic control in rural and urban children with type 1 diabetes mellitus", *Pediatric Diabetes,*Vol. 9(4), pp. 360-366. 2008.

Part 3

Perspectives of Diabetes Pathogenesis

9

Obesity in the Natural History of Type 1 Diabetes Mellitus: Causes and Consequences

Fernando Valente[1], Marília Brito Gomes[2]
and Sérgio Atala Dib[1]
[1]São Paulo Federal University, São Paulo
[2]State University of Rio de Janeiro, Rio de Janeiro
Brazil

1. Introduction

There has been a worldwide epidemic increasing in the prevalence of sedentary, overweight and obesity that comes with modernity and urbanization (Wang et al., 2002). The consequence is the development of insulin resistance (IR) and type 2 diabetes (T2D). This is classically defined as a metabolic disease that occurs due to a higher IR that leads to a slow setting of lower insulin production (more relative than absolute), in general in adult age. T2D is associated also with a genetic predisposition. The majority of T2D individuals are overweight or obese and the ones who do not, at least present increased abdominal adipose mass (ADA, 1997). The rising prevalence of overweight and obesity is happening also in children and adolescents (Pinhas-Hamiel et al., 1996; Willi & Egede, 2000; Rosenbloom et al., 1999). The metabolic syndrome (MS), which physiopathology is based on IR, shows the same trend in children and adolescents (Jago et al., 2008), as well as isolated pre-diabetes (Li et al., 2009).

In parallel, it has been seen an elevation in the number of type 1 diabetes (T1D) cases and its establishment at a younger age (EURODIAB ACE Study Group, 2000). T1D is characterized primarily by a pancreatic beta cell destruction, which may lead to ketosis. It can be classified as autoimmune (with positive anti-islet, anti-insulin, anti-GAD, anti-IA2 and/or anti-IA2 beta antibodies) or idiopathic, in which no autoantibodies can be detected, and occurs more frequently in individuals of African-American or Asian origin. Multiple genetic predisposition and environmental factors are involved with T1D (ADA, 1997). At least one of those autoantibodies is present in 85-90% of T1D on diagnosis. The treatment for T1D consists of multiple insulin injections, known as intensive treatment, to obtain adequate glycemic control and therefore prevent micro (The DCCT Research Group, 1993) and macrovascular (Nathan et al., 2005 and 2003) chronic complications. However, it can be followed by weight gain most of the times (Arai et al., 2008), which can amplify the risk of cardiovascular disease (CVD) in spite of good glycemic control. This weight gain can start on puberty and persist along adulthood (Särnblad et al., 2007). Therefore, some of these patients present clinical features of both T1D and T2D, confounding its classification. This phenotype was initially called double diabetes (DD) (Libman & Becker, 2003; Becker et al.,

2001), and is characterized by positive pancreatic autoantibodies in patients with clinical features of T2D, as IR and overweight and/or obesity (Pozzilli & Buzzetti, 2007; Gilliam et al., 2005; Reinehr et al., 2006), as shown in Table 1 (Pozzilli & Buzzetti, 2007) and in Figure 1.

	T1D	DD	T2D
Age at disease onset	Childhood +++ Adolescence +++ Adult +	Childhood ++ Adolescence ++ Adult (LADA) +	Childhood + Adolescence ++ Adult +++
Major genetics predisposition	MHC class I and II, *InsVNTR, CTLA-4, PTPN22*	?	*APM1, PPARγ 2, PtdCho-1, TCF7L2*
Environmental factors	Diet, viruses Cow´s milk in infancy	Life style (diet, sedentary life)	Life style (diet, sedentary life)
Circulating antibodies to β cells	+++	+	-
T cell-mediated immunity to β cells	+++	++	-
C-peptide secretion	-	+	+++
IR	-/+	++	+++
Inflammatory markers (cytokines, adipokines)	+	++	+++
Macrovascular complications	+	++	+++

Table 1. Clinical and pathogenic features of DD compared to T1D and T2D (Pozzilli & Buzzetti, 2007).

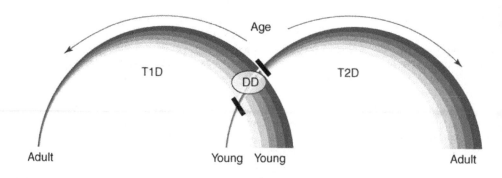

Fig. 1. Schematic representation showing where DD lies in respect to age and the two types of diabetes, as illustrated by two 'rainbows' (Pozzilli & Buzzetti, 2007).

2. Obesity as a accelerate factor to type 1 diabetes mellitus development

Studies with streptozotocin-induced diabetic baboons showed that to have an abnormal glucose tolerance it is necessary an isolated huge loss of beta-cell mass or a moderate loss of these cells associated to an IR (McCulloch et al., 1991), that could be in humans the physiologically IR of adolescence (Acerini et al., 2000) or gestation (Buschard et al., 1987), periods with higher incidence of T1D, or pathological situations like infection (usually one of the triggering factors of T1D) or weight gain.

Others studies suggest that the increase in the body mass index (BMI) and the consequent IR may accelerate the β cell destruction process in individuals predisposed to T1D, due to the release of obesity-related cytokines that show inflammatory and/or immunomodulatory properties (Aldhahi & Hamdy, 2003), triggering diabetes. This hypothesis may be reinforced by one study that correlated high anti-GAD levels with high BMI (Rolandsson et al., 1999). Two interesting data from studies with non-obese diabetic (NOD) mice are that hyperinsulinemia, an IR marker, precede clinical T1D (Armani et al., 1998) and that T1D incidence falls after treatment with rosiglitazone, an insulin sensitizer drug (Beales & Pozzili, 2002).

The IR, autoimmunity and apoptosis of the β cells constitutes the three factors of the called "accelerator hypothesis", proposed by Wilkin (Wilkin, 2001), that contemplate the factors presented in both more common types of diabetes, that is, T2D and T1D. There is a constitucional (intrinsic) high speed of apoptosis of β cells that is necessary to the development of diabetes, but rarely enough. The other two factors, extrinsic, that can speed the apoptosis of beta-cells are IR (result of weight gain and/or physical inactivity) and autoimmunity against beta-cells.

It is known that obese individuals have elevated serum levels of leptin, a cytokine secreted by adipocytes in proportion to adipose tissue mass and that is responsible, among other functions, for regulating food intake and thus BMI. Moreover, leptin controls the cellular immune response and is involved in the pathogenesis of autoimmune diseases (Lord, 2002). Studies have shown that administration of leptin in NOD mice promoted an early inflammatory infiltrate in the pancreatic islets, increased production of interferon gamma (IFN-gamma) by T lymphocytes, which accelerated the establishment of a T1D (Matarese, 2002 e 2005).

On the other hand, adiponectin, another important cytokine produced by adipose tissue, inversely proportional to its fat mass, can decrease the systemic and pancreatic islets inflammatory process, acting as a protective factor in the development of T1D, in addition to reducing IR (Kadowaki et al., 2006; Wellen & Hotamisligil, 2005).

However, development report (OECD, 2009) from 16 countries does not show any obvious relationship between national estimates of childhood obesity prevalence and incidence rates of T1D (Table 2). Therefore, obesity does not account for the wide between-country differences in T1D incidence, which range from 0.57 per 100 000 person-years in China to more than 48 per 100 000 person-years in Sardinia and Finland in the 0- to 14-year age group (Daneman, 2006).

On the other hand, in a meta-analysis of nine studies (eight case–control studies and one cohort study) comprising a total of 2658 cases (Verbeeten et al., 2011), seven reported a significant association between childhood obesity, BMI or %weight-for-height and increased risk for T1D. Four of these studies reported childhood obesity as a categorical exposure and produced a pooled odds ratio of 2.03 (95% CI 1.46–2.80) for subsequent T1D, but with age at obesity assessment varying from age 1 to 12 years (Figure 2). A dose–response relationship was supported by a continuous association between childhood BMI and subsequent T1D in a meta-analysis of five studies (pooled odds ratio 1.25 (95%CI 1.04–1.51) per 1 SD higher BMI) (Figure 3).

Country	T1D incidence rate in children aged 0-14 years (per 100.000 person-years)	% of children aged 11-15 years overweight or obese
Finland	57,4	15,8
Sweden	41	10,5
Norway	27,9	10
UK	24,5	12
Denmark	22,2	9,7
Canada	21,7	21,3
USA	20,8	29,8
Netherlands	18,8	8
Germany	18	12
Ireland	16,3	14,2
Iceland	14,7	14,5
Spain	13	16,7
Poland	12,9	11,2
France	12,2	10,5
Greece	9,9	18,8
Italy	8,4	18,3

Table 2. Relationship between Type 1 diabetes incidence and prevalence of childhood overweight or obesity in 16 Organization for Economic Co-Operation and Development (OECD) countries, from Health at a Glance 2009: OECD Indicators (OECD, 2009).

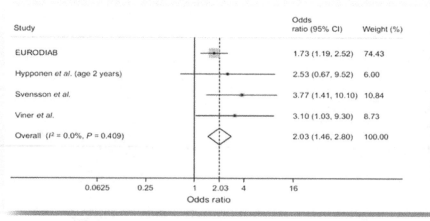

Fig. 2. Meta-analysis (fixed-effects inverse variance model) of studies of childhood obesity as a risk factor for subsequent T1D (Verbeeten et al., 2011).

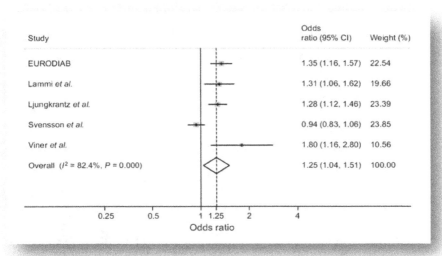

Fig. 3. Meta-analysis (random-effects inverse variance model) of studies of childhood BMI as a risk factor for subsequent T1D. Odds ratios correspond to a 1-unit increase in BMI standard deviation score (SDS)(Verbeeten et al., 2011).

3. Obesity after clinical Type 1 diabetes diagnostic

If on one hand intensive insulin prevents microvascular and macrovascular complications associated with poor glycemic control, the other brings an increased risk of severe hypoglycemia and weight gain, traditionally viewed as a normalization of weight, i.e. the correction of glycosuria, diuresis, and wasting with the initiation of insulin therapy. Insulin stimulates lipogenesis, inhibits protein catabolism, and slows basal metabolism. Other important aspect is the abnormal physiological route of insulin via its peripheral administration in those with T1D, which is also associated with reduced energy metabolism (Charlton & Nair, 1998). Classically normal or underweight, the phenotype of the T1D individuals is thus changing. A follow-up of 18 years of 589 individuals from the Pittsburgh Epidemiology of Diabetes Complications Study (EDC), a cohort of childhood-onset T1D, showed an increase in the prevalence of overweight by 47% (from 28.6% at baseline to 42%) and of obesity by sevenfold (from 3.4% at baseline to 22.7%), concomitantly with the highest prevalence of intensive insulin therapy - 7% and 82% were on intensive insulin therapy (≥ 3 insulin injections per day or on insulin pump) at baseline and 18 years after, respectively (Conway et al., 2010). Although injection frequency increased, total daily insulin dose decreased from 0.76 to 0.62 U/kg/day. Figure 4 shows the temporal patterns in the prevalence of being overweight and obese and the use of intensive insulin treatment, and these data was not influenced by the aging of the cohort and survivorship, as can be seen on Table 3. (age-group-specific prevalence for the 40–49-year-old age group by time period): overweight or obesity were present in 25% of the T1D individuals in 1986–1988 and in 68.2% in 2004–2007 (Conway et al., 2010).

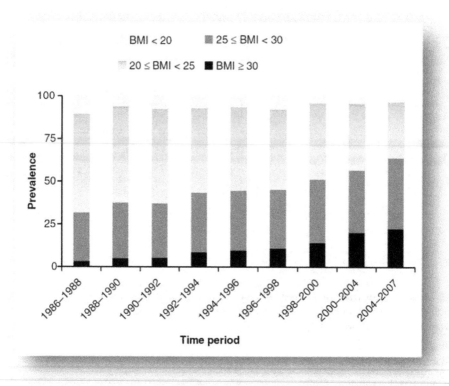

Fig. 4. Temporal patterns in overweight and obesity in Type 1 diabetes (Conway et al., 2010).

	BMI < 20 kg/m² (underweight)	20 ≤ BMI < 25 kg/m² (normal weight)	25 ≤ BMI < 30 kg/m² (overweight)	BMI ≥ 30 kg/m² (obese)
1986–1988	4 (9.1)	29 (65.9)	10 (22.7)	1 (2.3)
1988–1990	3 (5.8)	29 (55.8)	17 (32.7)	3 (5.8)
1990–1992	6 (8.5)	43 (60.6)	18 (25.4)	4 (5.6)
1992–1994	10 (12.2)	39 (47.6)	27 (32.9)	6 (7.3)
1994–1996	14 (11.9)	58 (49.2)	35 (29.7)	11 (9.3)
2004–2007	5 (2.9)	50 (28.9)	79 (45.7)	39 (22.5)

Table 3. Age-specific prevalence of underweight, normal weight, overweight, and obese for those aged 40-49 years in each time period, n (%)(Conway et al., 2010)

The prevalence of overweight/obesity in this T1D population was lower at baseline than general population (31.9 vs. 55.9%), although the incidence in both was similar after a mean of 7 years' follow-up (12%), and after 18 years' follow-up the prevalence of overweight in T1D people appear to have increased at a faster pace than in the general population.

Predictors of weight change were a higher baseline HbA1c, symptomatic autonomic neuropathy (inversely), overt nephropathy (inversely), and going onto intensive insulin therapy during follow-up. By the end of this study, 24% of the T1D people had died. Thus, as overt nephropathy and symptomatic autonomic neuropathy are associated with weight loss, the survivors are biased toward weight gain. The EDC Study also showed that, in T1D with a higher baseline HbA1c, moderate weight gain did not adversely affect the cardiovascular risk profile and favorably influenced the lipid profile in the setting of ameliorated glycemic control, but increased LDL cholesterol levels in the absence of a major improvement in glycemic control (Williams et al., 1999). Subjects who gained the least weight had the lowest LDL cholesterol levels at the follow-up period regardless of changes in HbA1 category. But when the weight gain after insulin was great, case of part of the patients who received intensive treatment in the Diabetes control and complications trial (DCCT) study and placed in the highest quartile of change in BMI, there was unmasking of central obesity or even MS in T1D (Purnell et al, 1998). These patients gained an average of 14 kg during the course of the study, about twice the weight gain equivalent to the third quartile of intensive care and the last quartile of patients on conventional treatment. Patients with the highest weight gain had the highest values of waist-hip ratio, blood pressure and insulin requirements when compared to the group with the same degree of glycemic control and also in intensive care, but who did not gain much weight. These youngsters also had a relatively atherogenic lipid profile, with elevations to levels of triglyceride, LDL cholesterol and apolipoprotein B (apoB) compared to their peers, also intensively treated, but without similar weight gain. The DCCT study (Purnell et al., 2003) also showed that the presence of family history of T2D was one of the strongest predictors for the weight gain in individuals with T1D who underwent intensive insulin therapy in the DCCT. In individuals with a family history of T2D, the weight gain, the final weight, the central fat distribution assessed by waist circumference, the insulin dose (units/kg/day) and degree of dyslipidemia were higher than in those without history familial T2D. Dyslipidemia included increases in triglycerides (TG) in VLDL particles and IDL (intermediate-density lipoprotein), which changes are common in individuals with central adiposity (Terry et al., 1989) and T2D (Brunzell & Chait, 1997). This could correspond to the expression of genes predisposing to T2D in this population. The findings of this study support the hypothesis that insulin treatment allows the expression of various components of MS in individuals with T1D who have family history of T2D, but also suggests that this group should be monitored more closely and earlier in relation to their potential of developing macrovascular complications, which is responsible for most of the increase in mortality found in patients with T1D (Laing et al., 1999), more than three times the general population.

4. Type 1 diabetes and Metabolic Syndrome

The insulin resistance is a soil to MS development and it is present during T1D evolution, even because of weight gain or because of the glucotoxicity – there was shown a proportion between fasting glycemic and IR, and improvement of glycemic control is linked to better insulin sensitivity, for example contributing to the so-called period of "honeymoon", the remission phase of diabetes, well known by clinicians, and may occur in up to 50% of patients during the first year of disease (DCCT Research Group, 1987). Yki-Jarvinen et al. (1986), studied insulin sensitivity using the hyperinsulinemic euglycemic clamp in 15 adult patients with T1D and normal BMI during the first 2 weeks, 3 months and 1 year after clinical diagnosis. In the first two weeks of diagnosis, they had a decrease in insulin sensitivity when compared to controls. However, three months after diagnosis, there was an improvement in insulin sensitivity in these patients, and it became similar to that of controls. Importantly, this improvement in insulin sensitivity coincided with the period of "honeymoon" in these patients, and showed a good correlation with HbA1c values and insulin doses in the treatment. Insulin sensitivity of patients who entered clinical remission was 40% greater than those who did not have this condition. Recently, our group performed a cohort and multicenter study (Gabbay et al, 2005; Dib, 2006) to determine the prevalence of MS in a group of patients with T1D and assessing their relation with the time of diagnosis. The study included 524 (276 females) T1D (according to the criteria of the Brazilian Diabetes Society and American Diabetes Association) with an average age of 20 ± 9 years and divided according to the time of T1D in 4 groups: GI, ≤ 5 years (n = 264), G-II, 6-10 years (n = 108), G III, 11-15 years (n = 96) and G IV,> 15 years (n = 56). In these groups were analyzed BMI (kg/m2), total daily doses of insulin for treatment (U/kg/day), HbA1c values and the prevalence of MS. The criterion used for characterization of MS was the one of the World Health Organization, that is, diabetes mellitus and 2 or more of the following: increase in waist circumference (criterion set for youth) (Freedman et al., 1999), TG ≥ 150 mg/dL or HDL-C < 40 mg/dL (males) and < 50 mg/dL (females), urinary albumin excretion (≥ 20 µg/min) and hypertension (according to criteria adjusted for age and sex) (Brazilian Hypertension, Heart and Nephrology , Societies 2002). The daily insulin dose and HbA1c values were significantly lower in G-I than in other groups (G-I: 0.7 ± 0.3, G-II: 1.1 ± 0.3, G-III: 1.0 ± 0.3 and G-IV: 0.8 ± 0.2 U/kg/day, p = 0.000) and (G-I: 8.7 ± 2.6, G-II: 9.5 ± 2.2, G-III, 9.5 ± 2.3 and G-IV: 9.4 ± 2.8%, p = 0.000), respectively. There was a significant increase in the values of waist circumference (G-I: 71.9 ± 2.2, G-II: 75.7 ± 11.1, G-III: 76.5 ± 8.4 and G-IV: 80.2 ± 7.5 cm, p = 0.000) and BMI (G-I: 20.6 ± 3.8, G-II: 22.4 ± 3.6, G-III: 22.5 ± 3.1 and G- IV: 23.1 ± 4.1 kg/m2, p = 0.000) after 5 years of diagnosis of T1D. However, it is important to note that the BMI values were not superior to classical criteria of obesity or even overweight. The prevalence of MS (G-I: 5.1, G-II: 11.2, G-III: 18.9 and G-IV, 31.5%, p = 0.000) increased with time of diagnosis (Figure 5). The odds ratio (OR) for the development of MS in the other groups in relation to G-I was significant G-III onwards, being equal to 3.59 and 7.18 for this for G-IV in relation to G-I, both with p = 0.001. That is, the odds for the development of MS in patients with T1D and over 15 years of diagnosis is 618% higher than under 5 years of disease. Similarly, the odds for the development of MS for patients with T1D between 11 and 15 years duration is 259% higher than those with less than 5 disease in this group of patients. Other factors related to insulin resistance, such as visceral fat, BMI and TG, even when considered separately, also increased with the duration of the disease.

In another study (Giuffrida et al., 2005), 500 T1D patients [age 19.7 ± 8.9 years (mean ± SD), 52% female], we observe that, also analyzed separately, the prevalence of microalbuminuria (GI: 24.1%, G-II: 25.0%, G-III: 31.0% and G-IV: 55.6%, p <0.05) and hypertension (GI, 8.3%;

G-II: 13.6%, G-III: 28.6% and G-IV: 44.4%, p = 0.000) increased with duration of disease. Data from these studies suggest that chronic glucotoxicity (elevated HbA1c) and factors involved in diabetic nephropathy (microalbuminuria and hypertension) may be one of the mechanisms for the development of MS in T1D, among many others.

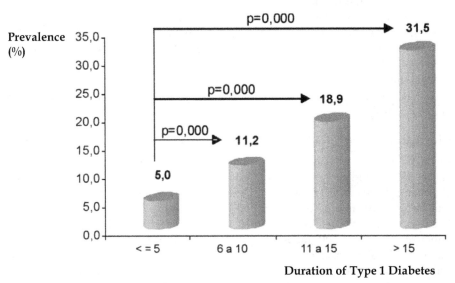

Fig. 5. Prevalence of MS in patients with T1D, according to disease duration. (Dib, 2006)

Aiming to compare the prevalence of MS using the ATP III criteria modified for age in our group of T1D, we studied 521 (51.2% female, age 20 ± 9 years; time of diagnosis of diabetes: 7.7 ± 6.9 years and HbA1c: 9.0 ± 2.4%) and found that this was equal to 12% (unpublished data).

The lowest concentration in the insulin in the liver causes a decrease in the synthesis of GHBP levels (Growth Hormone Binding Protein) (Bereket et al., 1999) that leads to a decrease in GH action, in the values of IGF-1 and in the inhibitory counter-regulation of this hormone, resulting in an exaggerated secretion of GH and increased insulin resistance.

The realization of a strict glycemic control in T1D, according to current guidelines, many often leads to use of supraphysiological doses of insulin, which could result in a stimulation of androgen synthesis, mediated by insulin, as occurs in cases of insulin resistance. Accordingly, the prevalence of Polycystic Ovary Syndrome (PCOS) and other symptoms and signs of hyperandrogenism were evaluated in a group of 85 patients with T1D (Escobar-Morreale et al., 2000). PCOS was defined by the presence of menstrual changes and clinical or laboratory evidence of hyperandrogenism. Other causes of elevated androgen hormones were excluded. Eighteen normal eumenorrheic women served as controls. Thirty-three patients (38%) presented with T1D changes associated with an androgen excess (16 with PCOS and 17 with hirsutism without menstrual abnormalities). The patients with T1D and PCOS had elevated total and free testosterone and androstenedione but normal levels of sex-hormone binding globulin (SHBG) and dehydroepiandrosterone sulfate (DHEAS). However, despite the finding of a high prevalence of hyperandrogenism (including PCOS and hirsutism), there was no difference between clinical variables such as duration of diabetes, age at diagnosis, conventional or intensive insulin treatment, average daily dose of insulin or glucose control between the T1D patients with and without hyperandrogenism in study.

The gold-standard method for evaluating IR is the hyperinsulinemic euglycemic clamp that directly measures the relationship between blood glucose and insulin levels, but it is difficult to be executed on a large scale since it is an invasive and expensive procedure. For this reason, HOMA-IR is used as a surrogate method to indirectly measure IR, calculated through fasting glycemia and insulinemia relationship. On the other hand, this calculation cannot be used for T1D as these patients do not produce endogenous insulin. So to evaluate the insulin sensitivity in these patients eGDR calculation (Equation 1) was developed that shown a good correlation with hyperinsulinemic euglycemic clamp (Chillarón et al., 2008):

$$\text{eGDR (mg.kg-1.min-1)} = 24{,}4 - 12{,}97 \ (W/H) - 3{,}39 \ (\text{Hypertension}) - 0{,}60 \ (\text{HbA1c}) \quad (E1)$$

In which W/H is the waist-hip ratio(cm), hypertension is the presence or absence of hypertension (0 = no and 1 = yes) and the value of HbA1c is represented in %. It is also a good predictor of mortality, coronary arterial disease (CAD), microalbuminuria - a precocious hallmark of endothelial dysfunction (Pambianco et al., 2007) – and MS for T1D individuals, according to IDF (International Diabetes Federation), WHO (World Health Organization) and NCEP/ATPIII modified by AHA (American Heart Association).

As we know the insulin resistance is linked to an ectopic store of fat in insulin sensitive tissues like liver and muscle, but it is not clear if this fat accumulation leads to a hyperinsulinemic state or if it is its consequence. In a study with T2D patients, the glycemic control obtained after 67 hours of insulin treatment caused an accrual in intramyocellular and intrahepatic lipid content measured by nuclear magnetic resonance (NMR) spectroscopy, without compromising insulin sensitivity (Anderwald et al., 2002). Like T2D individuals, the intramyocellular lipid content in T1D ones was increased compared to controls and there was a direct relation with the glycemic control (Sibley et al., 2003).

There has been also noted a clear association between IR and visceral fat store, that can take its content extended in consequence of intensive insulin treatment independently of the type of diabetes, aggravating the CVD risk. In the DCCT study, the subgroup of T1D individuals that received intensive insulin treatment had a higher growth in BMI compared to the ones who were treated conventionally and it was noted a stronger correlation of this BMI variation with visceral fat deposit than with subcutaneous fat (Sibley et al., 2003). In this study, there are also demonstrations of direct association between visceral fat content and hepatic lipase, which favors the emergence of atherogenic dyslipidemia in these intensive treated individuals that put on more weight, reaching lipid levels similar to those of the conventionally treated group, suggesting loss of the benefits of intensive insulin therapy on lipids in this group of patients who had an excessive weight gain.

In other study (Nadeau et al., 2010), lean T1D adolescents with short time of disease (average of 7.5 years) without any inflammatory, clinical or lipid abnormalities had a IR - measured by hyperinsulinemic euglycemic clamp - similar to non diabetic obese adolescents and a superior IR than control subjects matched for age, pubertal stage, physical activity level and BMI, despite normal waist and intramyocellular lipid content.

There was also a demonstrated association between fat mass and blood pressure levels in T1D children and adolescents – high fat content, identified by the bioimpedance (BIA), and BMI were related to higher systolic and diastolic blood pressure (Pietrzak et al., 2009). The BIA is an easy, noninvasive, portable, no risk, relatively inexpensive method to measure the percentage of fat and provides results comparable to dual energy X-ray absorptiometry (DXA) (Elberg et al., 2004; Völgyi et al., 2008), that is reliable but expensive, requiring trained operators, individuals exposed to ionizing radiation and is not portable (Thomson et al., 2007).

There are data indicating good correlation between BIA and DXA, including Brazilian (Braulio et al., 2010) and T1D subjects (Leiter et al., 1994). Although overestimating the percentage of fat in lean individuals and underestimate it in obese (Sun et al., 2005), proves useful for predicting metabolic risk (including IR) as well as BMI and waist circumference (Lee et al., 2008). Through the BIA, it is possible to calculate the CDI (central fat distribution index), which assesses the impact of subcutaneous fat in the central fat distribution, and can be measured by dividing the area of abdominal subcutaneous fat mass by total fat (Silva et al., 2009). This measure seems to be relevant in that, according to some studies (Silva et al., 2009; Van Harmelen et al., 1998), the main source of leptin is the abdominal subcutaneous adipose tissue, either by mass effect - the subcutaneous adipose tissue is the major fat depot - as to produce more leptin (larger cell size and leptin gene expression) that omental adipose tissue. However, depending on the impedance (eg the trunk), the results may vary according to position changes, skin temperature, variation in electrode impedance and errors in their placement (Scharfetter et al., 2001).

A new adipokine identified visfatin, increases in proportion to visceral fat mass (Fukuhara et al., 2005) and decreases after gastric band placement (Haider et al., 2006). It is high in individuals with T2D (Chen et al., 2006) and even more in T1D (López-Bermejo et al., 2006), suggesting that its rising is linked to deterioration of pancreatic β cells. In vitro, visfatin activates the insulin receptor regardless of fasting state, increasing glucose uptake in muscle and adipose tissue and reducing hepatic glucose production independently of insulin levels (Fukuhara et al., 2005).

Hyperhomocysteinemia, known risk factor for coronary atherosclerosis (Okada et al., 1999), has also been shown to be detrimental to pancreatic insulin secretion (Patterson et al., 2006). The C-reactive protein (CRP), an inflammatory marker that confers increased risk for atherosclerosis (Hayaishi-Okano et al., 2002), is increased in T2D patients (Nabipour et al., 2008) and obese subjects (Richardson et al., 2009), and also relates to the control of diabetes (King et al., 2003), i.e. may increase due to the weight gain caused by intensive control of diabetes (Schaumberg et al., 2005).

Ferritin is another acute phase inflammatory marker, correlate positively with CRP and BMI (Richardson et al., 2009), and also more specifically with visceral adiposity and insulin resistance (Iwasaki et al., 2005), leading to increased ferritin levels in T2D patients, concurrent with an augmentation of visfatin (Fernandez-Real et al., 2007).

Recently, several studies have indicated that the gene associated with fat mass and BMI (FTO) has an important genetic effect on BMI and risk of obesity through the rs9939609 polymorphism. This polymorphism is linked to an impaired responsiveness to satiety, ie have an effect on appetite (Wardle et al., 2008). The homozygous AA genotype results in an average gain of 3 kg or 1 unit of BMI over the TT genotype. There is evidence that this polymorphism is linked to BMI gain in subjects with T1D (Gu et al., 2010) and higher levels of leptin and CRP (Welsh et al., 2010).

5. Conclusion

Obesity may both contribute to the onset of T1D as being a consequence of intensive treatment with insulin, that is, good glycemic control in T1D can lead to excessive weight gain in predisposed individuals (eg relatives of T2D), IR and consequently MS. Thus, the current approach of patients T1D should happen as it is done in T2D, multifactorial with an early and intensive monitoring of lifestyle, blood glucose, blood pressure and lipids, with the aim of identifying, correcting these factors and potentially reduce the high risk for cardiovascular disease in these patients. So gain weight can accelerate the presentation and modify the initial TID phenotype as increase the cardiovascular risk factors during evolution do the disease .

6. References

Acerini CL, Vheetham TD, Ege JA, Dunger DB. Both insulin sensitivity and insulin clearance in children and young adults with type 1 (insulin-dependent) diabetes vary with growth hormone concentrations and with age. *Diabetologia* 2000; 43: 61-8.

Aldhahi, W. and Hamdy, O. Adipokines, inflammation and the endothelium in diabetes. *Curr. Diab. Rep.*2003, 3, 293-298.

American Diabetes Association. Report of the Expert Committee on the Diagnosis and Classification of Diabetes Mellitus. *Diabetes Care* 1997; 20: 1183-97.

Anderwald C, Bernroider E, Krssák M, Stingl H, Brehm A, Bischof MG, Nowotny P, Roden M and Waldhäusl W. Effects of Insulin Treatment in Type 2 Diabetic Patients on Intracellular Lipid Content in Liver and Skeletal Muscle. *Diabetes* 2002, 51: 3025-3032.

Arai K, Yokoyama H, Okuguchi F et al. Association between Body Mass Index and Core Components of Metabolic Syndrome in 1486 Patients with Type 1 Diabetes Mellitus in Japan (JDDM 13). *Endocrine Journal*, 2008, vol 55 (6), 1025-1032.

Armani A, Durant S, Throsby M, Coulad J, Dardenne M, Homo-Delarche F. Glucose homeostasis in the nonobese diabetic mouse at the pre-diabetic stage. *Endocrinology* 1998; 139: 1115-24.

Beales PE, Pozzili P. Thiazolidinediones for the prevention of diabetes in the non-obese diabetic (NOD) mouse: implications for human type 1 diabetes. *Diabetes Metab Res Rev* 2002; 18: 114-7.

Becker DJ, Libman I, Pietropaolo M, Dosch M, Arslanian S, LaPorte R. Changing phenotype of IDDM: is it type 1 or type 2? *Pediatr. Res.* 2001, 49, 93A.

Bereket A, Lang CH, Wilson TA. Alterations in the growth hormone-insulin-like growth factor axis in insulin dependent diabetes mellitus. *Horm Metab Res* 1999; 31: 172-81.

Braulio VB, Furtado VC, Silveira MG, Fonseca MH, Oliveira JE. Comparison of body composition methods in overweight and obese Brazilian women. *Arq Bras Endocrinol Metab.* 2010; 54/4.

Brunzell JD, Chait A. Diabetic dyslipidemia: pathology and treatment. In: Porte D, Sherwin J (eds.). *Ellenberg and Rifkin's Diabetes Mellitus*. 5th ed. Norwalk: Appleton and Lange; 1997. p.1077-98.

Buschard K, Buch I, Molsted-Pedersen L, Hougaard P, Kuhl C. Increased incidence of true type I diabetes acquired during pregnancy. *Br Med J (Clin Res Ed)* 1987; 294 (6567): 275-9.

Charlton M, Nair K. Role of hyperglucagonemia in catabolism associated with type 1 diabetes. Effects of leucine metabolism and the resting metabolic rate. *Diabetes* 1998; 47: 1748-1756.

Chen M-P, Chung F-M, Chang D-M, Tsai JC-R, Huang H-F, Shin S-J and Le Y-J. Elevated plasma level of visfatin/PBEF in patients with type 2 diabetes. *JCEM*, 2006, 91: 295-299.

Chillarón JJ, Goday A, Pedro-Botet J. Síndrome metabólico, diabetes mellitus tipo 1 y resistencia a la insulina. *Med Clin (Barc)* 2008, 130(12): 466-71.

Conway B, Miller RG, Costacou T, Fried L, Kelsey S, Evans RW and Orchard TJ. Temporal patterns in overweight and obesity in Type 1 diabetes. *Diabet. Med.* 27, 398-404 (2010).

Daneman D. Type 1 diabetes. Lancet 2006; 367: 847-858.

Dib, SA. Insulin Resistance and metabolic syndrome in Type 1 Diabetes Mellitus. *Arq Bras Endocrinol Metab* vol 50 n° 2 Abril 2006

Elberg J, McDuffie JR, Sebring NG, Salaita C, Keil M, Robotham D, Reynolds JC and Yanovski JA. Comparison of methods to assess change in children's body composition. *Am J Clin Nutr.* 2004 July; 80 (1): 64–69.

Escobar-Morreale HF, Roldan B, Barrio R, Alonso M, Sancho J, de Calle H, et al. High prevalence of the polycystic ovary syndrome and hirsutism in women with type 1 diabetes mellitus. *J Clin Endocrinol Metab* 2000; 85: 4182-7.

EURODIAB ACE Study Group. Variation and trends in incidence of childhood diabetes in Europe. EURODIAB ACE Study Group. *Lancet* 2000, 355, 873-876.

Fernandez-Real JM, Moreno JM, Chico B, López-Bermejo A and Ricart W (2007). Circulating Visfatin Is Associated With Parameters of Iron Metabolism in Subjects With Altered Glucose Tolerance. *Diabetes Care* 30: 616–621, 2007.

Freedman D, Serdula MK, Srinivasan SR, Berenson GS. Relation of circumference and skin fold thicknesses to lipid and insulin concentrations in children and adolescents: the Bogalusa Heart Study. *Am J Clin Nutr* 1999; 69: 308-17.

Fukuhara A, Matsuda M, Nishizawa M, Segawa K, Tanaka M, Kishimoto K, Matsuki Y, Murakami M, Ichisaka T, Murakami H, Watanabe E, Takagi T, Akiyoshi M, Ohtsubo T, Kihara S, Yamashita S, Makishima M, Funahashi T, Yamanaka S, Hiramatsu R, Matsuzawa Y, Shimomura I.Visfatin: a protein secreted by visceral fat that mimics the effects of insulin. *Science* 2005, 307, 426-430.

Gabbay MAL, Gomes MB, Pires AC, Dib SA. Prevalence and trends of metabolic syndrome in type 1 diabetes according to duration of the disease. *Diabetes* 2005; 54 (suppl.1): A176.

Gilliam LK, Brooks-Worrell BM, Palmer JP, Greenbaum CJ, Pihoker C. Autoimmunity and clinical course in children with type 1, type 2 and type 1.5 diabetes. *J Autoimmun.* 2005, 25, 244-250.

Giuffrida FMA, Gabbay MAL, Pires AC, Brito M, Dib SA. Desenvolvimento dos sinais da síndrome metabólica em pacientes com diabetes mellitus tipo 1 de acordo com o tempo de duração da doença. *Arq Bras Endocrinol Metab* 2005; 49: S96.

Gu HF, Alvarsson A and Brismar K. The Common FTO Genetic Polymorphism rs9939609 is Associated with Increased BMI in Type 1 Diabetes but not with Diabetic Nephropathy. *Biomarker Insights* 2010:5 29–32.

Haider DG, Schindler K, Schaller G, Prager G, Wolzt M and Ludvik B. Increased plasma visfatin concentration in morbidly obese subjects are reduced after gastric banding. *JCEM*, 2006, 91: 1578-1581.

Hayaishi-Okano R, Yamasaki Y, Katakami N, Ohtoshi K, Gorogawa S-I, Kuroda A, Matsuhisa M, Kosugi K, Nishikawa N, Kajimoto Y, Hori M. Elevated C-reactive protein associates with early-stage carotid atherosclerosis in young subjects with type 1 diabetes. *Diabetes Care* 2002, 25: 1432–1438.

Iwasaki T, Nakajima A, Yoneda M, Yamada Y, Mukasa K, Fujita K, Fujisawa N, Wada K and Terauch Y (2005). Serum Ferritin Is Associated With Visceral Fat Area and Subcutaneous Fat Area. *Diabetes Care* 28: 2486–2491, 2005.

Jago, R. et al. Studies to Treat or Prevent Pediatric Type 2 Diabetes (STOPP-T2D) Prevention Study Group * Prevalence of the metabolic syndrome Among a Racially/Ethnically Diverse Group of U.S. Eighth-Grade Adolescents and Associations With Fasting Insulin and Homeostasis Model Assessment of Insulin Resistance Levels. *Diabetes Care* 2008, 31(10): 2020-2025.

Kadowaki T, Yamauchi T, Kubota N, Hara K, Ueki K, Tobe K. Adiponectin and adiponectin receptors in insulin resistance, diabetes, and the metabolic syndrome. J. *Clin. Invest.* 2006, 116: 1784–1792.

King DE, Mainous AG, Buchanan TA and Pearson WS. C-reactive protein and glycemic control in adults with diabetes. *Diabetes Care* 2003, 26: 1535–1539.

Laing SP, Swerdlow AJ, Slater SD, Botha JL, Burden AC, Waugh NR, et al. The British Diabetic Association Cohort Study II: cause-specific mortality in patients with insulin treated diabetes mellitus. *Diabet Med* 1999;16:466-71.

Lee K, Song Y-M and Sung J. Which Obesity Indicators Are Better Predictors of Metabolic Risk? Healthy Twin Study. *Obesity* (2008) 16, 834–840.

Leiter LA, Lukaski HC, Kenny DJ. The use of bioelectrical impedance analysis (BIA) to estimate body composition in the diabetes control and complications trial (DCCT). *Int J Obesity* 1994; 18: 829–835.

Li C., Ford ES, Zhao G, Mokdad AH. Prevalence of Pre-Diabetes and Its Association With Clustering of Cardiometabolic Risk Factors and Hyperinsulinemia Among U.S. Adolescents National Health and Nutrition Examination Survey 2005–2006. *Diabetes Care* 2009, 32: 342–347.

Libman, I.M. and Becker, D.J. (2003). Coexistence of type 1 and type 2 diabetes mellitus: 'double' diabetes? *Pediatr. Diabetes* 2003, 4, 110-113.

López-Bermejo A, Chico-Julià B, Fernàndez-Balsells M, Recasens M, Esteve E, Casamitjana R, Ricart W, Fernández-Real JM Serum visfatin increases with progressive beta cell-deterioration. *Diabetes* 2006, 55, 2861-2875.

Lord, G. Role of leptin in immunology. *Nutr. Rev.* 2002, 60, S35-S38.

Matarese G, Moschos S, Mantzoros CS. Leptin in immunology. *J. Immunol.* 2005, 174, 3137-3142.

Matarese G, Sanna V, Lechler RI, Sarvetnick N, Fontana S, Zappacosta S, La Cava A. Leptin accelerates autoimmune diabetes in female NOD mice. *Diabetes* 2002, 51, 1356-1361.

McCulloch DK, Kahn SE, Schwartz MW, Koerker DJ, Palmer JP. Effect of nicotinic acid-induced insulin resistance on pancreatic B cell function in normal and streptozotocin treated baboons. *J Clin Invest* 1991; 40: 166-80.

Nabipour I, Vahdat K, Jafari SM, Beigi S, Assadi M, Azizi F, Sanjdideh Z. Elevated High Sensitivity C-Reactive Protein Is Associated with Type 2 Diabetes Mellitus: The Persian Gulf Healthy Heart Study. *Endocrine Journal*, 2008, vol 55 (4), 717-722.

Nadeau KJ, Regensteiner JG, Bauer TA, Brown MS, Dorosz JL, Hull A, Zeitler P, Draznin B. and Reusch JEB. Insulin Resistance in Adolescents with Type 1 Diabetes and Its Relationship to Cardiovascular Function. *Clin Endocrinol Metab*, February 2010, 95 (2): 513-521.

Nathan DM, Lachin JM, Cleary P., Pomar T., Brillon DJ, Backlund JY, O'Leary DH, Genuth SM. Diabetes Control and Complications Trial / Epidemiology of Diabetes Interventions and Complications Study Research Group. Intensive Diabetes therapy and carotid intima-media thickness in type 1 diabetes mellitus. *NEJM* 2003, 348: 2294-2303.

Nathan DM et al. Diabetes Control and Complications Trial / Epidemiology of Diabetes Interventions and Complications Study Research Group. Intensive Diabetes treatment and cardiovascular disease in patients with type 1 diabetes. *NEJM* 2005, 353: 2643-2653.

OECD. Health at a Glance 2009: OECD Indicators. Paris: Organization for Economic Co-Operation and Development Press, 2009: 38-51.

Okada E, Oida K, Tada H, Asazuma K, Eguchi K, Tohda G, Kosaka S, Takahashi S and Miyamori I. Hyperhomocysteinemia Is a Risk Factor for Coronary Arteriosclerosis in Japanese Patients With Type 2 Diabetes. *Diabetes Care* 1999, 22: 484-490.

Pambianco G, Costacou T, Orchard TJ. The Prediction of Major Outcomes of Type 1 Diabetes: a 12-Year Prospective Evaluation of Three Separate Definitions of the metabolic syndrome and Their Components and Estimated Glucose Disposal Rate - The Pittsburgh Epidemiology of Diabetes Complications Study experience. *Diabetes Care* 2007, 30: 1248-1254.

Patterson S, Flatt PR, Brennan L, Newsholme P, McClenaghan NH. Detrimental actions of metabolic syndrome risk factor, homocysteine, on pancreatic B-cell glucose metabolism and insulin secretion. Journal of Endocrinology 2006, 189: 301-10.

Pietrzak I, Mianowska B, Gadzicka A, Młynarski W, Szadkowska A. Blood pressure in children and adolescents with type 1 diabetes mellitus - the influence of body mass index and fat mass. *Pediatric Endocrinology, Diabetes and Metabolism* 2009, 15 (4): 240-5.

Pinhas-Hamiel O, Dolan LM, Daniels SR, Standiford D, Khoury PR, Zeitler P. Increased incidence of non-insulin-dependent diabetes mellitus among adolescents. *J Pediatr* 1996, 128, 608-15.

Pozzilli,P. and Buzzetti, R. A new expression of diabetes: double diabetes. *TRENDS in Endocrinology and Metabolism* 2007, 18 (2), 52-57.

Purnell JQ, Hokanson JE, Marcovina SM, Steffes MW, Cleary PA, Brunzell JD. Effect of excessive weight-gain with intensive therapy of type 1 diabetes on lipid levels and blood pressure: results from the DCCT. Diabetes Control and Complications Trial. *JAMA* 1998; 280: 140-6.

Purnell JQ, Dev RK, Steffes MW, Cleary PA, Palmer JP, Hirsch IB, et al. Relationship of family history of type 2 diabetes, hypoglycemia, and auto antibodies to weight gain and lipids with intensive and conventional therapy in the Diabetes Control and Complications Trial. *Diabetes* 2003; 52: 2623.

Reinehr T, Schober E, Wiegand S, Thon A, Holl R. DPV-Wiss Study Group. B-Cell autoantibodies in children with type 2 diabetes mellitus: subgroup or misclassification? *Arch. Dis. Child.* 2006, 91, 473-477.

Richardson MW, Richardson MW, Ang L, Visintainer PF, Wittcopp CA.The abnormal measures of iron homeostasis in pediatric obesity are associated with the inflammation of obesity. *Int J Pediatr Endocrinol.*; 2009:713269. Epub 2009 Oct 8.

Rolandsson O, Hägg E, Hampe C, Sullivan EP, Nilsson M, Jansson G, Hallmans G, Lernmark A. Glutamate decarboxylase (GAD65) and tyrosine phosphatase-like protein (IA-2) autoantibodies index in a regional population is related to glucose intolerance and body mass index. *Diabetologia* 1999, 42, 555-559.

Rosenbloom A, Joe JR, Young RS, Winter WE. Emerging Epidemic of Type 2 Diabetes in Youth. Diabetes Care 1999, 22: 345–354.

Särnblad S., Ingberg CM, Åman J, Schvarcz E. Body composition in young female adults with Type 1 diabetes mellitus. A prospective case-control study. *DIABETIC Medicine*, DOI: 10.1111/j.1464-5491.2007.02144.x

Scharfetter H, Schlager T, Stollberger R, Felsberger R, Hutten H and Hinghofer-Szalkay H. Assessing abdominal fatness with local bioimpedance analysis: basics and experimental findings. *International Journal of Obesity* (2001) 25, 502 ± 511.

Schaumberg DA, Glynn RJ, Jenkins AJ, Lyons TJ, Rifai N, Manson JE, Ridker PM, Nathan DM (2005). Effect of Intensive Glycemic Control on Levels of Markers of Inflammation in Type 1 Diabetes Mellitus in the Diabetes Control and Complications Trial. *Circulation* 2005; 111; 2446-2453.

Sibley SD, Palmer JP, Hirsch IB and Brunzell JD. Visceral Obesity, Hepatic Lipase Activity, and Dyslipidemia in Type 1 Diabetes. *J Clin Endocrinol Metab*, July 2003, 88 (7): 3379–3384.

Silva EA, Flexa F, Zanella MT. Impact of abdominal fat and insulin resistance on arterial hypertension in non-obese women. *Arq Bras Endocrinol Metab.* 2009; 53/3.

Sociedade Brasileira de Hipertensão. Sociedade Brasileira de Cardiologia e Sociedade Brasileira de Nefrologia 2002 IV. Diretrizes Brasileiras de hipertensão arterial. p.5-7.

Sun G, French CR, Martin GR, Younghusband B, Green RC, Xie Y, Mathews M, Barron JR, Fitzpatrick DG, Gulliver W and Zhang H. Comparison of multifrequency bioelectrical impedance analysis with dual-energy X-ray absorptiometry for assessment of percentage body fat in a large, healthy population. *Am J Clin Nutr* 2005; 81: 74–8.

Terry RB, Wood PDS, Haskell WL, Stefanick ML, Krauss RM. Regional adiposity patterns in relation to lipids, lipoprotein cholesterol, and lipoprotein subfraction mass in men. *J Clin Endocrinol Metab* 1989; 68: 191-9.

The Diabetes Control and Complications Trial (DCCT) Research Group. Effects of age, duration and treatment of insulin-dependent diabetes mellitus on residual betacell function: observations during eligibility testing for the Diabetes control and Complications Trial (DCCT). *J Clin Endocrinol Metab* 1987; 65: 30-6.

The Diabetes Control and Complications Trial Research Group. The effect of intensive treatment of diabetes on the development and progression of long-term complications in insulin-dependent diabetes mellitus. *NEJM*, 1993, 329 (14): 977-986.

Thomson R, Brinkworth GD, Buckley JD, Noakes M and Clifton PM. Good agreement between bioelectrical impedance and dual-energy X-ray absorptiometry for estimating changes in body composition during weight loss in overweight young women. *Clinical Nutrition* (2007) 26, 771–777.

Van Harmelen V, Reynisdottir S, Eriksson P, Thörne A, Hoffstedt J, Lönnqvist F and Arner P. Leptin Secretion From Subcutaneous and Visceral Adipose Tissue in Women. *Diabetes*, Vol. 47, June 1998.

Verbeeten KC, Elks CE, Daneman D, Ong KK. Association between childhood obesity and subsequent Type 1 diabetes: a systematic review and meta-analysis. *Diabetic Medicine* 2011 Jan: 28 (1): 10-8.

Völgyi E, Tylavsky FA, Lyytikäinen A, Suominen H, Alén M and Cheng S. Assessing Body Composition With DXA and Bioimpedance: Effects of Obesity, Physical Activity, and Age. *Obesity* (2008) 16, 700–705.

Wang, Y., Monteiro C., Popkin B.M. Trends of obesity and underweight in older children and adolescents in the United States, Brazil, China, and Russia1-3. *Am J Clin Nutr*; 75:971-7, 2002.

Wardle J, Carnell S, Haworth CMA, Farooqi IS, O'Rahilly S and Plomin R. Obesity Associated Genetic Variation in *FTO* Is Associated with Diminished Satiety. *J Clin Endocrinol Metab* 93: 3640–3643, 2008.

Wellen K., Hotamisligil G. Inflammation, stress, and diabetes. *J. Clin. Invest.* 2005, 115:1111–1119.

Welsh P, Polisecki E, Robertson M, Jahn S, Buckley BM, Craen AJM, Ford I, Jukema JW, Macfarlane PW, Packard CJ, Stott DJ, Westendorp RGJ, Shepherd J, Hingorani AD, Smith GD, Schaefer E and Sattar N. Unraveling the Directional Link between Adiposity and Inflammation: A Bidirectional Mendelian Randomization Approach. *J Clin Endocrinol Metab* 95: 93–99, 2010.

Wilkin TJ. The accelerator hypothesis: weight gain as the missing link between Type I and Type II diabetes. *Diabetologia* 2001;44:914-22.

Willi SM, Egede LE. Type 2 diabetes mellitus in adolescents. *Current Opinion in Endocrinology & Diabetes*, 2000, 7:71–76.

Williams KV, Erbey JR, Becker D, Orchard TJ. Improved glycemic control reduces the impact of weight gain on cardiovascular risk factors in type 1 diabetes. The Epidemiology of Diabetes Complications Study. *Diabetes Care* 1999; 22: 1084–1091.

Yki-Jarvinen H, Koivisto VA. Natural course of insulin resistance in type 1 diabetes. *N Engl J Med* 1986; 315: 224-30.

10

Meta-Analysis of Genome-Wide Association Studies to Understand Disease Relatedness

Stephanie N. Lewis, Elaine O. Nsoesie, Charles Weeks,
Dan Qiao and Liqing Zhang
Virginia Tech, Blacksburg, VA
USA

1. Introduction

Genome-wide association studies (GWAS) have become a popular method of surveying haplotype variations within populations. The recent explosion and success of these studies has allowed for identification of multiple gene variations and non-genetic risk factors that are often involved in pathogenesis of many diseases (Xavier&Rioux, 2008). Efforts to archive these single nucleotide polymorphisms (SNPs) and make the information publicly available have been made possible by the International Haplotype Map Project (HapMap) (The International HapMap Consortium, 2005; The International HapMap Consortium, 2007) and development of GWAS databases (Johnson&O'Donnell, 2009) such as Genomes.gov (Hindorff et al., 2009). The HapMap database of genetic variants and the ever progressing technology involved in identifying genetic disease susceptibility markers has allowed for identification of shared genetic associations that were undetectable with previous methods for identifying deleterious mutations effects for individual genes (Xavier&Rioux, 2008). We are now capable of detecting common susceptibility markers between previously unassociated diseases with the ability to assess combined association signals shared by biological pathways (Wang et al., 2011).

Research of immune-mediated disease susceptibility has benefited from the discovery of shared haplotypes. GWAS with a focus on autoimmune diseases, which included celiac disease, Crohn's disease, multiple sclerosis, rheumatoid arthritis, systemic lupus erythematosus, and type 1 diabetes (Lettre&Rioux, 2008), have shed light on shared genetic markers. Such markers can be exploited to identify biomedical traits that translate to improved diagnostic and treatment techniques (McCarthy et al., 2008). Under the common disease/common variant hypothesis (Wang et al., 2005), one would assume that shared variants result in shared disease phenotypes, and this commonality could serve as a global target for effective treatment options. It is under this assumption that many disease association studies are conducted. The Wellcome Trust Case Control Consortium (WTCCC) conducted a study in which nearly 2000 individuals were examined for coronary artery disease (CAD), hypertension, type II diabetes (T2D), rheumatoid arthritis (RA), Crohn's disease (CD), type I diabetes (T1D) and bipolar disorder (BD) susceptibility against a shared set of about 3000 controls (The Wellcome Trust Case Control Consortium, 2007). The study revealed several association loci for the seven diseases, with some of these indicating risk for more than one of the studied diseases (The Wellcome Trust Case Control Consortium, 2007).

Huang et al. used the data from the WTCCC study to see if associations could be made between the seven diseases given the loci and collections of other data regarding disease susceptibility (Huang et al., 2009). Huang et al. performed analyses at four levels (nucleotide, gene, protein, and phenotype) to determine the existence of overlap across SNPs associated with the seven diseases and constructed protein-protein interaction networks to visualize similarities between diseases (Huang et al., 2009). The group found strong associations across all four levels of analysis for the autoimmune group (CD, RA, and T1D), while no genetic associations were found at any level within the metabolic/cardiovascular group (CAD, hypertension and T2D) (Huang et al., 2009). These results reasserted some expectations derived from clinical literature in the case of the autoimmune group, and suggested inappropriate disease grouping in the case of the metabolic/cardiovascular group (Huang et al., 2009).

For this study, we proposed a large-scale disease and phenotype comparison based on the WTCCC and Huang et al. studies. To this end, we have combined data from GWAS with expression pattern data to determine if genetic and expression similarities exist between diseases. A total of 61 human diseases and phenotypes were assessed. Disease relatedness networks (DRNs) were constructed to visually assess associations on a larger scale. We also took advantage of high-throughput molecular assay technologies to incorporate mRNA expression profiles of diseases, and thus added another dimension of analysis toward assessing disease relationships. Gene expression is an indicator of cellular state, and gene expression profiles can be considered as quantitative traits that are highly heritable. The link between organismal complex traits, such as disease-related phenotype, and gene expression variation has been theoretically accepted (Goring et al., 2007; Moffatt et al., 2007; Chen et al., 2008; Emilsson et al., 2008). With the declining per-sample costs of high-throughput microarray experiments, the amount of gene expression data in international repositories has grown exponentially. The availability of these datasets for many different diseases provides an opportunity to use data-driven approaches to improve our understanding of disease relationships. Hu and Agarwal (Hu&P., 2009) determined disease-disease and disease-drug networks using large-scale gene expression data. Very recently, Suthram et al. (Suthram et al., 2010) presented a quantitative framework to compare and contrast diseases by combining both disease-related mRNA expression data and human protein interaction data. Although GWAS provide comprehensive views of disease interrelationships at the DNA level, the insights from the gene expression aspect, which reflects cellular phenotype, will further advance and strengthen the understanding of this issue. A large-scale disease comparison study such as this has the potential to uncover relationships between diseases and phenotypes that are often overlooked in single disease SNP data analysis.

2. Methods

2.1 SNP-based genetic analysis

Five populations were considered for this expansion study: Han Chinese (CHB), Japanese (JPT), a combined CHB and JPT population (CHB+JPT), Yoruba (YRI), and U.S. residents with northern and western European ancestry (CEU). SNP dataset 2009-02_rel24 (The International HapMap Consortium, 2005; The International HapMap Consortium, 2007) was downloaded from the HapMap site and the SNP set was expanded by means of linkage disequilibrium (LD). SNPs with an r^2 greater than or equal to 0.5 were included. SNPs were divided by associated disease or phenotype (listed in Table 1) and the divisions were maintained for each succeeding level of analysis. SNPs were divided into blocks based on an r^2 greater than or equal to 0.1. Gene names from Ensembl (Birney et al., 2004) were assigned to blocks if the genetic location was within 2 kilobases up- or downstream of the gene of interest or within the start and end bases for the gene. Gene data were cross-referenced against pathway-specific gene lists generated from the KEGG database (Kanehisa&Goto, 2000; Kanehisa et al., 2006; Kanehisa et al., 2010) in order to assign genes to identified pathways. Pairwise comparisons for each level were conducted to see if diseases and phenotpyes shared SNPs, blocks, genes, or pathway designations. Jaccard index values were calculated for each comparison at each level to assess similarity. Using the Jaccard indexes, DRNs were constructed to visualize the strength of relatedness between diseases. DRNs were visually inspected to identify the strongest relationships. Suggested associations were verified by principal components analysis (PCA) and minor data mining for clinical relevance. Complete details of these methods were previously described by Lewis et al (Lewis et al., 2011).

2.2 Gene expression dataset

The gene expression data used in this analysis was obtained from the NCBI Gene Expression Omnibus (GEO) (Barrett et al., 2009). Not all of the 61 diseases were represented by expression data on the GEO site. Data for a subset of diseases was found by scanning the experimental context of a collection of GEO data (or GEO Series, GSE) for microarrays that were assigned to human disease conditions. Only those microarrays that were curated and reported in the GEO Datasets (or GDS) were used in our analysis. The data set was also restricted to those GSEs in which both the disease and the corresponding control condition (from healthy tissue samples) were measured in the same tissue. For consistency, we further restricted the GSEs to only those datasets which used Affymetrix Gene Chip Human Genome U133 Array Set HG-U133A (GPL96), HG-U133B (GPL97) and HG-U133plus2 (GPL570), which are among the most commonly used platforms. Probes for these platforms were mapped to the current gene identifiers (Chen et al., 2007). This process yielded nineteen diseases for the final GEO analysis.

2.3 Expression measurement

To quantitatively compare expression data, we first normalized the data in each microarray sample using the Z-score transformation to make the expression values across various microarray samples and diseases comparable. Next, we performed an unpaired two-sample Student t-test to compute the t-test statistic and p-value of each gene between the disease and control groups. We only used the most appropriate Affymetrix probe set in which a single probe was representative of each gene. The most appropriate Affymetrix probe set was adopted from the work of Hu et al. (Hu&Agarwal, 2009) as many genes were represented by multiple probe sets in Affymetrix U133 microarray chips. This modification avoided correlation and scoring biases brought on by over-representation of those genes. 18,600 most appropriate probes/genes for each of nineteen diseases were identified. The genes were grouped with statistically significant high t-test statistics ($p<0.05$) as "up-regulated genes" and statistically significant low t-test statistics ($p<0.05$) as "down-regulated genes". Instead of using a p-value threshold as a cutoff to identify significantly changed genes, the 200 and 1000 most changed genes were designated as the disease-associated significantly changed genes for each disease state. The lowest p-values in each category

Abbreviation	Disease/Phenotype	Abbreviation	Disease/Phenotype	Abbreviation	Disease/Phenotype	Abbreviation	Disease/Phenotype
AD	Alzheimer's disease	EO	Early onset extreme obesity	LM	Lipid measurements	QT	Cardiac repolarization (QT interval)
AF	Atrial Fibrillation/Atrial Flutter	GCA	General cognitive ability	LOAD	Late-onset Alzheimer's disease	RA	Rheumatoid Arthritis
ALS	Amyotrophic Lateral Sclerosis	GD	Gallstone disease	LONG	Longevity and age-related phenotypes	RLS	Restless Leg Syndrome
BA	Brain aging	GLA	Glaucoma	MHA	Minor histocompatibility antigenicity	SA	Subclinical atherosclerosis
BC	Breast cancer	HAE	Hepatic adverse events with thrombin inhibitor ximelagatran	MI	Myocardial infarction	SALS	Sporadic Amyotrophic lateral Sclerosis
BD	Bipolar disorder	HBF	Adult fetal hemoglobin levels (HbF) by F cell levels	MS	Multiple sclerosis	SCP	Sleep and circadian phenotypes
BL	Blood lipids	HEI	Height	ND	Nicotine dependence	SLCL	Serum LDL cholesterol levels
BMG	Bone mass and geometry	HEM	Human episodic memory	NEU	Neuroticism	SLE	Systemic Lupus Erythematosus
BPAS	Blood pressure and arterial stiffness	HIV1	HIV-1 disease progression	OBE	Obesity-related traits	SP	Schizophrenia
CA	Childhood asthma	HT	Haematological (blood) traits	PA	Polysubstance addiction	SPBC	Sporadic post-menopausal breast cancer
CAD	Coronary Artery Disease	HYP	Hypertension	PC	Prostate cancer	SPM	Skin pigmentation
CC	Colorectal cancer	IC	Iris color	PD	Parkinson's disease	STR	Stroke
CD	Crohn's disease	IMAN	Immunoglobulin A nephropathy	PF	Pulmonary function phenotypes	T1D	Type I Diabetes
CDI	Celiac disease	IS	Ischemic stroke	PR	Psoriasis	T2D	Type II Diabetes
CS	Coronary spasm	KFET	Kidney function and endocrine traits	PSP	Progressive Supranuclear Palsy	TG	Triglycerides
CVD	Cardiovascular Disease outcomes						

Table 1. List of diseases and phenotypes considered for this study and the previous study (Lewis et al., 2011) with corresponding abbreviations.

(up-regulated, down-regulated, and combined) for the top 200 or 1000 genes were pooled for each disease. All of the genes with significant expression changes were grouped together and Jaccard index values were calculated. Gene lists for each disease were compared pair-wise for each of the three expression categories. Here, a high Jaccard index implied a high degree of commonality between diseases/phenotypes. The Jaccard indexes were normalized to produce Z-scores, which were then used as a measure of disease relatedness. The significantly changed genes shared by two diseases were also subjected to Gene Ontology (GO) term enrichment analysis using the web-based Gene Ontology enrichment analysis and visualization (GOrilla) tool (Eden et al., 2007; Eden et al., 2009).

2.4 Medical subject headings (MeSH) term mapping

MeSH is the National Library of Medicine's controlled vocabulary thesaurus (Bodenreider et al., 1998). It consists of sets of terms associated with descriptors in a hierarchical structure. For the nineteen GEO validation diseases (Table 2), the MeSH trees were downloaded and the first level of each tree was used as the disease category. The category that could best indicate the cause of the disease was taken as the disease category.

3. Results

3.1 Summary of significant disease associations for screening of 61 diseases and phenotypes

Jaccard index values were used to assess similarity between diseases and phenotypes within each level of analysis. Correlation between the levels was also assessed using the Spearman correlation method. High correlation was seen between the SNP and block data sets, while low correlation was seen between the pathway data and the other three levels of analysis. The progression from SNP to block, block to gene, and gene to pathway levels resulted in a grouping of susceptibility markers. Visualization of the associations by means of DRNs suggested the grouping translated to an increase in the strength of associations between diseases. This was also reflected in the distribution of Jaccard indexes for each level. Figure 1 shows a slight distribution shift to the right from SNP level to pathway level.

The DRNs suggested consistent association between several diseases for the SNP, block, and gene levels. The strongest associations seen for all populations were observed between (multiple sclerosis [MS], T1D, and RA), with noticeable association between (haematological traits [HT] and adult fetal hemoglobin levels [HBF]) and (serum low-density lipopolysaccharide cholesterol levels [SLCL] and lipid measurements [LM]). Several other less significant associations were suggested by the DRNs as well, but these associations were not consistent in significance for all populations. The qualitative assessments made by examining the DRNs were verified using PCA, which allowed for quantitative isolation of the strongest relationships. The PCA results matched the visual assessment for all levels, and suggested additional strong associations unique to specific populations were present. For example, an association between (LM and triglyceride levels [TG]) that was unique to the JPT population was suggested that was not outwardly apparent by visual inspection of the DRNs. This association was found in the CHB+JPT populations, but not the CHB population. JPT was also missing the (HBF and HT) association that was observed in the other populations. Further details regarding the results of this portion of the study were previously submitted for publication (Lewis et al., 2011).

Disease	platform	GEO record	Sample Size Disease	Sample Size Control	MeSH category
AD	GPL96	GSE1297	22	9	Nervous System Diseases [C10] Mental Disorders [F03]
ALS	GPL96 and 97	GSE3307	9	16	Nervous System Diseases [C10] Nutritional and Metabolic Diseases [C18]
BD	GPL96	GSE5388	30	31	Mental Disorders [F03]
BC	GPL96 and 97	GSE6883	6	3	Neoplasms [C04] Skin and Connective Tissue Diseases [C17]
CD	GPL96	GSE3365	59	42	Digestive System Diseases [C06]
IS	GPL96	GSE1869	6	10	Cardiovascular Diseases [C14]
OBE	GPL96	GSE474	16	8	Nutritional and Metabolic Diseases [C18]
PD	GPL96	GSE6613	50	22	Nervous System Diseases [C10]
PR	GPL96	GSE6710	13	13	Skin and Connective Tissue Diseases [C17]
SLE	GPL96 and 97	GSE11909	103	12	Skin and Connective Tissue Diseases [C17] Immune System Diseases [C20]
CAD	GPL96	GSE12288	110	120	Cardiovascular Diseases [C14]
T1D	GPL570	GSE10586	12	15	Nutritional and Metabolic Diseases [C18] Endocrine System Diseases [C19] Immune System Diseases [C20]
T2D	GPL96 and 97	GSE9006	12	24	Nutritional and Metabolic Diseases [C18] Endocrine System Diseases [C19]
CA	GPL570	GSE8052	268	136	Respiratory Tract Diseases [C08] Immune System Diseases [C20]
CC	GPL570	GSE9348	70	12	Neoplasms [C04] Digestive System Diseases [C06]
ND	GPL570	GSE11208	6	5	Disorders of Environmental Origin [C21] Mental Disorders [F03]
SP	GPL570	GSE4036	14	14	Mental Disorders [F03]
AF	GPL96 and 97	GSE2240	10	5	Cardiovascular Diseases [C14]
PSP	GPL96	GSE6613	6	22	Nervous System Diseases [C10] Eye Diseases [C11]

Table 2. List of nineteen diseases in gene expression analysis and their MeSH classification.

3.2 Clustering of genetic associations

Based on the observations made using the DRNs, agglomerative hierarchical clustering was used to find groups of diseases. At each level, the 61 diseases/phenotypes were clustered into ten groups. The number of clusters was set to ten based on visual inspection of the

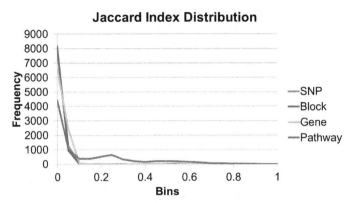

Fig. 1. Graphical representation of histogram data showing distribution of all Jaccard indexes for all populations at each level of analysis. Index values were grouped and then divided into twenty bins across the range zero to one. (N = 9150 for each analysis level)

hierarchical branching of the trees. Representative clustering results are shown for the CHB+JPT population in Figure 2. The CHB+JPT population showed a high correlation to most populations at all levels of analysis based on the Rand Index for similarity. The Rand Index for similarity was used to compare the clustering across populations at each level. The diseases within each cluster were least similar at the SNP level for all populations and most similar at the gene level across most of the populations. At the SNP level groupings, associations between (MS, RA, and T1D), (HBF and HT), and (breast cancer [BC] and sporadic post-menopausal breast cancer [SPBC]) were found for all populations (Figure 2A). The grouping of (RA and T1D), (BC and SPBC), (HBF and HT), (Amyotrophic Lateral Sclerosis [ALS] and Parkinson's disease [PD]) and (colorectal cancer [CC] and prostate cancer [PC]) were consistent at the block level for all populations (Figure 2B). At the gene level, the number of diseases/phenotypes included in each cluster increased with consistent groups again observed for all populations. These groups included (MS, RA, and T1D), (ALS, PD, CAD, Alzheimer's disease [AD] and T2D), and (neuroticism [NEU], brain aging [BA], and sleep and circadian phenotypes [SCP]) (Figure 2C). Clusters at the pathway level were also much larger than at the other levels. No consistent relationships were seen for the clusters containing a larger number of diseases, but the smaller groupings consistently showed relationships between (longevity and age-related phenotypes [LONG] and early onset extreme obesity [EO]), (cardiovascular disease outcomes [CVD], CD, and NEU) and (blood lipids [BL], LM, and Restless Leg Syndrome [RLS]) (Figure 2D). Four populations suggested clustering of (LONG, EO, and T1D), while one, YRI, showed a relationship between (LONG, EO, and SLCL).

3.3 Gene expression analysis

The gene expression profiles showed some patterns for the three expression categories (up-regulated, down-regulated, and combined), with the number of strong associations increasing with cutoff type (top 200 most changed genes, top 1000 most changed genes, and changes with a p-value less than 0.05). Jaccard indexes for each disease/phenotype pair were calculated and used to construct DRNs, which are shown in Figure 3. Strong associations between (PD, Progressive Supranuclear Palsy [PSP], and nicotine dependence

[ND]), (ischemic stroke [IS], CC, and CD), and (CAD and childhood asthma [CA]) were observed under all three cutoff scenarios for all three expression categories of analysis. Of these, the (CAD and CA) pair showed the most variation in association strength for all the variables considered.

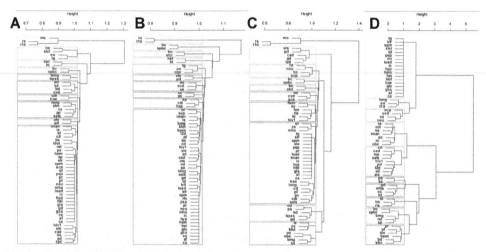

Fig. 2. Clustering dendrogram for 61 disease/phenotype comparisons at the (A) SNP, (B) block, (C) gene, and (D) pathway levels. Colored boxes indicate the clusters derived from Rand Index analysis. Results for the CHB+JPT population are shown as a representative data set for all populations.

Links between disease classifications were also seen. Connections between nervous system diseases and disorders of environmental origin (i.e., (PSP and ND) and (PD and ND)) were seen in all three expression categories and cutoff types. Associations between nervous system and mental disorders (e.g., AD and BD) were seen for the top 200 and top 1000 groups, but this association was masked in the p-value-derived group. For the p-value group, predominate associations between metabolic, cardiovascular, digestive, and immune system diseases were found. One unexpected classification association was the nervous system-metabolic disease link exemplified by (PSP and OBE) and (PD and OBE) for the down-regulation and subsequently combined expression groups with the top 1000 and p-value cutoffs.

As expected, the number of significant associations increased as the threshold criteria increased given that the quantity of data available for comparison was greater. Seemingly strong associations observed at the top 200 cutoff, such as the (AD and BD) and (BD and SP) associations were masked in the p-value cutoff data as other stronger associations were present. The increase in maximum Jaccard index for the combined expression data set from 0.44 to 0.81 agreed with this observation. Though we saw an increase in relationship strength with less stringent cutoff thresholds, the additional comparison data resulted in reduction in significant associations. Therefore, the expression categories for the p-value cutoff group were used to compare with the SNP-based data in order to avoid assigning an arbitrary cutoff for the expression data and to ensure enough data was available for the nineteen-disease comparison.

3.4 Comparison of the SNP and expression data for nineteen diseases

Correlation between data sets may have been influenced by the data sources. Both the SNP and block levels encompassed data from the HapMap site. The gene level data was obtained by cross referencing the HapMap data against the Ensembl database of gene names. The pathway data was obtained by cross referencing the Ensembl-derived data against the KEGG database. Given that the amount of data available through each of these sources is not consistent, there was loss of data in the transition from blocks to genes and genes to pathways. Of the reduced set of nineteen diseases and phenotypes compared, only atrial fibrillation/atrial flutter (AF) did not contain gene data for the SNP-based comparisons. The number of missing diseases/phenotypes increased to four at the pathway level (i.e., AF, CA, psoriasis [PR], and PSP). Despite the missing disease associations for AF, the gene level of analysis was used for comparison to the expression data. The range of Z-scores for this dataset was closest to the range seen for the expression data, and intuitively, the gene data should show some correlation to gene expression.

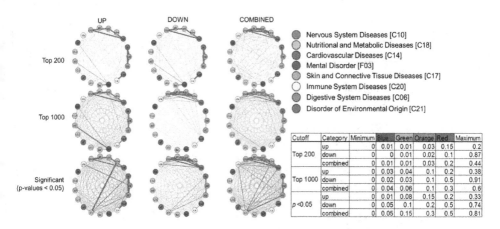

Fig. 3. DRNs for expression data for the three cutoff levels (top 200, top 1000, and significance with p-value < 0.05) and three expression categories (up-regulated, down-regulated, and combined). Disease nodes are color coded to show grouping of diseases based on MeSH classification. Edges are color coded according to increasing strength of disease association. Values for the color scale are listed in the inserted table.

DRNs comparing the gene level of analysis for the CEU, CHB+JPT, and YRI populations to the expression data are shown in Figure 4. The JPT and CHB populations are not shown since the CHB+JPT population is highly representative of the individual populations. A Spearman correlation was calculated between each population for the SNP-based data set and the expression data (Table 3). A weak negative correlation was observed between the genetic and expression data, suggesting no significant relationships were shared between the two data sets. A qualitative analysis of the networks and clustering from the SNP-based data analysis suggested a high degree of similarity between the predicted associations for all population. However, the strong associations observed in the genetic analysis were not seen in the expression data. Rather, a seemingly reciprocal relationship appeared between the genetic and expression DRNs. The strongest expression-based association was between ALS and obesity-related traits (OBE), which was in the weakest associations group for the SNP-based associations. An examination of the genetic DRNs suggested the strongest associations between (ALS and PD), (AD and T2D), and (T1D and SLE). These associations were weak for the expression data. Some associations near the middle of the Z-score range appeared more common between the data sets, such as the (IS and CC), (AD and BD), and (OBE and CC) pairs.

61 diseases	CEU	CHB	JPT	CHB+JPT	YRI
CEU	1	0.9599	0.9595	0.9574	0.9447
CHB		1	0.9779	0.9925	0.9726
JPT			1	0.9858	0.9556
CHB+JPT				1	0.9686
YRI					1
19 diseases					
GEO	-0.1367	-0.1228	-0.1278	-0.1254	-0.1176

Table 3. Spearman correlation coefficients between populations and between each population and the GEO data. The Spearman correlation is a comparison of the ranked Z-scores for each data set.

Despite the overall lack of correlation between the genetic and expression analyses, several unexpected links between neurological and cardiovascular/metabolic diseases were observed in both data sets (i.e., (AD and T2D) and (PD and OBE)). These potentially novel disease relationships may primarily rely on genetic similarity or genomic expression similarity instead of phenotypic classification, but this idea would need to be further explored.

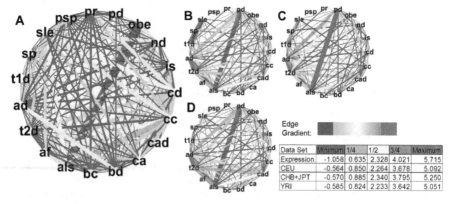

Fig. 4. DRNs based on Z-scores for three populations and expression data. DRNs for (A) combined expression data for significantly changed genes (p<0.05), (B) CEU gene level, (C) CHB+JPT gene level, and (D) YRI gene level are shown. Edge live color and width correspond to strength of association between disease pairs. The gradient and corresponding values are listed in the inserted table.

4. Discussion

The results from this study suggested it is possible to elucidate genetic similarities that can be overlooked during single disease GWAS. Several expected associations supported by literature were found (e.g. association between (SLE and RA) and (EO and SLCL)) while some unexpected associations were also observed. The unexpected neurological-cardiovascular/metabolic disease associations were observed for both the genetic analysis and the expression profile analysis. Though the origin and symptoms associated with diseases in each category may be different, the results suggest genetic similarities. Possible explanations for these associations cannot be elucidated solely from this study given the broad nature of the comparison. A detailed SNP-by-SNP and gene-by-gene examination may indicate the reason behind the neurological-cardiovascular/metabolic relatedness. Those relationships are particularly interesting and may indicate some common underlying molecular mechanism among these disease groups that has not yet been widely studied. Clinical evidence supports the strongest relationships identified from the expression data. PSP and PD share some common symptoms such as stiffness, and movement difficulties which could explain the common expression pattern indicating some degree of relatedness between the two. On the other hand, explaining the relationship between PSP and ND is more difficult. Several studies have shown that smokers have a lower risk of developing Parkinson's disease (Soto-Otero et al., 1998; Hernan et al., 2001; Quik, 2004). One recently published paper showed that smoking for a greater number of years may reduce the risk of the disease (Chen et al., 2010). An earlier study suggested that younger patients with CD might be under an increased risk of IS (Andersohn et al., 2010). Extensive studies have demonstrated a strong association between CD and CC (Gillen et al., 1994). The relationship between (IS and CC) and (CAD and CA) is also unclear, but shared immune-dependent responses may be the common link.

Similarities and differences were observed between the three categories (up-regulated, down-regulated and combined) of gene expression analysis (see Figure 3). The different association patterns may be due to the use of a single rule to identify disease associated genes for all kinds of diseases, which over simplifies the problem. Theoretically, variance of gene expression can be considered as a quantitative trait inherited from genetic variation. It is possible that a combined DNA variant and expression phenotype can better explain genetic architecture with reduced environmental and biological noise (Dermitzakis, 2008). However, the precise and reliable estimation of molecular link between functional genomic effects and complex organism phenotypes depends on a large number of pooled variant and gene expression data from corresponding tissues or cell types, since tissue-specific differences can be found widely (Dermitzakis, 2008). A combined genetic and gene expression profile study, as presented here, can shed light on disease relatedness from different perspectives. Parikh et al. performed a more direct comparison of GWAS and expression data in an effort to prioritize T2D susceptibility genes (Parikh et al., 2009). The group isolated SNPs from GWAS, searched for associated genes, and then found corresponding tissue-specific expression profiles for a subset of all the SNP-associated genes (Parikh et al., 2009). Parikh et al. were able to identify five genes common to individuals with T2D and twelve genes with differentiating expression patterns in individuals with versus without the disease (Parikh et al., 2009). Rather than focusing on a single disease to identify targets, we strove for a more global comparison of genetic and expression data.

Even though discrepancies between our data sets were observed, it is possible that the reduction in data between the gene and pathway level could have excluded some genes common to multiple diseases. With the increased density of GWAS and gene expression studies, the discrepancies and anomalies observed in this study might be better understood. We set out to support the idea that diseases potentially share phenotype similarity as a result of genetic factors, pathway associations, expression regulation, or some combination of these three ideas. Within the autoimmune disease group, we observed diseases that possessed some genetic similarity. We saw expected strong associations between T1D, MS, and RA, as well as less expected associations between AD and T2D. It would appear that systemic inflammation responses may be the key to shared susceptibility among many of the diseases and phenotypes for which we observed relatedness. Clinical studies suggested individuals with one immune-mediated disease, such as T1D, may be more susceptible to pathogenesis of another (Dorman et al., 2003; Nielson et al., 2006; Toussirot et al., 2006; Doran, 2007). It has also been clinically suggested that inflammation plays a role in neurological diseases like AD (Akiyama et al., 2000; Perry, 2004) and PD (Perry, 2004). We also know that cardiovascular and metabolic diseases, such as atherosclerosis, T2D, and OBE have links to chronic inflammatory responses (Stienstra et al., 2006; Tontonoz&Spiegelman, 2008). In all of these cases, our results suggest the clinical manifestations may have genetic relevance and the unexpected cardiovascular/neurological links may be important. Given the broad scope of this study, the conclusions made here are suggestions for where genetic commonality could be found without specific identification of the related targets. A more detailed disease-by-disease analysis similar to the study conducted by Parikh et al. (Parikh et al., 2009) would need to be conducted to identify specific genes of interest shared by diseases. The methods used in the Parikh et al. study can be specifically applied to the study of T1D by performing a detailed step-by-step comparison between this disease and other possibly related diseases in order to elucidate genetic commonalities to T1D. The results from our study and from one tailored specifically for T1D could influence current treatment options and suggest new approaches for managing and treating the disease. We feel our study is a strong example of how GWAS and expression data can be used conjunctively to predict significant disease associations relevant to improving and unifying diagnoses and treatment options for multiple immune-mediated diseases.

5. Acknowledgements

The authors would like to acknowledge the faculty and students of the Spring 2010 Genetics, Bioinformatics, and Computational Biology Problem Solving course for feedback regarding the progress of this study.

6. References

Akiyama, H., S. Barger, et al. (2000). "Inflammation and Alzheimer's." Neurobiology of Aging 21(3): 383-421.

Andersohn, F., M. Waring, et al. (2010). "Risk of ischemic stroke in patients with Crohn's disease: A population-based nested case-control study." Inflammatory Bowel Disease 16(8): 1387-1392.

Barrett, T., D. Troup, et al. (2009). "NCBI GEO: archive for high-throughput functional genomic data." Nucleic Acids Research 37: D885-D890.

Birney, E., T. D. Andrews, et al. (2004). "An overview of Ensembl." Genome Research 14(5): 925-928.

Bodenreider, O., S. Nelson, et al. (1998). Beyond synonymy: exploiting the UMLS semantics in mapping vocabularies. Annual Symposium of the American Medical Informatics Association, Orlando, FL, Hanley & Belfus, Inc.

Chen, H., X. Huang, et al. (2010). "Smoking, duration, intensity, and risk of Parkinson disease." Neurology 74(11): 878-884.

Chen, R., L. Li, et al. (2007). "AILUN: reannotating gene expression data automatically." Nature Methods 4(11): 879.

Chen, Y., J. Zhu, et al. (2008). "Variations in DNA elucidate molecular networks that cause disease." Nature 452(7186): 429-435.

Dermitzakis, E. T. (2008). "From gene expression to disease risk." Nature genetics 40(5): 492-493.

Doran, M. (2007). "Rheumatoid arthritis and diabetes mellitus: evidence for an association?" The Journal of Rhematology 34(3): 460-462.

Dorman, J. S., A. R. Steenkiste, et al. (2003). "Type 1 Diabetes and Multiple Sclerosis." Diabetes Care 26(11): 3192-3193.

Eden, E., D. Lipson, et al. (2007). "Discovering Motifs in Ranked Lists of DNA Sequences." PLoS Computational Biology 3(3): e39.

Eden, E., R. Navon, et al. (2009). "GOrilla: A Tool for Discovery and Visualization of Enriched GO Terms in Ranked Gene Lists." BMC Bioinformatics 10: 48.

Emilsson, V., G. Thorleifsson, et al. (2008). "Genetics of gene expression and its effect on disease." Nature 452(7186): 423-428.

Gillen, C. D., H. A. Andrews, et al. (1994). "Crohn's disease and colorectal cancer." Gut 35(5): 651-655.

Goring, H. H. H., J. E. Curran, et al. (2007). "Discovery of expression QTLs using large-scale transcriptional profiling in human lymphocytes." Nature Genetics 39: 1208-1216.

Hernan, M. A., S. M. Zhang, et al. (2001). "Cigarette Smoking and the Incidence of Parkinson's Disease in Two Prospective Studies." Annals of Neurology 50(6): 780-786.

Hindorff, L. A., P. Sethupathy, et al. (2009). "Potential etiologic and functional implications of genome-wide association loci for human diseases and traits." PNAS 106(23): 9362-9367.

Hu, G. and P. Agarwal. (2009). "Human disease-drug network based on genomic expression profiles." PLoS One 4(8): e6536.

Huang, W., P. Wang, et al. (2009). "Indentifying disease associations via genome-wide association studies." BMC Bioinformatics 10: 1-11.

Johnson, A. D. and C. J. O'Donnell (2009). "An Open Access Database of Genome-wide Association Results." BMC Medical Genetics 10: 1-6.

Kanehisa, M. and S. Goto (2000). "KEGG: Kyoto Encyclopedia of Genes and Genomes." Nucleic Acids Research 28(27-30).

Kanehisa, M., S. Goto, et al. (2010). "KEGG for representation and analysis of molecular networks involving diseases and drugs." Nucleic Acids Research 38: D355-D360.

Kanehisa, M., S. Goto, et al. (2006). "From genomics to chemical genomics: new developments in KEGG." Nucleic Acids Research 34: D354-D357.

Lettre, G. and J. D. Rioux (2008). "Autoimmune diseases: insights from genome-wide assocation studies." Human Molecular Genetics 17(2): R116-R121.

Lewis, S. N., E. Nsoesie, et al. (2011). "Prediction of Disease and Phenotype Associations from Genome-Wide Association Studies." PLoS One Submitted for Review.

McCarthy, M. I., G. R. Abecasis, et al. (2008). "Genome-wide Association Studies for Complex Traits: Consensus, Uncertainty and Challenges." Nature 9: 356-369.

Moffatt, M. F., M. Kabesch, et al. (2007). "Genetic variants regulating ORMDL3 expression contribute to the risk of childhood asthma." Nature 448(7152): 470-473.

Nielson, N. M., T. Westergaard, et al. (2006). "Type 1 Diabetes and Multiple Sclerosis: A Danish Population-Based Cohort Study." Archives of Neurology 63(7): 1001-1004.

Parikh, H., V. Lyssenko, et al. (2009). "Prioritizing genes for follow-up from genome wise assocation studies using information on gene expression in tissues relevant for type 2 diabetes mellitus." BMC Medical Genetics 2(72).

Perry, V. H. (2004). "The influence of systemic inflammation on inflammation in the brain: implications for chronic neurodegenerative disease." Brain, Behavior, and Immunity 18(5): 407-413.

Quik, M. (2004). "Smoking, nicotine and Parkinson's disease." Trends in Neurosciences 27(9): 561-568.

Soto-Otero, R., E. Mendez-Alvarez, et al. (1998). "Studies on the interaction between 1,2,3,4-tetrahydro-B-carboline and cigarette smoke: a potential mechanism of neuroprotection for Parkinson's disease." Brain Research 802(1-2): 155-162.

Stienstra, R., C. Duval, et al. (2006). "PPARs, Obesity, and Inflammation." PPAR Research 2007: 1-10.

Suthram, S., J. T. Dudley, et al. (2010). "Network-Based Elucidation of Human Disease Similarities Reveals Common Functional Modules Enriched for Pluripotent Drug Targets." PLoS Computational Biology 6(2): 1-10.

The International HapMap Consortium (2005). "A Haplotype Map of the Human Genome." Nature 437(7063): 1299-1320.

The International HapMap Consortium (2007). "A second generation human haplotype map of over 3.1 million SNPs." Nature 449: 851-861.

The Wellcome Trust Case Control Consortium (2007). "Genome-wide association study of 14,000 cases of seven common diseases and 3,000 shared controls." Nature 447: 661-678.

Tontonoz, P. and B. M. Spiegelman (2008). "Fat and Beyond: The Diverse Biology of PPARγ." Annual Review of Biochemistry 77: 289-312.

Toussirot, E., E. Pertuiset, et al. (2006). "Association of Rheumatoid Arthritis with Multiple Sclerosis: Report of 14 Cases and Discussion of Its Significance." The Journal of Rhematology: Correspondence 33(5): 1027-1028.

Wang, L., P. Jia, et al. (2011). "An efficient hierarchical generalized linear mixed model for pathway analysis of genome-wide assocation studies." Bioinformatics 27(5): 686-692.

Wang, W. Y. S., B. J. Barratt, et al. (2005). "Genome-Wide Association Studies: Theoretical and Practical Concerns." Nature Reviews Genetics 6: 109-118.

Xavier, R. J. and J. D. Rioux (2008). "Genome-wide association studies: a new window into immune-mediated diseases." Nature Reviews Immunology 8: 631-643.

11

Fulminant Type 1 Diabetes Mellitus in IRS-2 Deficient Mice

Toshiro Arai, Nobuko Mori and Haruo Hashimoto
Nippon Veterinary and Life Science University
Japan

1. Introduction

Type 1 diabetes mellitus (T1DM), one of two major forms of diabetes, results from nearly complete destruction of pancreatic beta (β) cells. According to the classification of diabetes made by the American Diabetes Association, T1DM is divided into two subtypes: immune-mediated (type 1A) and idiopathic (type 1B) (American Diabetes Association, 2008). Fulminant type 1 diabetes mellitus (FT1DM), which was first reported by Imagawa et al. in 2000, is thought to be a unique subtype of type 1B diabetes. The initial reports of FT1DM were exclusively in Japanese population and accounted for about 20% of their T1DM (Imagawa et al., 2000; 2003). Outside Japan, Cho et al. (2007) reported prevalence for FT1DM of 7.1% in the newly diagnosed Korean T1DM patients. However, epidemiological study of FT1DM is lacking in other Asian populations and its incidence and pathogenesis remain to be elucidated. While a search for FT1DM was reported to be negative in the Caucasian population, case reports on FT1DM had surfaced in different ethnic groups, predominantly from Asian origins (Jung et al., 2004; Taniyama et al., 2004; Moreau et al., 2008). However, the causative mechanism of FT1DM is currently unknown. On the other hand, insulin receptor substrate (IRS) disorders are associated with onset of insulin resistance and diabetes mellitus (Withers et al., 1998; Kido et al., 2000). A small population of male IRS-2 deficient mice showed hyperglycemia associated with markedly diminished pancreatic islet size, and these extremely hyperglycemic IRS-2 deficient mice exhibited 1) abrupt onset of diabetes and 2) very short duration of diabetic symptoms, such as polyuria, thirst, and body weight loss. These symptoms resembled the features of human nonautoimmune FT1DM (Hashimoto et al., 2006). Characteristics of abrupt onset of hyperglycemia associated with marked diminished islet mass in IRS-2 deficient mice were investigated to analyze the onset mechanism of FT1DM.

2. Characteristics of fulminant type 1 diabetes mellitus

2.1 Onset of fulminant type 1 diabetes mellitus

Fulminant type 1 diabetes mellitus (FT1DM) is a novel clinical entirely within diabetes mellitus and accounts for 20% of T1DM in Japan. Since its initial description by Imagawa et al. (2000), many cases have been reported predominately in Japan and Korea. FT1DM shows clinical characteristics of (1) remarkably abrupt onset of disease; (2) very short (< 1 week) duration of diabetic symptoms, such as polyuria, thirst and body weight loss; (3) acidosis at diagnosis; (4) negative status of islet-related antibodies, islet cell antibodies (ICA), anti-glutamic acid decarboxylase antibodies (GADAb), insulin autoantibodies (IAA) or anti-islet antigen 2 antibodies (IA-2); (5) virtually no C-peptide secretion (< 10 μg/day in urine); and (6) elevated serum pancreatic enzyme level. Fas and Fas ligand expression are lacking and the mechanism of β cell destruction differs from that in autoimmune T1DM. However the degradation mechanism of β cell in FT1DM of humans is unknown. Recently, it has been reported that the onset of FT1DM may be attributed to certain HLA subtype, to viral infection, or to pregnancy (Imagawa et al., 2003; Imagawa et al., 2005; Shimizu et al., 2006; Kawabata et al., 2009). In recent study, macrophages and T cells - but not natural killer cells – had infiltrated the islets and the exocrine pancreas and Toll-like receptor (TLR) 3, a sensor of viral components, was detected in most of macrophages and T cells in FT1DM patients (Shibasaki et al., 2010). Their study showed remarkably decreased numbers of pancreatic beta and alpha cells, macrophage-dominated insulitis and the expression of TLRs, a signature of viral infection, in FT1DM soon after the disease onset. These results suggest a new mechanism of virus-induced macrophage-dominated inflammatory process, rather than autoimmune T cell response, plays a major role in β cell destruction in FT1DM.

2.2 FT1DM associated with viral infection

Causative mechanism for accelerated β cell destruction in FT1DM is unclear. To date, viral infection has been the most popular speculated cause of acute destruction of the pancreatic β cell as many patients reported flu-like symptoms prior to the disease onset (Zheng et al., 2011). Tanaka et al (2009) investigated islet cell status, including the presence of enterovirus and chemokine/cytokline/major histocompatibility complex (MHC) expression in the pancreata using immunohistochemical analyses in three subjects with FT1DM. Immunohistochemical analyses revealed the presence of enterovirus-capsid protein in all three affected pancreata. Extensive infiltration of CXCR3 receptor-bearing T-cells and macrophages into islets was observed. Dendritic cells were stained in and around the islets. Interferon-γ and CXC chemokine ligand 10 (CXCL10) were strongly coexpressed in all subtypes of islet cells, including β cell and α cells. No CXCL10 was expressed in exocrine pancreas. Serum levels of CXCL10 were increased. Expression of MHC class II and hyper-expression of MHC class I was observed in some islet cells. These observations strongly suggest the presence of a circuit for destruction of β cells in FT1DM. Enterovirus infection of the pancreata initiates coexpression of interferon-γ and CXCL10 in β cells. CXCL10 secreted from β cells activates and attracts autoreactive T-cells and macrophages to the islets via CXCR3. These infiltrating autoreactive T-cells and macrophages release inflammatory cytokines including interferon-γ in the islets, not only damaging β cells but also accelerating CXCL10 generation in residual β cells and thus further activating cell-mediated autoimmunity until all β cells have been destroyed. On the other hand, Shibasaki et al (2010) investigated pathogenesis of FT1DM with special reference to insulitis and viral infection using pancreatic autopsy samples from three patients. Both β and α cell area were significantly decreased in comparison with those of normal controls. Macrophages and T cells – but not natural killer cells – had infiltrated the islets and the exocrine pancreas. Toll-like receptor (TLR) 3, a sensor of viral components, was detected in 84.7% of macrophages and 62.7% of T cells in all three patients. TLR7 and TLR9 were also detected in the pancreas of all three patients. Enterovirus RNA was detected in β cells positive islets in one of the three patients by *in situ* hybridization. These results suggest that macrophage-dominated inflammatory process, rather than autoimmune T cell response, plays a major role in β cell destruction in FT1DM.

2.3 FT1DM associated with pregnancy

FT1DM associated with pregnancy is very rare. However if it occurs, the rapid onset is associated with an extremely high risk of fetal death. Therefore, it is important for physicians to make an appropriate diagnosis as early as possible and to begin immediate treatment of both the mother and the fetus (Murabayashi et al., 2009). Shimizu et al. (2006) characterized the clinical and immunogenetic features of Japanese pregnancy-associated FT1DM (PF). A group of patients with PF was compared with a group of patients of child-bearing age with FT1DM that was not associated with pregnancy (NPF) in a nationwide survey conducted from 2000-2004. The criteria used for inclusion of FT1DM were 1) ketosis or ketoacidosis within 1 week after the onset of hyperglycemic symptoms; 2) urinary C peptide excretion less than 10 μg/day, fasting serum C peptide levels less than 0.3ng/ml, or serum C peptide levels less than 0.5 ng/ml after glucagon injection or a meal load soon after the onset of the disease; and 3) hemoglobin A_{1c} levels less than 8.5% on the first visit. Twenty two PF patients showed increased plasma amylase values and negative for GADab except one with transient increase in GADab (12U/ml). In 22 PF patients, 18 developed disease during pregnancy, whereas four cases occurred immediately after delivery. Twelve cases that developed during pregnancy resulted in stillbirty, and five of the six fetal cases that survived were delivered by cesarean section. The haplotype frequency of HLA DRB1*0901-DQB1*0303 in PF was significantly higher than those in NPF and controls, whereas that of DRB1*0405-DQB1*0401 in NPF was significantly higher than those in PF. The type 1 diabetes-susceptible HLA class II haplotype is distinct in PF and NPF patients, suggesting that different HLA haplotypes underlie the presentation of PF or NPF. Moreau et al. (2008) reported three cases of FT1DM in Caucasian French women. HLA phenotyping of these Caucasian patients did not find the specific HLA haplotype (DRB1*0405-DQB1*0401) found to be linked to FT1DM in Japanese patients. Two cases of FT1DM associated with pregnancy was reported from Malaysia (Tan & Loh, 2010), and FT1DM as subtype of type1B diabetes with severe and persistent β cell failure may be an important subtype in the young adult Asian populations. More international collaborative epidemiological studies are warranted in order to better understand and characterize FT1DM associated with pregnancy.

3. Metabolic disorders in IRS-2 deficient mice

3.1 IRS-2 deficient mouse

Insulin receptor substrate (IRS) disorders are associated with onset of insulin resistance and diabetes mellitus. IRS-1 deficient mice are growth-retarded and show skeletal muscle insulin resistance but do not develop diabetes because the hyperinsulinemia associated with the β cell hyperplasia in these mice efficiently compensates for the insulin resistance (Withers et al., 1998; Kido et al., 2000). IRS-2 deficient mice develop diabetes, presumably due to inadequate β cell proliferation combined with insulin resistance, and the insulin resistance in IRS-2 deficient mice is ameliorated by reduction of adiposity. IRS-2 deficient mice are widely used for analysis of pathophysiology of human type 2 diabetes mellitus (T2DM). In male IRS-2 deficient mice (C57BL/6 x CBA hybrid background) generated by Kubota et al. (2000) with C57BL/6J:Jcl mice established an inbred line of IRS-2 deficient mice, serious T1DM accompanied by abrupt and marked increase of their plasma glucose concentrations and ketonuria was sometimes observed (Hashimoto et al., 2006). The symptoms observed in IRS-2 deficient mice with serious T1DM with insulin-deficient hyperglycemia resembled those of human nonautoimmune FT1DM reported by Imagawa et al. (2000). Analyses of plasma metabolite, insulin, C-peptide, hepatic enzyme activities related to energy metabolism and histopathological changes in pancreas and islet-related antibodies may clarify the mechanism of β cell destruction and onset of FT1DM in animals.

3.2 Metabolic characteristics in IRS-2 deficient mice

We established an inbred line of mice deficient in insulin receptor substrate-2 (IRS-2) that have a C57BL/6J genetic background (B6J-IRS2-/- mice). At 6 week of age, there was no difference in body weight between wild-type (control) and IRS-2 deficient mice, but IRS-2 deficient mice showed remarkable impaired glucose tolerance and insulin resistance (Hashimoto et al., 2006). IRS-2 deficient mice showed significant increases in plasma glucose, free fatty acid (FFA), triglyceride (TG), total cholesterol (TC) and insulin concentrations compared to wild-type (control) mice at 6-week-old. In the livers of male IRS-2 deficient mice, the activities of cytosolic pyruvate kinase (PK), glucose-6-phosphate dehydrogenase (G6PD), ATP citrate lyase (ACL), fatty acid synthase (FAS) and malic enzyme (ME) were significantly higher than those of control mice (Table 1). Increase in activities of G6PD, ACL, FAS and ME, which are crucial enzymes for fatty acid synthesis, means activation of lipid synthesis in liver of IRS-2 deficient mice. Insulin resistance observed in IRS-2 deficient mice tends to deteriorate with aging. On the other hand, two of eight male IRS-2 deficient mice each at the ages of 14 and 24 week suddenly showed extreme hyperglycemia, similar to that in case of FT1DM. Another 2 male IRS-2 deficient mice developed extreme hyperglycemia at the age of 11 and 12 week and died. Plasma glucose and FFA concentrations in the extremely hyperglycemic IRS-2 deficient mice showed abnormal increases compared with moderately hyperglycemic IRS-2 deficient mice. Plasma insulin concentrations in extremely hyperglycemic IRS-2 deficient mice were below the detection limit. On histopathologic examination, the pancreatic islets of extremely hyperglycemic IRS-2 deficient mice were either absent or decreased in size and number compared with those of moderately hyperglycemic IRS-2 deficient mice. The islets of extremely hyperglycemic IRS-2 deficient mice showed karyorrhexis, cytoplasmic swelling, and partial necrosis. In addition, the liver of one extremely hyperglycemic IRS-2 deficient mouse showed collagen fibrinoid degeneration and macrophages.

In conclusion, at 6 week of age, IRS-2 deficient mice showed profiles compatible with several features of metabolic syndrome, including hyperglycemia, hyperinsulinemia, insulin resistance, hypertriglyceridemia, and high FFA concentrations. Therefore even young IRS-2 deficient mice are useful animal models for studying T2DM. Moreover, hyperglycemia and insulin resistance in these mice progressed to their highest levels when the animals were 14 week of age. A small population of male IRS-2 deficient mice developed abrupt onset of hyperglycemia associated with markedly diminished islet mass, resembling the features of human nonautoimmune FT1DM. The IRS-2 deficient mice may also serve as an animal model for studying FT1DM.

			Wild-type (n=8)	IRS-2 deficient (n=8)
Plasma	Glucose (mg/dl)		152 (8)	223 (23)*
	Free fatty acid (mEq/l)		0.26 (0.03)	0.49 (0.09)*
	Triglyceride (mg/dl)		55.4 (2.5)	75.8 (8.4)*
	Total cholesterol (mg/dl)		54.8 (2.6)	88.0 (8.1)*
	Insulin (ng/ml)		0.74 (0.10)	2.01 (0.35)*
Liver	Cytosol	HK	5.6 (0.3)	6.0 (0.6)
		GK	1.4 (0.1)	1.6 (0.2)
		PK	11.1 (1.5)	14.8 (1.4)*
		G6PD	6.0 (0.7)	8.5 (0.8)*
		LDH	1658 (75)	1633 (83)
		MDH	4340 (211)	4342 (162)
		AST	546 (60)	577 (57)
		ACL	4.4 (0.4)	5.9 (0.4)*
		FAS	7.7 (0.6)	10.8 (1.1)*
		ME	10.1 (1.2)	20.1 (2.0)*
		PEPCK	20.9 (2.2)	22.3 (2.8)
	Microsomes	G6Pase	424 (11)	440 (22)
	Mitochondria	GLDH	1264 (96)	1462 (78)
		MDH	3985 (216)	4247 (349)
		AST	1008 (110)	981 (55)

Data are presented as mean (SE).
*P<0.05 (Student's t test) versus value for wild-type mice.
Hepatic enzyme activities are presented as nmol/min/mg protein.
HK, hexokinase; GK, glucokinase; PK, pyruvate kinase; G6PD, glucose-6-phosphate dehydrogenase; LDH, lactate dehydrogenase; MDH, malate dehydrogenase; AST, aspartate aminotransferase; ACL, ATP citrate lyase; FAS, fatty acid synthase; ME, malic enzyme; PEPCK, phosphoenolpyruvate carboxykinase; G6Pase, glucose-6-phosphatase; GLDH, glutamate dehydrogenase

Table 1. Plasma metabolite concentrations and hepatic enzyme activities in 6-week-old male wild-type and IRS-2 deficient mice

3.3 Obesity with insulin resistance in IRS-2 deficient mice with high-fat diet feeding

Type 2 diabetes mellitus (T2DM) appears to be increasing mainly in the United States, Africa and Asia. In 2000 there were one hundred and fifty million T2DM patients, but they are predicted to increase substantially to two hundred and twenty million world-wide in 2010. Since World War II (WWII), T2DM patients have increased markedly with dramatic changes of lifestyle in Japan. Typical changes of the lifestyle include the increases in high fat diets, sedentary habit and driving. Especially, the level of fat in modern Japanese diets increased from 20.0 g/day in 1953 to 59.9 g/day in 1995 according to the nation-wide nutrition monitoring survey in Japan. Japanese population is predisposed to develop T2DM due to insufficient insulin secretion in spite of no predisposition to obesity. IRS-2 deficient mice show at 6 weeks of age showed profiles compatible with several features of the metabolic syndrome, including hyperglycemia, hyperinsulinemia, insulin resistance, hypertriglyceridemia, and high FFA. To investigate the characteristics in energy metabolism in IRS-2 deficient, three kinds of diets with different lipid concentrations were supplied to IRS-2 deficient mice (4 weeks old) for 2weeks. Total calories of diets were calculated as 395.1

kcal/100g for Modern American diet, 365.0 kcal/100g for Modern Japanese diet and 328.9 kcal/100g for Japanese diet after WWII. Each diet contained 15.5% (American diet, Ad), 10.1% (Japanese diet, Jd) and 3.9% (WWII diet) as crude fat, respectively. Regular diet (Rd) for laboratory animals (390kcal/100g) contained 5.0% as crude fat were based on human Japanese diet after WWII. Male IRS-2 deficient mice (4 weeks old) were provided with

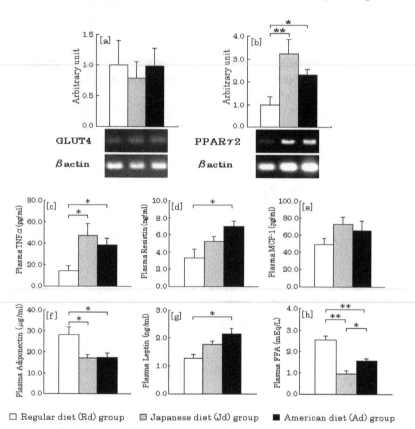

□ Regular diet (Rd) group   ▨ Japanese diet (Jd) group   ■ American diet (Ad) group

Fig. 1. Effects of modern Japanese and American diets on RNA expression of GLUT4 and PPARγ2 of adipose tissues and plasma adipocytokines concentrations in IRS-2 deficient mice fed with three kinds of diets with different lipid levels.

regular and Japanese and American diets as well as tap water *ad libitum* for 2 weeks, and used for glucose tolerance test, insulin tolerance test, and harvests of blood, liver, femoral muscles, white adipose tissue (WAT), and pancreas for chemical analysis at the age of 6 weeks (Hashimoto et al., 2009). Average body weight of Rd, Jd and Ad group at 6 week of age were 20.8, 22.7 and 22.9g each. Japanese and American diet increased significantly the body weight of IRS-2 deficient mice when compared with regular diet. Ad group showed severely impaired glucose tolerance, and Jd and Ad group showed deterioration of insulin resistance. Expression of SREBP-1c mRNA in the livers of Ad group was increased with Rd group (p<0.05). In addition, expression of PPARγ2 mRNA and GLUT2 mRNA in the Ad group were higher than in other groups (p<0.05). Cytosolic ACL and ME activities in the

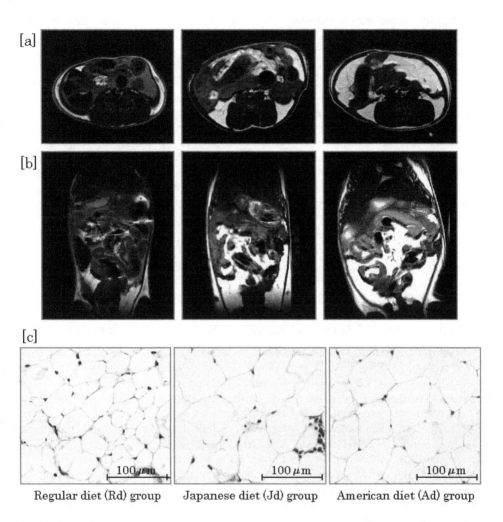

Fig. 2. Effects of modern Japanese and American diets on intraperitoneal white adipose tissues, (a) Axial views, (b) Coronal views of MRI, and (c) Adipocytes in white adipose tissues of IRS-2 deficient mice with three kinds of diets with different lipid levels.

livers of the Jd and Ad groups increased when compared with the Rd group (p<0.05). Expression of GLUT4 mRNA in the skeletal muscle of the Jd and Ad groups were lower than that in the Rd group (p<0.01). Figure 1 shows expression of mRNA in WAT and plasma cytokine concentrations in IRS-2 deficient mice. Expression of GLUT4 mRNA was not changed in WAT of each group. Expression of PPARγ2 mRNA in the Jd and Ad groups was higher than that in the Rd group (p<0.05). Both the Jd and Ad groups showed increased plasma TNF-α concentrations compared with the Rd group (p<0.05). In addition, the Ad group showed increased plasma resistin concentrations compared with other groups (p<0.05). However, plasma MCP-1 concentrations were not altered. On the other hand, both of Jd and Ad groups showed decreased plasma adiponectin concentrations compared with the Rd group (p<0.05). The Ad group showed increased plasma leptin concentrations compared with the Rd group (p<0.05). Both the Jd and Ad groups showed decreased plasma FFA concentrations compared with the Rd group (p<0.05). MRI showed the effects of Japanese and American diets on intraperitoneal WAT in IRS-2 deficient mice. Peritoneal WAT was accumulated in mice fed on Japanese and American diets. WAT around the kidney and testes in the Jd and Ad groups increased in proportion to fat concentrations of diets when compared with the Rd group. In addition, adipocytes of the Jd and Ad groups were corpulent when compared with those of the Rd group (Figure 2c). Expression of GLUT2 mRNA in pancreas of the Ad group was the lowest among all groups (p<0.05). The Jd and Ad groups showed hyperinsulinemia when compared with Rd group (p<0.05). On histopathologic examination of islets, insulin secretion was observed in all three groups.

In conclusion, high-fat diet feeding induced rapid accumulation of fat intraperitoneal cavity of IRS-2 deficient mice. Obese IRS-2 deficient mice showed higher activities of lipid synthesis in their livers and the increase in TNF-α of corpulent adipocyte origin further aggravated insulin resistance and the increase in resistin also aggravated the impaired glucose tolerance, leading to aggravation of T2DM. Plasma adiponectin concentrations decreased significantly in obese IRS-2 deficient mice fed on high-fat diet, and decreased adiponectin concentrations might worsen T2DM to severe diabetic condition.

4. Fulminant type 1 diabetes mellitus (FT1DM) in IRS-2 deficient mice

4.1 Onset of FT1DM in IRS-2 deficient mice

Two of eight male IRS-2 deficient mice each at 14 and 24 weeks of age suddenly showed extreme hyperglycemia associated with markedly diminished pancreatic islet size. These extremely hyperglycemic mice had greatly diminished activities of hepatic ACL, FAS, and ME. In these mice, plasma ALT activities were elevated and histochemical analysis of the liver confirmed inflammation. These cases of extreme diabetes resemble the human nonautoimmune FT1DM (Hashimoto et al., 2006). Occurrence rate of FT1D appears to be ~20% in male IRS-2 deficient mice after the age of 8 weeks, and is not observed in the female mice. FT1DM mice showed clinical characteristics of (1) remarkably abrupt onset of disease; (2) very short (< 1 week) duration of diabetic symptoms; (3) acidosis at diagnosis; (4) negative status of islet-related antibodies, ICA, GADAb, IAA or IA-2; (5) virtually no C-peptide secretion; and (6) elevated serum pancreatic enzyme level.

4.2 Characteristics of plasma metabolite and hormones in IRS-2 deficient mice with FT1DM

Because over 50% of male IRS-2 deficient mice after 10 weeks of age tended to show glycosuria with obesity, male IRS-2 deficient mice (8 weeks old) without glycosuria according to Diasticks (Bayer Medical Ltd., Tokyo, Japan) were used as the control. Eight IRS-2 deficient mice (8-20 weeks old) with abrupt increase of blood glucose concentrations over 450 mg/dl (25 mmol/l) within a week and ketonuria with ketosticks (Bayer Medical Ltd.) were determined as FT1DM. Plasma glucose, FFA, TG, TC, insulin and C-peptide concentrations and hepatic enzyme activities were compared between control and diabetic mice. The body weights of the diabetic mice were 26.0 ± 4.6 g (mean ± SD), smaller than those of the control mice (29.6 ± 3.8 g). As the diabetic mice (8-24 weeks old) were older than the control mice (8 weeks old), the reduction of body weights in the diabetic mice was significant. All the diabetic mice showed ketonuria. In the diabetic mice, the plasma glucose and TC concentrations were significantly higher than those in the controls, whereas plasma insulin and C-peptide concentrations decreased significantly under one third of the control values. There were no significant differences in FFA and TG concentrations between the diabetic and control mice (Table 2).

4.3 Activities of hepatic enzymes related to glucose and lipid metabolism

Activities of HK and GK as rate-limiting enzymes in glycolysis, G6PD as rate-limiting in pentose-phosphate pathway, LDH as cytosol marker enzyme, MDH and AST as crucial enzymes in the malate-aspartate shuttle, PEPCK and FBPase as rate-limiting enzymes in gluconeogenesis, ACL, ME and FAS as rate-limiting enzymes in fatty acid synthesis, PC as oxaloacetate-supplying enzyme to the tricarboxylic acid (TCA) cycle, GLDH as mitochondrial marker enzyme and 3HBD as rate-limiting enzyme in ketone body synthesis were measured. Removed pancreas from the control and the diabetic mice (12 weeks old, plasma glucose 560 mg/dl, plasma insulin <0.2 ng/ml) were examined histopathologically. Existence of the islet-related antibodies was investigated immunohistochemically in sera of NOD mice as autoimmune type 1 diabetic model and IRS2-deficient mice using pancreatic sections prepared from mice before (control mice) and after (diabetic mice) onset of FT1DM. Activities of HK and GK in glycolysis and MDH in the malate-aspartate shuttle in cytosolic fraction of liver in the diabetic mice were significantly lower than those of the control mice. Activities of FBPase in gluconeogenesis and ME in fatty acid synthesis in liver of the diabetic mice were significantly higher than those of the controls. In the mitochondrial fraction of liver of the diabetic mice, activities of 3-HBD were significantly higher than the controls, whereas activities of AST and PC were significantly lower than those of the controls. In the liver of the diabetic mice, activities of cytosolic LDH, G6PD, AST and mitochondrial GLDH were lower than those of the control mice. The clinical symptoms of FT1DM observed in male IRS-2 deficient mice are significant increase in plasma glucose and cholesterol concentrations and a significant decrease in plasma insulin and C-peptide concentrations. All diabetic mice showed reduction of body weight, glycosuria and ketonuria and they were considered to fall into complete insulin deficiency. In the diabetic mice with insulin deficiency, their plasma TG and FFA concentrations were expected to increase generally, however those concentrations were not changed in IRS-2 deficient diabetic mice. In our previous report (Hashimoto et al., 2006), plasma TG and FFA concentrations decreased significantly notwithstanding plasma glucose and cholesterol concentrations increased significantly in the diabetic IRS-2 deficient mice at 14 weeks old. Liver-specific insulin receptor knockout (LIR-KO) mice with remarkable insulin resistance showed a significant decrease in their plasma TG and FFA concentrations. As IRS-2 deficient mice seemed to have unique regulation mechanism of plasma TG and FFA concentrations, their characteristics in lipid metabolism should be further studied in more IRS-2 deficient mice.

In livers of the diabetic IRS-2 deficient mice, activities of enzymes in glycolysis and the malate-aspartate shuttle were significantly decreased, whereas those in gluconeogenesis and ketone body synthesis were significantly elevated. Decreased activities of pyruvate carboxylase, supplying oxaloacetate to the TCA cycle, suggested depression of citrate synthesis, the rate limiting reaction of TCA cycle, and activation of ketone body synthesis. Moreover, depression in the malate-aspartate shuttle means decreased ATP production. Decrease in glycolysis or increase in gluconeogenesis and ketone body synthesis may be typical metabolic changes induced by complete insulin deficiency. Decreased activities of LDH, MDH, AST and GLDH in the diabetic IRS-2 deficient mice reflected depression of liver function frequently observed in the diabetic animals.

			Control (n=8)	Diabetic (n=8)
Plasma	Glucose (mg/dl)		223 (20)	569 (77)*
	Free fatty acid (mEq/l)		0.60 (0.02)	1.20 (0.30)*
	Triglyceride (mg/dl)		79.7 (8.9)	97.5 (17.7)
	Total cholesterol (mg/dl)		88.9 (7.7)	162.3 (27.1)*
	Insulin (ng/ml)		1.32 (0.16)	0.28 (0.05)*
	C-peptide (ng/ml)		3.4 (0.4)	1.1 (0.3)*
Liver	Cytosol	HK	6.9 (0.5)	4.7 (0.4)*
		GK	4.2 (0.6)	1.3 (0.3)*
		G6PD	5.1 (0.5)	4.6 (0.3)
		LDH	1294 (86)	1108 (163)
		MDH	4288 (160)	3499 (250)*
		AST	653 (75)	615 (40)
		PEPCK	26 (3)	31 (3)
		FBPase	68 (8)	101 (6)*
		ACL	3.5 (0.4)	3.5 (0.3)
		FAS	4.7 (0.5)	4.9 (0.8)
		ME	17 (2)	30 (2)*
	Mitochondria	GLDH	1834 (116)	1635 (124)
		MDH	2480 (101)	2524 (334)
		AST	1684 (62)	1354 (52)*
		3-HBD	4.1 (0.2)	8.6 (1.4)*
		PC	153 (8)	66 (6)*

Data are presented as mean (SE).
Control means 8-week-old male IRS-2 deficient mice without glycosuria according to Diasticks.
*p<0.05 vs. controls
Hepatic enzyme activities are presented as nmol/min/mg protein.
FBPase, fructose-1,6-bisphophatase; 3-HBD, 3-hydroxybutyrate dehydrogenase; PC, pyruvate carboxylase

Table 2. Plasma metabolite concentrations and hepatic enzyme activities in control and diabetic IRS-2 deficient mice

4.4 Pathology and islet antibodies in IRS-2 deficient mice with FT1DM

On histopathological examination, the pancreatic islets of the diabetic mice were significantly decreased in size and number compared to those of the control mice. In particular, size and number of insulin secreted β cells in the diabetic mice decreased significantly compared to those in the controls, whereas number of glucagon secreted α cells decreased a little. Remarkable insulitis by autoimmunity was not observed in pancreatic sections in the diabetic mice (Figure 3). In the sera of the diabetic NOD mice, the islet-related antibodies reacted with their own islets (Figure 4, B1) and IRS2-deficient mouse islets before (Figure 4, B2) and after (Figure 4, B3) onset of FT1DM. In the serum of the control NOD mouse without glycosuria, the islet-related antibodies were not observed (Figure 4, A1-3). In sera of control and diabetic IRS2-deficient mice, the islet-related antibodies were not observed (Figure 4, C1-3 and D1-3). We also noted observed fatty degeneration in the liver of FT1DM mice. The cause of this degeneration might be increased adiposity due to increased activities of lipogenic enzymes (such as ACL, FAS, and ME) before the change of glucose tolerance in IRS-2 deficient mice. We consider that macrophages noted on histopathologic examination likely appeared to phagocytize the degraded collagen fibrinoid induced by fatty degeneration.

In the diabetic IRS-2 deficient mice, hepatic steatosis is frequently observed. The finding of severe, selective destruction of pancreatic β cells was considered to be one of the characteristics in FT1DM in IRS-2 deficient mice. The diabetic IRS-2 deficient mice did not show the islet-related antibodies observed in the diabetic NOD mice as autoimmune T1DM model. The destruction mechanism of pancreatic islet cells in IRS-2 deficient mice may differ clearly from that in the diabetic NOD mice. IRS-2 deficient mice develop diabetes because of insulin resistance in the liver and failure to undergo β cells hyperplasia. Progress of changes in islet mass should be further studied to investigate pancreatic β cells destruction. At the moment abrupt increase in plasma concentrations and appearance of ketonuria are available indicators to decide complete insulin deficiency caused by pancreatic β cells destruction in diabetic mice. In IRS-2 deficient mice, the sterol regulatory element binding protein (SREBP)-1 downstream genes, such as ATP citrate lyase and fatty acid synthase genes, are significantly increased and an excess amount of lipid is accumulated in their tissues. Accumulated lipid is also considered to be one of the causes of injury to their pancreatic islets. As FT1DM in IRS-2 deficient resembles human FT1DM, IRS-2 deficient mice are a good animal model for T2DM of human and some IRS-2 deficient mice with FT1DM may be a useful animal model for studying the destruction mechanism of pancreatic β cells in progressing to FT1DM.

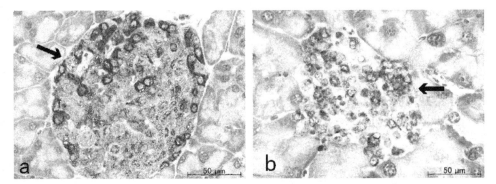

Fig. 3. Histopathological examinations of pancreatic islet cells of IRS-2 deficient mice. Pancreatic islets (arrowheads) in a control mouse (a) and a diabetic mouse (b). Pancreas sections were pretreated with 0.03% H_2O_2 in methanol to block endogenous peroxidase activity, and incubated for 60 min at room temperature with guinea pig anti-swine insulin (Dako Cytomation), followed by 30 min incubation with peroxidase-conjugate rabbit anti-guinea pig immunoglobulin. Then, the sections were incubated for 60 min at room temperature with rabbit anti-human glucagon (Dako Cytomation), followed by 30 min incubation with alkaline phosphatase-labelled polymer conjugated goat anti-rabbit antibody (Nichirei). For double staining, peroxidase (brown, DAB) and alkaline phosphatase (red, New Fuchsin) were used, respectively. Magnification, x 200

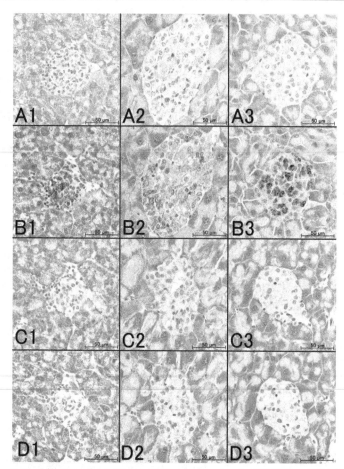

Fig. 4. Observation of islet-associated autoantibodies in serum of NOD and IRS-2 deficient mice. All pancreas specimens were fixed in 10% buffered formalin and embedded paraffin, mounted on amino-silane coated glass slide and stained using the indirect immunoperoxidase method. For each mouse, sera were treated with 0.03% H_2O_2 in methanol to measure the endogenous peroxidase activity. After pre-incubation with the 10% normal rabbit serum (Dako Cytomation) for 10 min at room temperature, sections were then incubated with preclinical NOD/shi mice sera, diabetic NOD/shi mice sera, control IRS-2 mice sera and diabetic IRS-2 mice sera, followed by incubation overnight at 4℃. Sections were serially incubated with polyclonal rabbit anti-mouse IgG/HRP antibodies (Dako Cytomation) for 60 min at room temperature. The peroxidase activity was visualized by incubation in a 0.05M Tris-HCl buffer (pH 7.6) containing 0.02% 3,3′-diaminobenzidine (DAB) and 0.006% H_2O_2 solution for 5 min. Immunostained sections were counterstained with hematoxylin for visualization of nuclei. Column 1, 2 and 3 present diabetic NOD, control IRS-2 deficient and diabetic IRS-2 deficient mouse pancreatic sections, respectively. Control NOD mouse serum (A) reacted with diabetic NOD (A1), control IRS-2 deficient (A2) and diabetic IRS-2 deficient mouse (A3) pancreatic sections. Diabetic NOD (B1-3), control IRS-2 (C1-3) and diabetic IRS-2 (D1-3) mouse sera reacted with pancreatic sections, respectively.

5. Onset mechanism of obesity and diabetes in IRS-2 deficient mice

5.1 Onset mechanism of FT1DM in IRS-2 deficient mice

Figure 5 summarizes onset mechanism of obesity and diabetes in IRS-2 deficient mice. IRS-2 deficient mice tend to fall in insulin resistance. Excess calorie and physical inactivity induce hyperglycemia followed by increased insulin secretion, which accelerates fatty acid synthesis via activation of transcriptional factor, SREBP-1c etc. Acceleration of fatty acid synthesis induces heterotopic accumulation of lipid, and visceral fat accumulation is increased. This situation is defined as obesity. Adiponectin exerts antidiabetic effects on muscles and the liver through AMP-activated protein kinase (AMPK) activation (Yamauchi et al., 2002) and antiatherosclerotic effects by inhibiting monocyte adhesion to endotherial cells and lipid accumulation into macrophages (Ouchi et al., 2001). Thus adiponectin increases glucose uptake and fatty acid oxidation in muscles via the type 1 adiponectin receptor (Yamauchi et al., 2003), and hepatic gluconeogensis via type 2 adiponectin receptor. Moreover adiponectin protects against oxidative stress in skeletal muscle by activating nuclear factor (NF)-κB target genes, manganese superoxide dismutase and inducible nitric oxide synthase (Ikegami et al., 2009). Decreased adiponectin secretion and increased inflammatory cytokines secretion from swelling adipose tissue deteriorate insulin resistance in obese animals (1st stage). Decreased adiponectin causes depression of activity of AMPK which increases glucose utilization and fatty acid β-oxidation in skeletal muscle and adipose tissues (Whitehead et al., 2006). Then hyperglycemia, hyperinsulinemia and accelerated lipid synthesis are maintained and hyper-secretion of insulin force excessively heavy work on pancreatic β cells. In over functional pancreatic islets, β-oxidation of fatty acid is accelerated resulting in excess amount of reactive oxygen species (ROS) production, which induces ROS stress leading to mitochondrial dysfunction and apoptosis of β-cells with low scavenging activity of ROS (2nd stage). It has been reported that adiponectin inhibits fatty acid-induced apoptosis by suppression of ROS generation via both the cAMP/PKA and AMPK pathway in endothelial cells (Kim et al, 2010). Macrophages (but not T cells) infiltration is observed frequently in FT1DM (Shibasaki et al., 2010). In IRS-2 deficient mice with FT1DM macrophage infiltration induced by MCP-1 was observed. Infiltrated macrophages may participate in destruction process of pancreatic islets leading to T1DM. The β cell deficit is believed to be due to autoimmune induced β cell apoptosis mediated by the release of inflammatory cytokines, such as IL-1β and TNF-α, from T lymphocytes and macrophages (Donath et al., 2003). Cytokine-induced β cell death preferentially affects newly forming beta cells, which implies that replicating beta cells might be more vulnerable to cytokine destruction. Efforts to expand beta cell mass in type 1 diabetes by fostering β cell replication are likely to fail unless cytokine-induced apoptosis is concurrently suppressed (Meier et al., 2006). Inflammatory cytokines from corpulent adipocytes appear to participate in destruction of islets β cells leading to T1DM. In autoimmune T1DM, β cells are assumed to be destroyed through a long-standing autoimmune process, whereas in FT1DM, β cells seem to be destroyed very rapidly, probably by a destructive process triggered by viral infection (Hanafusa & Imagawa, 2008). Since IRS-2 deficient mice were maintained under specific pathogen free conditions (Hashimoto et al., 2006), viral infection was deleted from the causes of β cell destruction. Adipocyte-secreted factors associate the pancreatic β cells destructions. Chronic exposure of human islets to leptin leads to β cell apoptosis (Donath et al., 2003). TNFα, in combination with other cytokines, accelerates dysfunction and destruction of the β cell (Eizirik & Mandrup-Poulsen, 2001). IL-6 released by adipocytes may be responsible for the increases in plasma IL-6 concentrations observed in obesity and at least in combination with other cytokines, IL-6 has cytotoxic effects on β cell (Eizirik et al., 1994). Increased FFA levels are known to be toxic for β cell, leading to the concept of lipotoxicity (McGarry & Dobbins, 1999). The toxic effect of FFA is mediated via formation of ceramide, increased nitric oxide production and activation of the apoptotic mitochondrial pathway (Maedler et al., 2001). Elevated glucose concentrations induced β cell apoptosis at higher concentration in rodent islet (Efanova et al., 1998). In human islets glucose-induced β cell apoptosis and dysfunction are mediated by β cell production and secretion of IL-1β. Chronic hyperglycemia increases production of ROS, which may cause oxidative damage in β cell (Matsuoka et al., 1997; Laybutt et al., 2002). IL-1β and ROS activate the transcription factor nuclear transcription factor (NF) κB, which plays a critical role in mediating inflammatory responses. A series of inflammatory reaction appear to have important roles in the β cell destruction process in IRS-2 deficient mice with insulin resistance.

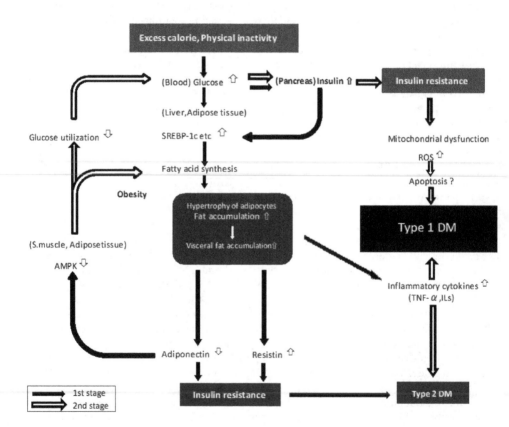

SREBP, sterol regulatory element binding protein; AMPK, AMP-activated protein kinase; ROS, reactive oxygen species;
TNF, tumor necrosis factor; IL, interleukins

Fig. 5. Onset mechanism of obesity and diabetes in IRS-2 deficient mice

5.2 Comparison of pathology of FT1DM between IRS-2 deficient mice and human patients

IRS-2 deficient mice with FT1DM show remarkable body weight loss, polydipsia, polyuria, glycosuria and ketonuria as typical symptoms of T1DM as reported in human FT1DM patients. Laboratory data in IRS-2 deficient mice with FT1DM reveal hyperglycemia, hyperlipidemia and remarkable decrease in insulin secretion as in human FT1DM patients (Table 3). The above symptoms of T1DM were onset abruptly after hyperglycemia was observed in IRS-2 deficient mice. Insulitis with macrophage dominant infiltration was observed in IRS-2 deficient mice and human FT1DM. Destruction mechanism of β cells associated HLA, viral infection and pregnancy were investigated in detail in human FT1DM patients (Kawabata et al., 2009; Murabayashi et al., 2009; Tan & Loh, 2010), whereas association with MHC was not investigated in IRS-2 deficient mice. Since FT1DM was observed in only male IRS-2 deficient mice, pregnancy is not associated with onset of FT1DM. Inflammatory cytokines play a major role in destruction process of pancreatic β cell in both IRS-2 mice and human FT1DM patients. Trigger of the β cell destruction process is different between IRS-2 mice and human. Insulin resistance by increase in inflammatory cytokines seemed to be main cause to lead β cell destruction in IRS-2 deficient mice, whereas viral infection may be a trigger for destruction mechanism in human FT1DM patients.

	IRS-2 deficient mice	Human patients	References
Clinical characteristics			
Body weight loss	Remarkable	Remarkable	Imagawa et al. (2003)
Polydipsia	Positive	Positive	Imagawa et al. (2003)
Polyuria	Positive	Positive	Imagawa et al. (2003)
Glycosuria	Positive	Positive	Imagawa et al. (2003)
Ketonuria	Positive	Positive	Imagawa et al. (2003)
Laboratory data			
Fasting plasma glucose (mg/dl)	570 (480 – 640)	711 (300 – 1293)	Shimizu et a. (2006)
Fasting plasma C peptide (ng/ml)	1.1 ± 0.3*	< 0.5	Shibasaki et al. (2010)
Serum triglyceride (mmol/l)	1.1 ± 0.2*	2.0 ± 1.8**	Imagawa et al. (2003)
Serum total cholesterol (mmol/l)	4.2 ± 0.7*	5.1 ± 1.6**	Imagawa et al. (2003)
Insulitis	Macrophages dominant infiltration	Macrophages as the main cell type in insulitis lesion, followed by T lymphocytes	Hanafusa & Imagawa (2008)
Islet related autoantibodies	Negative	Negative	Imagawa et al. (2003)

*Mean ± SE, **Mean ± SD

Table 3. Characteristics of FT1D in IRS-2 deficient mice and human patients

Type 1 diabetes is a polygenic disease. Approximately 50% of the genetic susceptibility can be explained by allele in HLA class II region, in particular certain DQ alleles. More than 95%

of type 1 diabetic patients carry these predisposing alleles, but the occurrence of these alleles in the background population is high, approximately 50%. It is believed that the diabetes predisposing DQ antigens have a shape of the antigen presenting groove of the molecule that leads to more efficient presentation of β cell associated autoantigens (Donath et al., 2003). HLA comment should be in the text. In FT1DM patients, the haplotype frequency of HLA DRB1*0901-DQB1*0303 was significantly higher than those in controls (Moreau et al., 2008). HLA phenotyping of these Caucasian patients did not find the specific HLA haplotype (DRB1*0405-DQB1*0401) found to be linked to FT1D in Japanese patients. More investigation about haplotype frequency of MHC was necessary for IRS-2 mice in the destruction process of pancreatic β cells.

6. Conclusion

IRS-2 mice tend to become obese accompanying insulin resistance after 8 weeks of age. IRS-2 deficient mice develop diabetes, presumably due to inadequate β cell proliferation combined with insulin resistance compared to IRS-1 deficient mice with the β cell hyperplasia to compensate for the insulin resistance. Heterotopic accumulation of lipid observed frequently in obese IRS-2 mice, and corpulent adipocytes secrete various inflammatory cytokines, such as TNF-α and ILs, whereas production of adiponectin as antidiabetic agent is decreased significantly. About 20% of male IRS-2 deficient mice showed clinical characteristics of (1) remarkably abrupt onset of disease; (2) very short (< 1 week) duration of diabetic symptoms; (3) acidosis at diagnosis; (4) negative status of islet-related antibodies; (5) virtually no C-peptide secretion; and (6) elevated serum pancreatic enzyme level. These symptoms resembled the features of human nonautoimmune FT1DM. In IRS-2 deficient mice with FT1DM, insulitis with macrophage dominated infiltration to islet β cell area was observed frequently as in human FT1DM patients. Inflammatory cytokines appear to have important roles in the process of β cell destruction leading to FT1DM. IRS-2 deficient mice are considered to be useful animal model for studying the mechanism of β cell destruction leading to FT1DM.

7. References

American Diabetes Association. (2008). Diagnosis and classification of diabetes. *Diabetes Care* Vol. 31 (Suppl. 1): S55-S60. ISSN 0149-5992

Cho, Y.M., Kim, J.T., Ko, K.S., Koo, B.K., Yang, S.W., Park, M.H., Lee, H.K. & Park, K.S. (2007). Fulminant type 1 diabetes in Korea: highprevalence among patients with adult-onset type 1 diabetes. *Diabetologia* Vol. 50 (No. 11): 2276-2279. ISSN 0012-186x

Donath, M.Y., Storling, J., Maedler, K. & Mandrup-Poulsen, T. (2003). Inflammatory mediators and islet β-cell failure: a link between type 1and type 2 diabetes. *Journal of Molecular Medicine* Vol. 81 (No. 8): 455-470. ISSN 0946-2716

Efanova, I.B., Zaitsev, S.V., Zhivotovsky, B., Kohler, M., Efendic, S., Orrenius, S & Berggren, P.O. (1998). Glucose and tolbutamide induce apoptosis in pancreatic beta-cells. A process dependent on intracellular Ca2+ concentration. *Journal of Biological Chemistry* Vol.273 (No. 50): 33501-33507. ISSN 0021-9258

Eizirik, D.L., Sandler, S., Welsh, N., Cetkovic-Cvrlje, M., Nieman, A., Geller, D.A., Pipeleers, D.G., Bendtzen, K. & Hellerstrom, C. (1994).Cytokines suppress human islet function irrespective of their effects on nitric oxide generation. *Journal of Clinical Investigation* Vol. 93 (No. 5): 1968-1974. ISSN 0021-9738

Eizirik, D.L. & Mandrup-Poulsen, T. (2001). A choice of death-the signal-transduction of immune-mediated beta-cell apoptosis. *Diabetologia* Vol. 44 (No. 12): 2115-2133. ISSN 0021-186x

Hanafusa, T. & Imagawa, A. (2008). Insulitis in human type 1 diabetes. *Annals of the New York Academy of Science* Vol. 1150: 297-299. ISSN 0077-8923

Hashimoto, H., Arai, T., Takeguchi, A., Hioki, K., Ohnishi, Y., Kawai, K., Ito, M., Suzuki, R., Yamauchi, T., Ohsugi, M., Saito, M., Ueyama, Y., Tobe, K., Kadowaki, T., Tamaoki, N. & Kosaka, K. (2006). Ontogenetic characteristics of enzyme activities and plasma metabolites in C57BL/6J:Jcl mice deficient in insulin receptor substrate 2. *Comparative Medicine* Vol. 56 (No. 3): 176-187. ISSN 1532-0820

Hashimoto, H., Arai, T., Mori, A., Kawai, K., Hikishima, K., Ohnishi, Y., Eto, T., Ito, M., Hioki, K., Suzuki, R., Ohsugi, M., Saito, M., Ueyama, Y., Okano, H., Yamauchi, T., Kubota, N., Ueki, K., Tobe, K., Tamaoki, N., Kadowaki, T. & Kosaka, K. (2009). Reconsideration of insulin signals induced by improved laboratory animal diets, Japanese and American diets, in IRS-2 deficient mice. *Experimental and Clinical Endocrinology & Diabetes* Vol. 117(No. 2): 577-586. ISSN 0947-7349

Ikegami, Y., Inukai, K., Imai, K., Sakamoto, Y., Katagiri, H., Kurihara, S., Awata, T. & Katayama, S. (2009). Adiponectin upregulates ferritin heavy chain in skeletal muscle cell. *Diabetes* Vol. 58 (No. 1): 61-70. ISSN 0012-1797

Imagawa, A., Hanafusa, T., Miyagawa, J. & Matsuzawa, Y. (2000). A novel subtype of type 1 diabetes mellitus characterized by a rapid onset and an absence of diabetes-related antibodies. *The New England Journal of Medicine* Vol. 342 (No. 5): 301-307. ISSN 0028-4793

Imagawa, A., Hanafusa, T., Uchigata, Y., Kanatsuka, A., Kawasaki, E., Kobayashi, T., Shimaka, A., Shimizu, I., Toyoda, T., Maruyama, T. & Makino, H. (2003). Fulminant type 1 diabetes. A nationwide survey in Japan. *Diabetes Care* Vol. 26 (No. 8): 2345-2352. ISSN 0149-5992

Imagawa, A., Hanafusa, T., Uchigata, Y., Kanatsuka, A., Kawasaki, E., Kobayashi, T., Shimada, A., Shimizu, I., Maruyama, T. & Makino, H. (2005). Different contribution of class II HLA in fulminant and typical autoimmune type 1 diabetes mellitus. *Diabetologia* Vol. 48 (No. 2): 294-300. ISSN 0012-186x

Jung, T.S., Chung, S.I., Kim, S.J., Park, M.H., Kim, D.R., Kang, M.Y. & Hahm, J.R. (2004). A Korean patient with fulminant autoantibody-negative type 1 diabetes. *Diabetes Care* Vol. 27 (No. 12): 3023-3024. ISSN 0149-5992

Kawabata, Y., Ikegami, H., Awata, T., Imagawa, A., Maruyama, T., Kawasaki, E., Tanaka, S., Shimada, A., Osawa, H., Kobayasahi, T.,Hanafusa, T., Tokunaga, K., Makino, H. & the Committee on Type 1 Diabetes, Japan Diabetes Society. (2009).Differential association of HLA with three subtypes of type 1 diabetes: fulminant, slowly progressive and acute-onset.*Diabetologia* Vol. 52 (No. 12): 2513-2521. ISSN 0021-186x

Kido, Y., Burks, D.J., Withers, D., Bruning, J.C., Kahn, C.R., White, M.E. & Accili, D. (2000). Tissue-specific insulin resistance in mice withmutations in the insulin receptor, IRS-1, and IRS-2. *Journal of Clinical Investigation* Vol. 105 (No. 2): 199-205. ISSN 0021-9738

Kim, J-E., Song, S.E., Kim, T-W., Kim, J-Y., Park, S-C., Park, Y-K., Baek, S-H., Lee, I.K. & Park, S-Y. (2010). Adiponectin inhibits palmitate-induced apoptosis through suppression of reactive oxygen species in endothelial cells: involvement of cAMP/protein kinase A and AMP-activated protein kinase. *Journal of Endocrinology* Vol. 207(No. 1): 35-44. ISSN 0022-0795

Kubota, N., Tobe, K., Terauchi, Y., Eto, K., Yamauchi, T., Suzuki, R., Tsubamoto, Y., Komeda, K., Nakano, R., Miki, H., Satoh, S., Sekihara, H., Sciacchitano, S., Lesniak, M., Aizawa, S., Nagai, R., Kimura, S., Akanuma, Y., Taylor, S.I. & Kadowaki, T. (2000). Disruption of insulin receptor substrate 2 causes type 2 diabetes because of liver insulin resistance and lack of compensatory beta-cell hyperplasia. *Diabetes* Vol. 49 (No. 11): 1880-1889. ISSN 0012-1797

Laybutt, D.R., Kaneto, H., Hasenkamp, W., Grey, S., Jonas, J.C., Sgroi, D.C., Groff, A., Ferran, C., Bonner-Weir, S., Sharma, A. & Weir, G.C. (2002). Increased expression of antioxidant and antiapoptotic genes in islets that may contribute to beta-cell survival during chronic hyperglycemia. *Diabetes* Vol. 51 (No. 2): 413-423. ISSN 0012-1797

Maedler, K., Spinas, G.A., Dyntar, D., Moritz, W., Kaiser, N. & Donath, M.Y. (2001). Distict effects of saturated and monosaturated fatty acids on beta-cell turnover and function. *Diabetes* Vol. 50 (No. 1): 69-76. ISSN 0012-1797

Matsuoka, T., Kajimoto, Y., Watada, H., Kaneto, H., Kishimoto, M., Umayahara, Y., Fujitani, Y., Kamada, T., Kawamori, R. & Yamasaki, Y. (1997). Glycation-dependent, reactive oxygen species-mediated suppression of the insulin gene promoter activity in HIT cell. *Journal of Clinical Investigation* Vol. 99 (No. 1): 144-150. ISSN 0012-9738

McGarry, J.D. & Dobbins, R.L. (1999). Fatty acid, lipotoxicity and insulin secretion. *Diabetologia* Vol. 42 (No. 1): 128-138. ISSN 0012-186x

Meier, J.J., Ritzel, R.A., Maedler, K., Gurlo, T. & Butler, P.C. (2006). Increased vulnerability of newly forming beta cells to cytokine-induced cell death. *Diabetologia* Vol. 49 (No. 1): 83-89. ISSN 0012-186x

Moreau, C., Drui, D., Arnault-Ouary, G., Charbonnel, B., Chaillous, L. & Cariou, B. (2008). Fulminant type 1 diabetes in Caucasians: a report of three cases. *Diabetes and Metabolism* Vol. 34 (No. 5): 529-532. ISSN 1262-3636

Murabayashi, N., Sugiyama, T., Kihara, C., Kusaka, H., Sugihara, T. & Sagawa, N. (2009). A case of fulminant type 1 diabetes mellitus associated with pregnancy. *Journal of Obstetrics and Gynaecology Research* Vol. 35 (No. 6): 1121-1124. ISSN 1341-8076

Ouchi, N., Kihara, S., Arita, Y., Nishida, M., Matsuyama, A., Okamoto, Y., Ishigami, M., Kurihara, H., Kishida, K., Nishizawa, H., Hotta, K., Muraguchi, M., Ohmoto, Y.,

Yamashita, S., Funahashi, T. & Matsuzawa, Y. (2001). Adipocyte-derived plasma protein, adiponectin,suppresses lipid accumulation and class A scavenger receptor expression in human monocyte-derived macrophages. *Circulation* Vol. 103 (No. 8): 1057-1063. ISSN 0009-7322

Shibasaki, S., Imagawa, A., Tauriainen, S., Iino, M., Oikarinen, M., Abiru, H., Tamaki, K., Seino, H., Nishi, K., Takase, I., Okada, Y., Uno, S., Murase-Mishiba, Y., Terasaki, J., Makino, H., Shimomura, I., Hyoty, H. & Hanafusa, T. (2010). Expression of Toll-like receptors in the pancreas of recent-onset fulminant type 1 diabetes. *Endocrine Journal* Vol. 57 (No. 1): 211-219. ISSN 0918-8959

Shimizu, I., Makino, H., Imagawa, A., Iwahashi, H., Uchigata, Y., Kanatsuka, A., Kawasaki, E., Kobayashi, T., Shimada, A., Maruyama, T.& Hanafusa, T. (2006). Clinical and immunogenetic characteristics of fulminant type 1 diabetes associated with pregnancy.*Journal of Clinical Endocrinology & Metabolism* Vol. 91 (No. 2): 471-476. ISSN 0021-972x

Tanaka, S., Nishida, Y., Aida, K., Maruyama, T., Shimada, A., Suzuki, M., Shimura, H., Takizawa, S., Takahashi, M., Akiyama, D., Arai-Yamashita, S., Furuya, F., Kawaguchi, A., Kaneshige, M., Katoh, R., Endo, T. & Kobayashi, T. (2009). Enterovirus infection, CXC chemokine ligand 10 (CXCL10), and CXCR3 circuit. A mechanism of accelerated β cell failure in fulminant type 1 diabetes.*Diabetes* Vol. 58 (No. 10): 2285-2291. ISSN 0012-1797

Tan, F. & Loh, K. (2010). Fulminant type 1 diabetes associated with pregnancy: A report of 2 cases from Malaysia. *Diabetes Research and Clinical Practice* Vol. 90: e30-e32. ISSN 0168-8227

Taniyama, M., Katsumata, R., Aoki, K., Suzuki, S. (2004). A Filipino patient with fulminant type 1 diabetes. *Diabetes Care,* Vol. 27(No. 3): 842-843, ISSN 0149-5992

Whitehead, I.P., Richards, A.A., Hickman, I.J., Macdonald, G.A. & Prins, J.B. (2006). Adiponectin – a key adipokine in the metabolic syndrome. *Diabetes, Obesity and Metabolism* Vol. 8 (No. 2): 264-280, ISSN 1462-8902

Withers, D.J., Gutierrez, J.S., Towery, H., Burks, D.J., Ren, J.M., Previs, S., Zhang, Y., Bernal, D., Pons, S., Shulman, G.I., Bonner-Weir, S., & White, M.E. (1998). Disruption of IRS-2 causes type 2 diabetes in mice. *Nature* Vol. 391: 900-904. ISSN 0028-0836

Yamauchi, T., Kamon, J., Minokoshi, Y., Ito, Y., Waki, H., Uchida, S., Yamashita, S., Noda, M., Kita, S., Ueki, K., Eto, K., Akanuma, Y., Froguel, P., Foufelle, F., Ferre, P., Carlin, D., Kimura, S., Nagai, R., Kahn, B.B. & Kadowaki, T. (2002). Adiponectin stimulates glucose utilization and fatty-acid oxidation by activating AMP-activated protein kinase. *Nature Medicine* Vol. 8: 1288-1295. ISSN 1078-8956

Yamauchi, T., Kamon, J., Ito, Y., Tsuchida, A., Yokomizo, T., Kita, S., Sugiyama, T., Miyagishi, M., Hara, K., Tsunoda, M., Murakami, K., Ohzeki, T., Uchida, S., Takekawa, S., Waki, H., Tsuno, N.H., Shibata, Y., Terauchi, Y., Froguel, P., Tobe, K., Koyasu, S., Taira, K., Kitamura, T., Shimizu, T., Nagai, R. & Kadowaki, T. (2003). Cloning of adiponectin receptors that mediate antidiabetic metabolic effects. *Nature* Vol. 423: 762-769. ISSN 0028-0836

Zheng, C., Zhou, Z., Yang, L., Huang, G., Li, X., Zhou, W., Wang, X. & Liu, Z. (2011). Fulminant type 1 diabetes mellitus exhibits distinct clinical and autoimmunity features from classical type 1 diabetes mellitus in Chinese. *Diabetes Metabolism Research and Reviews* Vol. 27 (No. 1): 70-78. ISSN 1520-7552

12

Cytokine-Induced β-Cell Stress and Death in Type 1 Diabetes Mellitus

Lisa Vincenz[1], Eva Szegezdi[1], Richard Jäger[1],
Caitriona Holohan[1], Timothy O'Brien[2] and Afshin Samali[1]
[1]*Apoptosis Research Centre*
[2]*Regenerative Medicine Institute,*
National University of Ireland Galway
Ireland

1. Introduction

1.1 Pathophysiology of type I diabetes mellitus: Role of pro-inflammatory cytokines

Type 1 diabetes mellitus (T1DM) is an autoimmune disease characterised by the destruction of insulin-producing β-cells in the pancreatic islets of Langerhans (Fig.1), which is mediated by autoreactive T cells, macrophages and pro-inflammatory cytokines (Fig.2). This leads to an inability to produce sufficient insulin resulting in elevated blood glucose levels and pathological effects (Eizirik & Mandrup-Poulsen, 2001).

T1DM is believed to be initiated by physiological β-cell death or islet injury triggering the homing of macrophages and dendritic cells that in turn launch an inflammatory reaction. The infiltrating macrophages secrete pro-inflammatory cytokines, namely interleukin-1β (IL-1β) and tumour necrosis factor α (TNFα) as well as various chemokines that attract immune cells such as dendritic cells, macrophages and T lymphocytes. T cells recognising β-cell-specific antigens become activated, infiltrate the inflamed islets and attack the β-cells (Baekkeskov et al., 1990, Elias et al., 1995, Lieberman et al., 2003, Nakayama et al., 2005). In a normally functioning immune system, T cells with a high affinity for self-antigens are eliminated during their differentiation resulting in immune 'tolerance'. Autoreactive cells that have escaped these mechanisms are subject to 'peripheral immune regulation' that blocks their activation and clonal expansion, preventing development of an autoimmune disease (Mathis & Benoist, 2004). For reasons we do not fully understand, these immune regulatory mechanisms either fail to launch, or are ineffective in stopping the immune attack against the β-cells in T1DM, and a positive feedback cycle is established (Mathis & Benoist, 2004). This forward-feeding process of T cell- and cytokine-mediated β-cell killing can be ongoing for years progressively destroying the β-cells. When over 80 % of the β-cells are deleted by this continuous T lymphocyte and inflammatory cytokine-driven attack the insulin secretory capacity falls below a certain threshold and the disease manifests itself.

Activated T cells induce death of a target cell by (1) secreting perforin and granzymes, (2) releasing pro-inflammatory cytokines including interferon-γ (IFNγ) and TNFα or (3) activation of Fas receptors on the surface of target cells. All these factors have also been described to contribute to β-cell killing in T1DM (Kägi et al., 1997, D. Liu et al., 2000, Petrovsky et al., 2002, Suk et al., 2001). In particular, recent evidence suggests that the

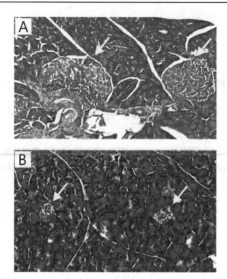

Fig. 1. β-cell islets in the pancreas of (A) pre-diabetic and (B) diabetic NOD mice. The yellow arrows indicate the islets in the haematoxylin-eosin stained tissue section (original magnification 200X).

cytokines IL-1β, TNFα and IFNγ that are secreted by macrophages and T cells have a broader role in the development of T1DM than previously thought. They are the main inducers of β-cell stress responsible for significant levels of β-cell death in both rodent (Iwahashi et al., 1996, Rabinovitch et al., 1994) and human (Delaney et al., 1997) experimental models of T1DM.

Underlining the importance of the cytokines, it has been shown that neutralisation of the pro-inflammatory cytokines by antibodies and/or soluble cytokine receptors against IL-1β, IFNγ, IL-6 and TNFα can inhibit the development of T1DM in NOD mice or BB rats (Mandrup-Poulsen, 1996). Transgenic mice expressing IFNγ in β-cells develop severe insulitis (pre-diabetes) and destruction of β-cells. Treatment of these mice with anti-IFNγ antibody prevents the development of T1DM. IFNγ-deficient mice as well as mice injected with neutralising anti-IFNγ receptor antibodies were resistant to development of experimentally-induced T1DM (Cailleau et al., 1997, Seewaldt et al., 2000, B. Wang et al., 1997). Similar to IFNγ, genetic or pharmacological abrogation of IL-1β action also reduces disease development in animal models of T1DM (Mandrup-Poulsen et al., 2010).

Although many factors contribute to β–cell destruction during T1DM, in this book chapter we review current knowledge regarding the role of cytokines mediating β–cell stress and death in T1DM.

1.2 Signal transduction of pro-inflammatory cytokines in β-cells

IL-1β, IFNγ and TNFα exert a variety of effects on β-cells. They sensitise β-cells to apoptosis by increasing the expression of pro-apoptotic proteins, such as the Fas receptor (Stassi et al., 1997). They drive and stabilise the autoimmune response by triggering the secretion of chemokines (e.g. CXCL9 and CXCL10) by β-cells (Frigerio et al., 2002), which results in constant recruitment of autoreactive T cells. Finally, pro-inflammatory cytokines directly

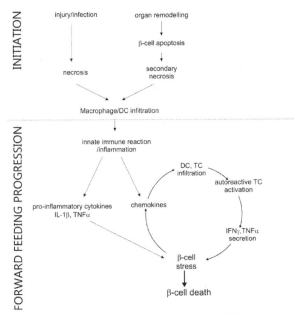

Fig. 2. Cytokine-induced β-cell death. Initial β-cell death caused by injury, infection or physiologically during development can activate an autoimmune response that leads to activation and infiltration of cytokine-secreting macrophages, dendritic cells (DC) and T cells (TC). Pro-inflammatory cytokines IL-1β, TNFα and IFNγ secreted by macrophages and TCs cause β-cell stress and death and secretion of chemokines that further stimulate autoimmune cell infiltration.

cause stress in β-cells which eventually activates the cell's death machinery. The signal transduction pathways activated by these pro-inflammatory cytokines leading to chemokine secretion, β-cell stress and death are detailed below (also see Fig. 3).

It is very important to note that any of the above pro-inflammatory cytokines alone has limited effects in terms of cell stress or death, on β-cells. However, combinations of IL-1β/IFNγ or TNFα/IFNγ have very strong, synergistic effects that trigger serious levels of stress culminating in cell death.

1.2.1 IL-1β signalling

The main mediator of IL-1β signalling is the transcription factor nuclear factor kappa B (NF-κB) (Flodström et al., 1996, Kwon et al., 1995). The pathway by which IL-1β activates NF-κB has been delineated in a number of cell types and experimental models (Fig.3). It is thought that the same mechanisms are involved in pancreatic β-cells. IL-1β, secreted by activated macrophages and T cells, binds to the IL-1 receptor 1 (IL-1R1) on the surface of target cells. IL-1R1 then recruits IL-1 receptor accessory protein (IL-1RAcP) (Dinarello, 1997). This allows binding of the adaptor protein myeloid differentiation factor 88 (MyD88) and recruitment of IL-1R1 activated kinase 1 (IRAK1) and/or IRAK2 (Burns et al., 1998, Muzio et al., 1997, Wesche et al., 1997). IRAK proteins are in complex with a protein named Tollip prior to recruitment to the receptor (Burns et al., 2000). Tollip associates with IL-1RacP when the IRAK/Tollip complex is recruited to the activated receptor. TNF-receptor-associated

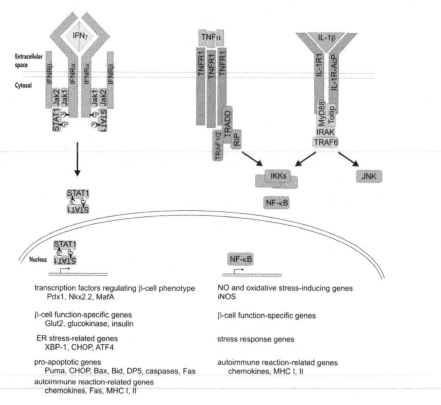

Fig. 3. Cytokine-signalling in pancreatic β-cells. IL-1β, TNFα and IFNγ activate receptors on the surface of β-cells inducing a signalling cascade leading to the activation of transcription factors STAT1 and NF-κB that control numerous genes involved in β-cell function, inflammation, stress responses and apoptosis.

factor-6 (TRAF6) is recruited to IRAK1 and IRAK2 (Muzio et al., 1997, Yamin & Miller, 1997) leading to the activation of inhibitor of NF-κB (IκB) kinase (IKK) *via* NF-κB inducing kinase (NIK). IKK then phosphorylates IκB which triggers its degradation and the release of the transcription factor NF-κB from the inhibitory interaction.

In addition, phosphatidyl inositol-3 kinase (PI3K) is recruited to the activated IL1-R1 complex where it becomes activated (Reddy et al., 1997, Reddy et al., 2004). PI3K activity is required, but not sufficient for NF-κB activation (Reddy et al., 1997).

NF-κB can regulate the transcription of numerous target genes (for review see (Pahl, 1999)). The target genes include cytokines (e.g. IL-1β, TNFα, IFNγ), chemokines, immunoreceptors, proteins involved in antigen presentation, cell adhesion molecules, stress response genes, regulators of apoptosis (both pro- and anti-apoptotic), growth factors and other transcription factors. The effects of NF-κB signalling are highly cell type-specific. In most cell types the net effect of NF-κB activation is to promote cell survival. In contrast, in β-cells NF-κB activation has a pro-apoptotic effect (Eldor et al., 2006, Ortis et al., 2008). These studies demonstrate that inhibition of NF-κB protects rodent pancreatic β-cells from the damaging effects of cytokine-exposure *in vitro* and prevents streptozocin-induced diabetes *in vivo*.

A large number of NF-κB target genes were identified using DNA microarray technology in cytokine-treated primary rat β-cells (Cardozo et al., 2001a). Cytokines induced NF-κB-dependent up-regulation of genes involved in stress responses (including CHOP, C/EBPβ and δ, Hsp27 and MnSOD), immune responses (e.g. MHC-II-associated invariant chain γ and MHC-I) and down-regulation of genes involved in β-cell function (glucose transporter-2 (Glut-2)), insulin production (Isl-1), insulin processing (PC-1), insulin release (PLD-1, CCKA-receptor) and Ca^{2+} homeostasis (SERCA2, IP 3-kinase) (Cardozo et al., 2001a). Inducible nitric oxide synthase (iNOS) is strongly induced and is the best characterised NF-κB target in both rat β-cells (Cardozo et al., 2001a, Kutlu et al., 2003) and human pancreatic islets (Flodström et al., 1996). Induction of iNOS increases nitric oxide (NO) production in β-cells, resulting in the generation of reactive oxygen species (ROS) and oxidative stress. The cellular stress triggered by NO in rodent and human cells will be discussed later in this chapter (under section 2.2).

In addition to NF-κB, IL-1β signalling also activates the mitogen activated protein kinase (MAPK) extracellular signal-regulated kinase (ERK) 1/2 and induces suppressor of cytokine signalling-3 (SOCS-3) (Emanuelli et al., 2004). Signal transduction pathways induced by MAPKs and SOCS-3 are interlinked with the NF-κB-regulated pathways; MAPK activation potentiates IL-1β-dependent NF-κB activation and subsequent iNOS induction, and (ERK)1/2 activation was shown to contribute to cytokine-induced apoptosis in rat pancreatic β-cells (Pavlovic et al., 2000). While MAPKs positively affect NF-κB signalling and enhance β-cell death, SOCS-3 has a negative effect. SOCS-3 belongs to a family of proteins that provide a negative feedback for cytokine-induced signalling. It was also identified as an inhibitor of insulin signalling (Emanuelli et al., 2000) as SOCS-3 can bind to the insulin receptor and block its insulin-induced autophosphorylation and activation (Emanuelli et al., 2004). SOCS-3 inhibits IL-1β signalling upstream and thus negatively regulates nearly all effects of IL-1β. SOCS-3 suppresses the expression of several IL-1β-induced pro-apoptotic genes, many of them known to be NF-κB-dependent (Karlsen et al., 2004) and protects rat β-cells from IL-1β- and TNFα-induced cell death (Bruun et al., 2009).

As mentioned above, over 200 genes have been identified to be NF-κB-regulated in β-cells treated with pro-inflammatory cytokines. However, which of these genes are targets of IL-1β signalling, or to what extent their expression is regulated by IL-1β alone is currently unknown. Determining the individual targets of the cytokines would lead to a better understanding of how the cytokines synergise to cause β-cell stress and death.

1.2.2 TNFα signalling

TNFα was also shown to lead to activation of NF-κB in pancreatic β-cells (Ortis et al., 2006). TNFα binds to and activates the TNF receptor (TNFR1), which is present on the surface of β-cells (Kägi et al., 1999). TNFα binding to TNFR1 leads to the latter's trimerisation and activation (Fig. 3). Upon activation, the cytosolic death domain of TNFR1 recruits TNF receptor-associated death domain (TRADD) (Hsu et al., 1995), TRAF2 (Hsu et al., 1996b) and the death domain kinase receptor interacting protein (RIP) (Hsu et al., 1996a). TRAF2, in turn, recruits IκB kinase (IKK) and induces its activation in a RIP-dependent manner via activation of an IKK kinase (e.g. NIK) (Devin et al., 2000). Activated IKK phosphorylates IκB proteins leading to their proteasomal degradation and release of NF-κB. The activation of NF-κB by both TNFα and IL-1β has a pro-apoptotic effect in rat pancreatic β-cells (Ortis et al., 2008). This effect was more pronounced in response to IL-1β than TNFα.

TNFα signalling can lead to RIP-dependent activation of three MAPKs (c-Jun N-terminal kinase JNK, p38 and ERK) in a cell type-specific manner (Devin et al., 2003). In rat pancreatic β-cells, TNFα treatment induced activation of JNK and p38 which has been suggested to contribute to an inhibitory effect of TNFα on glucose-stimulated insulin secretion (H.-E. Kim et al., 2008) and hence β-cell dysfunction in response to TNFα.

1.2.3 IFNγ signalling

IFNγ is a homodimeric cytokine. It binds to two IFNγ receptor α (IFNγRα) chains (Fig. 3). A third unit of IFNγRα and two molecules of IFNγ receptor β (IFNγRβ, also termed accessory factor 1, AF-1) bind to the IFNγRα (Thiel et al., 2000). This leads to the activation and transphosphorylation of Janus tyrosine kinase 1 and 2 (JAK1 and JAK2) which are associated with IFNγRα and IFNγRβ, respectively, and are brought together upon receptor oligomerisation (Igarashi et al., 1994, Kotenko et al., 1995). JAK1 and JAK2 phosphorylate IFNγR leading to the recruitment of two molecules of the transcription factor, signal transducer and activator of transcription-1 (STAT-1). After phosphorylation and activation by JAK2, STAT-1 homodimerises and translocates to the nucleus where it stimulates the expression of target genes (Takeda & Akira, 2000). Islet cells isolated from STAT-1-/- non-obese diabetic (NOD) mice were resistant to apoptosis induced by combined treatment with IFNγ and TNFα or IFNγ and IL-1β (S. Kim et al., 2007). In support of this, blockade of STAT-1 protected against diabetes induced by injection of multiple low doses of streptozotocin in mice (Callewaert et al., 2007, C.A. Gysemans et al., 2005). A recent gene expression analysis showed that nearly two thousand genes are regulated by STAT-1 in response to cytokine exposure (IL-1β and IFNγ) in β-cells (Moore et al., 2011). STAT-1 was found to regulate the IL-1β/IFNγ-mediated induction of chemokines, including CXCL9, CXCL10, CXCL11 and CCL20 (Moore et al., 2011) and islets from STAT-1-/- mice have decreased production of CXCL10 upon cytokine exposure both *in vitro* and *in vivo* (C.A. Gysemans et al., 2005).

STAT-1 also down-regulates several genes specific to β-cell functions, such as insulin, glucokinase, Glut2, prohormone convertases, as well as many transcription factors involved in the differentiation and maintenance of β-cell phenotype (e.g. Pdx1, MafA, Nkx2.2) (Moore et al., 2011, Perez-Arana et al., 2010).

Finally, STAT-1 is an important regulator of genes mediating intracellular stress and apoptotic pathways. Several apoptosis-related genes such as Puma, CHOP, Bax, Bid, caspase-3, -4, -7, DP5/Hrk and endoplasmic reticulum stress-transducing genes (XBP1, ATF4) are regulated by STAT-1 (Eizirik & Darville, 2001, Moore et al., 2011, Anastasis Stephanou et al., 2000). IFNγ has been found to profoundly accelerate IL-1β-mediated iNOS induction and thus cause oxidative stress. We have demonstrated that treatment of a rat insulinoma cell line (RIN-r) with a combination of IL-1β and IFNγ induces the mitochondrial apoptotic pathway in an iNOS-dependent manner (Holohan et al., 2008). This is in line with reports from other groups (Gurzov et al., 2009).

The inflammatory effects of IFNγ are controlled by negative feedback regulation, exerted by interferon regulated factor-1 (IRF-1) (Moore et al., 2011) and SOCS-1 and -3 (Alexander, 2002). IRF-1 is likely to exert its STAT-1 regulatory role by up-regulation of SOCS-1 (Moore et al., 2011). IRF-1 expression reduces chemokine expression in β-cells and resulting T cell infiltration in Langerhans islets (C. Gysemans et al., 2008, Moore et al., 2011), however the effect of IRF-1 on STAT-1-mediated β-cell de-differentiation (loss of β-cell function) and β-cell stress is minor (Moore et al., 2011). In line with this, transgenic expression of SOCS-1 in β-cells reduced diabetes development in non-obese diabetic (NOD) mice (Flodström-

Tullberg et al., 2003) and protected β-cells against infiltrating autoreactive T cells (Chong et al., 2004). In summary, the effect of IFNγ in β-cells is primarily mediated by STAT-1 through which IFNγ controls key processes culminating in loss of β-cell function, stress and finally death. IFNγ regulates a number of genes that increase the sensitivity of β-cells to apoptotic stimuli and intracellular stress.

2. Cytokine-induced β-cell death

2.1 Mechanisms of cytokine-induced β-cell death

During the development of T1DM, there are two waves of β-cell death. It is believed that β-cell death is the initial trigger for the autoimmune attack. While autoimmune attack was thought to be initiated by cytolytic activity or immune-stimulation of viruses (Jun & Yoon, 2003), it is also possible that physiological β-cell death might be a trigger. Instead of an exogenous impact, or environmental effect, induction of diabetes might be initiated during physiological tissue remodelling of the pancreas peaking at age 2-3 weeks in rodents. At this time, an increased level of β-cell death occurs in the islets and might be the primary trigger of the autoimmune attack (Turley et al., 2003). Programmed cell death associated with normal tissue remodelling does not induce inflammation. However, if the dead cells are not removed promptly by phagocytosis they can disintegrate and release cellular contents in a manner similar to pathological tissue damage which can trigger inflammation. In fact, accumulation of dead cells has been noticed in NOD mice and similarly, disintegrating, so called secondary necrotic cells were sufficient to induce inflammation, macrophage infiltration and pre-diabetic insulitis in NOD mice (H.S. Kim et al., 2007).

The second wave of β-cell death is driven by the autoimmune reaction. This is an ongoing process gradually killing the β-cells and culminating in the disease phenotype. The mechanism of β-cell death induced by the autoreactive leukocytes has been extensively examined with consensus that the major form of β-cell death is apoptosis, however, under certain conditions and especially in rodent experimental models of T1DM, necrotic β-cell death can also contribute to β-cell loss.

Apoptosis is a physiological form of cell death involved in the elimination of cells that have served their function, are no longer needed or are damaged. It is an active, highly ordered and rapid process characterised by the detachment of the dying cell from its neighbours, cell shrinkage, condensation of chromatin, fragmentation of the nucleus and finally fragmentation of the cell into membrane bound particles, called apoptotic bodies which are engulfed by neighbouring cells or professional phagocytic cells (Samali et al., 1996). By this means, cells are eliminated without leakage of otherwise inflammatory cellular material.

The morphological changes typical of apoptosis are orchestrated by the caspase family of proteases (Samali et al., 1999). Caspases are activated by two distinct mechanisms. The extrinsic pathway is triggered by an extracellular pro-apoptotic stimulus, usually a cytokine that belongs to the death ligand subfamily of the TNF superfamily. Upon engagement of the death ligand with its cognate death receptor on the cell surface of the target cell, the receptors trimerise and induce the formation of a protein complex, called the death-inducing signalling complex (DISC). The DISC is an activation platform for caspases-8 and/or -10 (Peter & Krammer, 2003). Once these initiator caspases are activated they activate downstream effector caspases, which leads to a burst of caspase activity and subsequent proteolysis that dismantles the cells.

The second, so called intrinsic pathway is initiated at the level of mitochondria. Upon intracellular stress these organelles release cytochrome c that associates with the adaptor protein APAF-1 to build a multimeric cytoplasmic protein complex termed the apoptosome, which functions to activate another initiator caspase, caspase-9 (Riedl & Salvesen, 2007). Mitochondrial release of cytochrome c, and thus activation of the intrinsic apoptosis pathway, is controlled by members of the Bcl-2 family of proteins (see section 2.3). Once cytochrome c is released and caspase-9 is activated, the same caspase cascade is triggered as during the extrinsic apoptotic pathway that leads to the final demise of the cell.

Interestingly, TNFα was shown to induce expression of an endogenous caspase inhibitor in β-cells that prevents apoptosis, the X-linked inhibitor of apoptosis protein (XIAP). This NF-kB-mediated induction of XIAP is inhibited by IFNγ signalling, providing a mechanism for synergistic cytoxicity of TNFα and IFNγ in β-cells (H.S. Kim et al., 2005).

Apoptosis is distinguished from **necrosis**, a pathological, mostly uncontrolled mode of cell death. During necrosis cells swell, their membranes disintegrate and their content is released, inducing inflammation. Recently, an active mode of necrosis, termed necroptosis, has been described that can be induced upon activation of TNFR1 when caspase-8 activation is blocked (Vandenabeele et al., 2010). A possible role of necroptosis in initiation of diabetes seems worthy of further investigation in light of the known involvement of TNFR1 signalling in diabetes and of a recent study that provided evidence of necrotic β-cell death playing a role in initiating autoimmune-type diabetes (Steer et al., 2006).

2.2 The role of nitric oxide in cytokine-mediated β-cell loss

It is thought that cytokine-induced β-cell stress and death is partly caused by intracellular production of ROS and NO. NO is a gaseous hydrophobic signalling molecule that readily diffuses through membranes and plays an essential role in various neurological, immunological and cardiovascular processes. The biosynthesis of NO is catalysed by nitric oxide synthases (NOS). In β-cells IL-1β signals up-regulation of iNOS and subsequent generation of NO. The main physiological effect of NO is mediated via the direct activation of guanylyl cyclase by NO leading to production of cyclic GMP (cGMP) and activation of cGMP-dependent signal transduction pathways. However, if present for a prolonged period or in high quantities, NO can nitrosylate specific cysteine residues of various proteins (S-nitrosylation) forming nitrosothiols and thereby affect the protein's activity, stability and localisation (Hess et al., 2005). In most cases this leads to rapid degradation of the nitrosylated proteins but a small subgroup of proteins have been shown to gain stability after nitrosylation (Paige et al., 2008). NO can have anti-apoptotic and cytoprotective effects in some cell types (McCabe et al., 2006), but can become toxic if present at high levels due to formation of ROS and protein nitrosylation which, amongst other things, also causes mitochondrial damage.

It has been shown that NO can induce both necrotic and apoptotic cell death (Bonfoco et al., 1995). With respect to β-cell destruction, it has been shown that endogenous levels of NO are sufficient to induce β-cell injury in rodent models of T1DM (Thomas et al., 2002) and increased levels of NO caused by cytokine-mediated iNOS induction cause cell death by both necrosis (Hoorens et al., 2001, Welsh et al., 1994) and apoptosis (Holohan et al., 2008). The relative involvement of NO in the destruction of β-cells in human and rodent islets is not fully elucidated. Several studies have shown that a combination of IL-1β with IFNγ or TNFα induces cell death in rodent pancreatic islet cells, predominantly by induction of apoptosis but also partly by necrosis (D. Liu et al., 2000, Saldeen, 2000). In rodent β-cells the cytokine-induced induction of necrosis seems to be dependent on iNOS-induced production of NO as the level of necrotic cell death was greatly reduced in purified β-cells from iNOS-deficient mice (D. Liu et al., 2000). Another study found that inhibition of iNOS in rat islets reduced both necrosis and apoptosis induction (Saldeen, 2000). In any case, the cytokine-induced production of NO seems to play a major role in mediating β-cell death in rodent experimental models of T1DM. Additionally, we recently demonstrated that a combination of IL-1β and IFNγ induces the intrinsic apoptosis pathway in a synergistic manner in a rat insulinoma cell line (RIN-r) and showed that iNOS-mediated production of NO was both required and sufficient for apoptosis induction (Holohan et al., 2008). This is in agreement with previous findings that showed that apoptosis induced by a combination of IL-1β and IFNγ is NO-dependent in a rat insulinoma cell line (Storling et al., 2005).

Human islets have been shown to be less sensitive to NO-induced damage compared to rodent cells. As such, inhibition of iNOS could not protect human islets from cytokine-induced cell death suggesting a NO-independent cytotoxicity. (Delaney et al., 1997, Eizirik & Mandrup-Poulsen, 2001, Hoorens et al., 2001). The resistance of human islets towards NO compared to rodent islets is speculated to be due to higher levels of heat shock protein 70 (Hsp70) in human β-cells (Burkart et al., 2000) which protects cells from the oxidative stress inflicted by NO (Welsh et al., 1994).

2.3 Role of the Bcl-2 family proteins

Cytokines can modulate the expression and/or activity of several members of the Bcl-2 family (Gowda et al., 2008, A. Stephanou et al., 2000, P. Wang et al., 2009, L. Zhang et al., 2008). The various interactions between the pro- and anti-apoptotic members of this family of proteins lie at the heart of the intrinsic pathway of apoptosis (Youle & Strasser, 2008). Bcl-2 family members are characterised by up to four conserved regions termed Bcl-2 homology (BH) domains. The pro-apoptotic multidomain family members Bax and Bak contain three BH domains and can be activated to form oligomeric structures in the outer mitochondrial membrane that trigger cytochrome c release, which then initiates the intrinsic pathway of caspase activation. Activation proceeds through interaction with BH3-only family members (harbouring only the third BH domain) that are induced or activated by cellular stress signals. Activation of Bax or Bak is counteracted by anti-apoptotic multidomain Bcl-2 family members (such as Bcl-2, Bcl-xL, or Mcl-1), which bind and sequester the BH3-only proteins.

Viral transduction of Bcl-2, the prototype member of the family, was shown to protect human islet cells from cytokine-induced apoptosis, giving a first indication that regulation of Bcl-2 family proteins by cytokines might contribute to β-cell apoptosis (Rabinovitch et al., 1999). Likewise, adenoviral transduction of Bcl-X$_L$ prevented cytokine-mediated apoptosis of RIN-r cells (Holohan et al., 2008).

Several recent studies have addressed the involvement of Bcl-2 family proteins in cytokine-induced β-cell death in more detail. Treatment of human or rat islets with inflammatory cytokines resulted in activation of the intrinsic pathway of apoptosis and involved activation of the pro-apoptotic BH3-only protein Bad by dephosphorylation (Grunnet et al., 2009). Dephosphorylation of Bad was also found in a second study analysing cytokine-treated rat islets, and in addition up-regulation of pro-apoptotic BH3-only proteins Bim and Bid was also detected (Mehmeti et al., 2011). In a different study it was shown that in primary rat β-cells cytokines as well as ER stress lead to increased expression of the pro-apoptotic BH3-only protein DP5/Hrk in a JNK-dependent manner (Gurzov et al., 2009). Up-regulation of DP5 in β-cells is mediated by the transcription factor STAT-1 which is regulated by IFNγ (Moore et al., 2011). In addition, inflammatory cytokines led to up-regulation of the pro-apoptotic BH3-only protein PUMA in primary rat β-cells as well as in human islets through a pathway involving NF-κB signalling, iNOS activation and ER stress (Gurzov et al., 2010). Furthermore, down-regulation of the anti-apoptotic multidomain Bcl-2 family member Mcl-1 turned out to be critically involved in the cytokine-induced apoptosis of the rat insulinoma cell line INS-1E (Allagnat et al., 2011). In summary, exposure to cytokines leads to alterations in expression of several Bcl-2 family members in β-cells in a manner that favours activation of the intrinsic pathway of apoptosis.

3. β-cell stress in type 1 diabetes

3.1 Endoplasmic reticulum stress

It has been suggested that endoplasmic reticulum (ER) stress is involved in β-cell destruction. Pancreatic β-cells are specialised cells that rapidly synthesise and secrete insulin in response to fluctuations in blood glucose levels (Pirot et al., 2007). This imparts a heavy burden on the ER and, consequently, β-cells are particularly susceptible to cellular conditions that impair the ER's ability to correctly fold nascent proteins. Under such conditions, the resultant accumulation of unfolded or damaged proteins within the ER lumen triggers the unfolded protein response (UPR), an adaptive signalling pathway that increases the folding capacity of the ER and restores homeostasis (Szegezdi et al., 2006). Although the initial UPR is a protective response, prolonged ER stress can lead to the initiation of apoptosis. Thus while under physiological conditions the UPR acts as a pro-survival mechanism in β-cells, chronic ER stress can lead to redirection of the UPR towards pro-apoptotic signalling.

Three ER-localized transmembrane proteins sense the accumulation of unfolded proteins in the ER lumen and initiate the UPR, PKR-like ER kinase (PERK), inositol-requiring enzyme 1 α (IRE1α) and activating transcription factor 6 (ATF6). These proteins transduce information from the ER to the nucleus by activating transcription factors that control genes involved in restoring ER function (Szegezdi et al., 2006). The PERK arm of the UPR has been the main focus of studies with regard to β-cell stress in diabetes, therefore this chapter will focus on PERK signalling in more detail. Upon accumulation of unfolded proteins, PERK is activated and induces a translational block by phosphorylating eukaryotic initiation factor 2 α (eIF2α). Phosphorylation of eIF2α by PERK leads to inhibition of cap-dependent protein synthesis. This reduces the protein load of the ER while allowing cap-independent translation to persist and leads to preferential translation of the transcription factor ATF4. One target gene induced by ATF4 (in conjunction with ATF6) is C/EBP homologous protein CHOP, a transcription factor that is known to promote apoptosis (Zinszner et al., 1998).

3.1.1 The role of PERK in β-cell function

The PERK signalling branch of the UPR appears to be essential for the regulation of β-cell function. Stimulation of insulin production in mouse pancreatic islets leads to dephosphorylation of eIF2α (P. Zhang et al., 2002) reversing the translational block caused by PERK signalling and allowing for increased biosynthesis of insulin. Studies with knockout mice showed that PERK is essential for β-cell function and survival (Harding et al., 2001, P. Zhang et al., 2002). Pancreatic β-cells of PERK⁻/⁻ mice degenerated within the first four weeks after birth, and a diabetic phenotype could be observed (Harding et al.,

2001, P. Zhang et al., 2002). β-cell loss was associated with damaged rough ER and high levels of apoptosis in the pancreas (P. Zhang et al., 2002). However, a subsequent study discovered that the onset of diabetes in PERK$^{-/-}$ mice is due to developmental defects during β-cell proliferation and differentiation leading to a reduction in β-cell mass (W. Zhang et al., 2006). At the molecular level, down-regulation of PERK in rat β-cells was shown to induce deregulation of ER chaperones Grp78 and ERp72 and disruption of ER function leading to reduced insulin production and reduced cell proliferation (Feng et al., 2009).

3.1.2 Involvement of the UPR in cytokine-induced β-cell death

There is some evidence to suggest that cytokines induce β-cell apoptosis by stimulating pro-apoptotic signalling of the UPR. Ca^{2+} levels in the ER are about four times higher than in the cytosol as high Ca^{2+} levels are required for ER function in aiding protein folding and posttranslational processing. Disruption of Ca^{2+} homeostasis causes severe ER stress resulting in accumulation of unfolded proteins in the ER and activation of the UPR. It was shown that cytokine-exposure leads to elevated basal cytosolic Ca^{2+} levels selectively in mouse pancreatic β-cells compared to glucagon-secreting α-cells and this was associated with cytokine-induced apoptosis (L. Wang et al., 1999). In line with these results, it was shown that increased production of NO in rodent β-cells leads to depletion of ER Ca^{2+} levels (Oyadomari et al., 2001). Furthermore, overexpression of the ER-located Ca^{2+}-binding protein, calreticulin increased levels of Ca^{2+} in the ER and made cells more resistant to NO-induced apoptosis (Oyadomari et al., 2001). This suggests that NO-induced apoptosis in rodent β-cells is at least partly caused by ER stress induced by NO-mediated Ca^{2+} depletion. Some evidence suggests that NO may regulate Ca^{2+} levels in β-cells through down-regulation of the sarcoendoplasmic reticulum Ca^{2+} ATPase 2b (SERCA2b) (Cardozo et al., 2005). SERCA pumps Ca^{2+} from the cytoplasm into the ER thus maintaining ER Ca^{2+} levels. Rodent and human islet cells have been reported to express the isoforms SERCA2b and SERCA3 (Varadi et al., 1996). Treatment of rodent pancreatic β-cells with a combination of IL-1β and IFNγ induced transcriptional down-regulation of SERCA2b and this was partially prevented by inhibition of iNOS. Furthermore, after inhibition of SERCA, the effect of cytokine exposure on ER Ca^{2+} was abolished (Cardozo et al., 2005). This suggests that NO-induced depletion of ER Ca^{2+} is at least in part mediated by SERCA down-regulation. The SERCA isoform SERCA2a has been shown to be specifically inactivated by peroxynitrite (ONOO-)-mediated nitration of a tyrosine residue within the channel-like domain *in vitro* (Viner et al., 1999). Peroxynitrite is produced in cells by a reaction between NO and the free radical superoxide (Pacher et al., 2007). SERCA2a differs from SERCA2b only in regions of the C-terminus (Dode et al., 1998) and it could be hypothesised that cytokine-induced NO production inhibits SERCA2b Ca^{2+}-ATPase activity by peroxynitrite-mediated nitration in the same way. Another possible mechanism by which NO might mediate reduction of ER Ca^{2+} levels is via activation of the ryanodine receptor-2. Ryanodine receptor-2 is a calcium channel located in the ER membrane that releases Ca^{2+} from the ER into the cytosol and has been reported to be expressed in mouse pancreatic β-cells (Islam et al., 1998). NO-induced poly-S-nitrosylation enhances the activity of this calcium channel (Xu et al., 1998) but whether this mechanism is relevant to cytokine-exposed β-cells remains to be determined. Treatment of rodent β-cells with a combination of IL-1β and IFNγ induces the expression of CHOP in an NO-dependent manner (Fig. 4). This is in line with a number of other reports (Cardozo et al., 2001b, Cardozo et al., 2005). Inhibition of iNOS by N5-(1-iminoethyl)-L-ornithine (L-NIO) or N^G-methyl-L-arginine (LMA) blocked cytokine-induced NO production and expression of CHOP. In addition to CHOP, the UPR marker proteins Grp78 and phosphorylated eIF2α were also found to be up-regulated after cytokine treatment, without affecting expression of spliced X-box binding protein 1 (sXBP-1) which is induced downstream of IRE1α (Fig. 4). Overexpression of iNOS alone was sufficient for CHOP expression (Fig. 4) and treatment with the NO-donor molecule S-nitroso-N-acetyl-D,L-penicillamine (SNAP) induced expression of Grp78 and CHOP (Oyadomari et al., 2001). This suggests that NO is sufficient to activate the UPR in rodent pancreatic β-cells. Pancreatic islet cells from CHOP-/- mice were shown to be resistant to cytokine- and NO-mediated apoptosis compared to cells from CHOP+/+ and CHOP+/- mice (Oyadomari et al., 2001). Together these results suggest that the apoptotic effects of cytokine-induced NO are mediated by activation of CHOP.

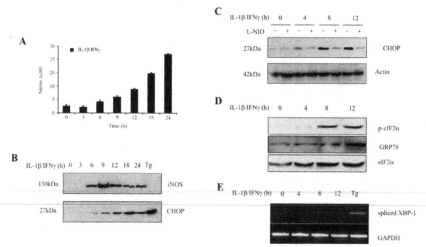

Fig. 4. IL-1β/IFNγ induced the expression of the pro-apoptotic transcription factor CHOP and other UPR markers. (A) A time-course cytokine treatment (IL-1β and IFNγ, 60 U/ml of each) was carried out and samples assayed for NO production. (B) The same samples were then analysed by Western blotting for iNOS and CHOP expression. This data demonstrates an increase in NO production, iNOS expression and CHOP induction occurring at 6 h post cytokine treatment, although CHOP is not strongly expressed until 9 h. (C) Samples were assayed for CHOP expression following cytokine treatment in the presence and absence of the iNOS inhibitor L-NIO. Cytokine-induced CHOP expression was decreased in the presence of L-NIO indicating that this is an NO-dependent process. (D) Alterations in the expression of ER stress-associated proteins after cytokine treatment were analysed by Western blotting. The expression of UPR markers Grp78 and phosphorylated eIF2α (p-eIF2α) were up in response to cytokine treatment. (E) Production of spliced XBP-1 mRNA after cytokine treatment was determined by RT-PCR. Thapsigargin (Tg) treatment was used as a positive control. Cytokine treatment did not show an effect on the level of spliced XBP-1 mRNA. The images presented are representative of three independent experiments.

Conversely, another study suggested that although cytokine signalling induces ER stress as demonstrated by activation of PERK and JNK, induction of CHOP is not required for β-cell death in rodents (Åkerfeldt et al., 2008). In support of these findings, a recent study suggests that CHOP is not required for β-cell death and the development of diabetes in NOD mice (Satoh et al., 2011). However, CHOP$^{-/-}$ NOD mice showed delayed production of insulin autoimmune antibodies (Satoh et al., 2011) suggesting a role for CHOP in the early onset of the autoimmune reaction leading to β-cell destruction. Therefore, cytokine-induced β-cell death may be partly mediated by induction of CHOP.

While a functional UPR (at least the PERK branch) appears to be essential for β-cell function and development, its downstream target CHOP has been associated with cytokine-induced β-cell destruction suggesting that PERK signalling regulates β-cell function and survival under physiological conditions but may switch towards pro-death signalling under conditions of cytokine-induced β-cell stress.

3.2 Oxidative stress

Cytokines induce multiple stress pathways in β-cells. Oxidative stress is induced by increased production of ROS and an imbalanced, low level of antioxidant enzymes (Sies, 1997). IL-1β, TNFα and IFNγ induce the production of ROS and NO by inducing iNOS (Rabinovitch & Suarez-Pinzon, 1998). Free oxygen and nitrogen radicals generated can react to form peroxynitrite, which is a very strong oxidant. Oxygen free radicals, nitrogen free radicals as well as the radical peroxynitrite can react with and damage a range of cellular proteins and in this way block metabolic functions and induce β-cell death (Azevedo-Martins et al., 2003). β-cells have been shown to be especially susceptible to such oxidative stress because they have particularly low levels of antioxidant enzymes (Lenzen et al., 1996, Tiedge et al., 1998).

4. Therapeutic strategies

The number of people affected by T1DM is approximately 20 million worldwide and is rapidly rising (Chabot, 2002). While exogenous administration of insulin is an effective treatment for acute hyperglycaemia in T1DM, it does not prevent secondary complications (White et al., 2008) and can in some cases lead to hypoglycaemia (Kort et al., 2011). Alternative therapeutic strategies include pancreas transplantation and islet transplantation. While whole pancreas transplantation is an invasive surgical method associated with major complications, islet transplantation is less invasive and associated with significantly lower morbidity and mortality. Successful islet transplantation would result in insulin independence, protection from hypoglycaemia, improvement of microvascular complications, improved patient survival and enhanced quality of life (Kort et al., 2011). The method is currently in clinical trials and has been used to treat around 1,000 individuals worldwide (Kort et al., 2011). Islet transplantation has many limitations, including limited availability of suitable islet graft donors, high cost and high rate of partial or total graft failure. Islet graft failure can be caused by allorejection, toxicity of immunosuppressive drugs that are required to reduce immune rejection, glucotoxicity, and recurrence of autoimmunity (Kort et al., 2011).

An approach to reduce β-cell death in islet grafts is the transfer of therapeutically useful genes into islet cells prior to transplantation (McCabe et al., 2006). The development of gene therapy techniques that can protect β-cells from autoimmune destruction may not only improve outcomes after islet transplantation but may also lead to preventive therapies for patients at high risk of developing T1DM (McCabe et al., 2006).

Various candidate transgenes are being examined for their potential in protecting β-cells under various stresses including cytokine-exposure and oxidative stress. The rational choice of therapeutic genes is helped by understanding the mechanism of β-cell destruction which has been the subject of this chapter. Potential targets will be reviewed in this section. Target genes studied to date encode regulators of the cytokine signal transduction pathways, molecules that inhibit β-cell apoptosis, antioxidant enzymes, immunoregulatory proteins and pro-survival cytokines (McCabe et al., 2006).

4.1 Anti-apoptotic gene transfer

Apoptosis plays a major role in β-cell death in T1DM (see section 2.). The transfer of anti-apoptotic genes as a strategy to counteract islet destruction has been explored. Candidate genes include those expressing cytoprotective and anti-apoptotic heat shock proteins (Hsps) and anti-apoptotic Bcl-2 family proteins. Hsp70 is one of the major heat shock proteins in mammals and is thought to be responsible for the relative resistance of human β-cells to cytokine-induced stress and death (Burkart et al., 2000). Hsp70 can protect cells under conditions of stress by directly inhibiting the transduction of the apoptotic signal, by decreasing the amount of oxidative stress and also by reducing ER stress via its chaperone activity. It has been shown that pre-conditioning by heat shock could protect pancreatic islet cells from insults by NO, ROS and the cytotoxic drug streptozocin and this increased resistance correlated with induced expression of Hsp70 (Bellmann et al., 1995). Another Hsp that is potentially capable of protecting β-cells is heme oxygenase (HO-1), also known as Hsp32. HO-1 exerts its cytoprotective effects mainly by reduction of oxidative stress (McCabe et al., 2006) and overexpression of HO-1 could protect cytokine-exposed islet cells from apoptosis (Pileggi et al., 2001, Ye & Laychock, 1998). Bcl-2 family proteins, such as the anti-apoptotic Bcl-2, are major regulators of the apoptotic signalling cascade. It has been suggested that an impaired induction of anti-apoptotic Bcl-2 plays a role in cytokine-induced dysfunction and cell death of human islet cells relative to porcine islets (Piro et al., 2001). Moreover, overexpression of Bcl-2 was shown to protect β-cells from cytokine-induced apoptosis (Y. Liu et al., 1996) and increase the longevity of islet grafts after transplantation (Contreras et al., 2001). Several mechanisms by which Bcl-2 might exert β-cell protection have been suggested (McCabe et al., 2006). These include inhibition of cytochrome c release from mitochondria, inhibition of ER stress-induced apoptosis and blocking of Ca^{2+} release from the ER. It was shown that Bcl-2 overexpression can reduce ER stress-induced apoptosis in islet cells (Contreras et al., 2003). Both of these mechanisms have been associated with cytokine-induced β-cell death. Another candidate transgene may be the gene encoding the cellular FADD-like IL-1β-converting enzyme (FLICE)-like inhibitory protein (cFlip) as its overexpression has been shown to inhibit the activation of caspase-8 in β-cells exposed to TNFα (Cottet et al., 2002).

4.2 Anti-cytokine gene transfer

Inhibition of NF-κB, a main effector of cytokine-signalling, was shown to reduce cytokine-induced apoptosis in rodent β-cells *in vitro* (Baker et al., 2001, Heimberg et al., 2001) and *in vivo* (Eldor et al., 2006) and Fas-induced apoptosis in human islet cells (Giannoukakis et al., 2000). It should be noted that active NF-κB has been shown to be an essential factor in mediating glucose-stimulated insulin secretion (Norlin et al., 2005) and while NF-κB inhibition may protect β-cells from apoptosis it may also interfere with insulin secretion.

JNK is another candidate target for anti-cytokine gene therapy. Inhibition of JNK has been shown to protect pig islet cells from apoptosis and loss of JNK function after isolation and also after transplantation suppresses IL-1β induced apoptosis in insulin-secreting rodent cell lines (Nikulina et al., 2003, Noguchi et al., 2005). Other potential transgenes interfering with cytokine signalling include feedback inhibitors, e.g. SOCS (Yasukawa et al., 2000). It is thought that a compromised ability to up-regulate SOCS in response to cytokine exposure makes β-cells particularly susceptible to cytokine-induced damage (Karlsen et al., 2001, Yasukawa et al., 2000). The overexpression of SOCS-3 in response to IL-1β was shown to be slower in β-cells compared to other cell lines (Karlsen et al., 2001). It was also demonstrated that SOCS-3 overexpression can protect rodent β-cells from cytokine-induced death (Karlsen et al., 2001).

4.3 Anti-oxidant gene transfer

The protective effects of several antioxidant enzymes including catalase, glutathione peroxidase and the superoxide dismutases (SODs) MnSOD and CuZnSOD have been investigated. While results have not been entirely consistent, many studies have demonstrated that activation or overexpression of these enzymes can protect β-cells against oxidative stress or cytokine-induced destruction at least to some extent (Benhamou et al., 1998, Bertera et al., 2003, Hohmeier et al., 1998, Lortz & Tiedge, 2003, Lortz et al., 2000). These studies have shown that antioxidant gene transfer is a promising strategy in prolonging islet graft longevity. However, it has also been observed that transfer of antioxidant genes alone could not protect β-cells long term against toxicity caused by cytokine exposure and oxidative stress.

5. Conclusion

In recent years basic biomedical research has delivered a wealth of knowledge about the pathways by which inflammatory cytokines sensitise β-cells to cell death during the course of T1DM pathogenesis. Although the picture is still incomplete, we have learned about the major stresses to which β-cells are exposed. Some of the molecular players mediating these stresses have been identified. In particular, pro-inflammatory cytokines IL-1β, TNFα and IFNγ have been implicated as main mediators of β-cell stress and death during T1DM. It emerges that these cytokines synergistically activate transcriptional programs that lead to NO signalling, oxidative stress, ER stress, as well as modulation of Bcl-2 family protein expression. How these pathways precisely intersect has not yet been fully clarified. Studies elucidating these mechanisms may provide the knowledge to improve therapy. Islet transplantation, a therapeutic approach that would overcome the need of continuous insulin administration, is still in its infancy. Modern gene transfer techniques offer a huge potential for improvement to islet transplantation as it can help overcoming the cellular and autoimmune-mediated stress transplanted islets are exposed to. The experiments mentioned at the end of this chapter are encouraging that the accumulating knowledge of the molecules and pathways mediating β-cell stress will help to develop gene therapeutic approaches alleviating these stresses, thus improving survival of transplanted islets.

6. Acknowledgement

We are grateful to Dr. Sandra Healy for critical reading of this manuscript and Anna McCormick for providing the microscopy images of mouse pancreatic tissue sections. LV is funded by an Irish Cancer Society Scholarship (CRS10VIN). Our work is in part supported by a grant from Science Foundation Ireland (09/RFP/BIC2371).

7. References

Åkerfeldt, M.C., Howes, J., Chan, J.Y., Stevens, V.A., Boubenna, N., McGuire, H.M., King, C., Biden, T.J. & Laybutt, D.R. (2008). Cytokine-Induced B-Cell Death Is Independent of Endoplasmic Reticulum Stress Signaling. *Diabetes*, Vol. 57, No.11, (Nov), pp.(3034-3044), 1939-327X (Electronic), 0012-1797 (Linking)

Alexander, W.S. (2002). Suppressors of Cytokine Signalling (Socs) in the Immune System. *Nat Rev Immunol*, Vol. 2, No.6, (Jun), pp.(410-416), 1474-1733

Allagnat, F., Cunha, D., Moore, F., Vanderwinden, J.M., Eizirik, D.L. & Cardozo, A.K. (2011). Mcl-1 Downregulation by Pro-Inflammatory Cytokines and Palmitate Is an Early Event Contributing to Beta-Cell Apoptosis. *Cell Death Differ*, Vol. 18, No.2, (Feb), pp.(328-337), 1476-5403 (Electronic), 1350-9047 (Linking)

Azevedo-Martins, A.K., Lortz, S., Lenzen, S., Curi, R., Eizirik, D.L. & Tiedge, M. (2003). Improvement of the Mitochondrial Antioxidant Defense Status Prevents Cytokine-Induced Nuclear Factor-Kb Activation in Insulin-Producing Cells. *Diabetes*, Vol. 52, No.1, (Jan), pp.(93-101), 0012-1797

Baekkeskov, S., Aanstoot, H.-J., Christgai, S., Reetz, A., Solimena, M., Cascalho, M., Folli, F., Richter-Olesen, H. & Camilli, P.-D. (1990). Identification of the 64k Autoantigen in Insulin-Dependent Diabetes as the Gaba-Synthesizing Enzyme Glutamic Acid Decarboxylase. *Nature*, Vol. 347, No.6289, (Sep 13), pp.(151-156), 0028-0836

Baker, M.S., Chen, X., Cao, X.C. & Kaufman, D.B. (2001). Expression of a Dominant Negative Inhibitor of Nf-[Kappa]B Protects Min6 [Beta]-Cells from Cytokine-Induced Apoptosis. *Journal of Surgical Research*, Vol. 97, No.2, (May 15), pp.(117-122), 0022-4804 (Print), 0022-4804 (Linking)

Bellmann, K., Wenz, A., Radons, J., Burkart, V., Kleemann, R. & Kolb, H. (1995). Heat Shock Induces Resistance in Rat Pancreatic Islet Cells against Nitric Oxide, Oxygen Radicals and Streptozotocin Toxicity in Vitro. *The Journal of Clinical Investigation*, Vol. 95, No.6, (Jun), pp.(2840-2845), 0021-9738

Benhamou, P.Y., Moriscot, C., Richard, M.J., Beatrix, O., Badet, L., Pattou, F., Kerr-Conte, J., Chroboczek, J., Lemarchand, P. & Halimi, S. (1998). Adenovirus-Mediated Catalase Gene Transfer Reduces Oxidant Stress in Human, Porcine and Rat Pancreatic Islets. *Diabetologia*, Vol. 41, No.9, (Sep), pp.(1093-1100), 0012-186X

Bertera, S., Crawford, M.L., Alexander, A.M., Papworth, G.D., Watkins, S.C., Robbins, P.D. & Trucco, M. (2003). Gene Transfer of Manganese Superoxide Dismutase Extends Islet Graft Function in a Mouse Model of Autoimmune Diabetes. *Diabetes*, Vol. 52, No.2, (Feb), pp.(387-393), 0012-1797

Bonfoco, E., Krainc, D., Ankarcrona, M., Nicotera, P. & Lipton, S.A. (1995). Apoptosis and Necrosis: Two Distinct Events Induced, Respectively, by Mild and Intense Insults with N-Methyl-D-Aspartate or Nitric Oxide/Superoxide in Cortical Cell Cultures. *Proceedings of the National Academy of Sciences of the United States of America*, Vol. 92, No.16, (Aug 1), pp.(7162-7166), 0027-8424 (Print), 0027-8424 (Linking)

Bruun, C., Heding, P.E., Rønn, S.G., Frobøse, H., Rhodes, C.J., Mandrup-Poulsen, T. & Billestrup, N. (2009). Suppressor of Cytokine Signalling-3 Inhibits Tumor Necrosis Factor-Alpha Induced Apoptosis and Signalling in Beta Cells. *Molecular and Cellular Endocrinology*, Vol. 311, No.1-2, (Nov 13), pp.(32-38), 1872-8057 (Electronic), 0303-7207 (Linking)

Burkart, V., Liu, H., Bellmann, K., Wissing, D., Jäättelä, M., Cavallo, M.G., Pozzilli, P., Briviba, K. & Kolb, H. (2000). Natural Resistance of Human Beta Cells toward Nitric Oxide Is Mediated by Heat Shock Protein 70. *Journal of Biological Chemistry*, Vol. 275, No.26, (Jun 30), pp.(19521-19528), 0021-9258

Burns, K., Clatworthy, J., Martin, L., Martinon, F., Plumpton, C., Maschera, B., Lewis, A., Ray, K., Tschopp, J. & Volpe, F. (2000). Tollip, a New Component of the Il-1ri Pathway, Links Irak to the Il-1 Receptor. *Nat Cell Biol*, Vol. 2, No.6, (Jun), pp.(346-351), 1465-7392

Burns, K., Martinon, F., Esslinger, C., Pahl, H., Schneider, P., Bodmer, J.-L., Di Marco, F., French, L. & Tschopp, J. (1998). Myd88, an Adapter Protein Involved in Interleukin-1 Signaling. *Journal of Biological Chemistry*, Vol. 273, No.20, (May 15), pp.(12203-12209), 0021-9258

Cailleau, C., Diu-Hercend, A., Ruuth, E., Westwood, R. & Carnaud, C. (1997). Treatment with Neutralizing Antibodies Specific for Il-1beta Prevents Cyclophosphamide-Induced Diabetes in Nonobese Diabetic Mice. *Diabetes*, Vol. 46, No.6, (Jun 1), pp.(937-940), 0012-1797

Callewaert, H.I., Gysemans, C.A., Ladrière, L., D'Hertog, W., Hagenbrock, J., Overbergh, L., Eizirik, D.L. & Mathieu, C. (2007). Deletion of Stat-1 Pancreatic Islets Protects against Streptozotocin-Induced Diabetes and Early Graft Failure but Not against Late Rejection. *Diabetes*, Vol. 56, No.8, (Aug), pp.(2169-2173), 1939-327X (Electronic), 0012-1797 (Linking)

Cardozo, A.K., Heimberg, H., Heremans, Y., Leeman, R., Kutlu, B., Kruhøffer, M., Ørntoft, T. & Eizirik, D.L. (2001a). A Comprehensive Analysis of Cytokine-Induced and Nuclear Factor-Kb-Dependent Genes in Primary Rat Pancreatic B-Cells. *Journal of Biological Chemistry*, Vol. 276, No.52, (Dec 28), pp.(48879-48886), 0021-9258

Cardozo, A.K., Kruhoffer, M., Leeman, R., Orntoft, T. & Eizirik, D.L. (2001b). Identification of Novel Cytokine-Induced Genes in Pancreatic Beta-Cells by High-Density Oligonucleotide Arrays. *Diabetes*, Vol. 50, No.5, (May), pp.(909-920), 0012-1797

Cardozo, A.K., Ortis, F., Storling, J., Feng, Y.-M., Rasschaert, J., Tonnesen, M., Van Eylen, F., Mandrup-Poulsen, T., Herchuelz, A. & Eizirik, D.L. (2005). Cytokines Downregulate the Sarcoendoplasmic Reticulum Pump Ca2+ Atpase 2b and Deplete Endoplasmic Reticulum Ca2+, Leading to Induction of Endoplasmic Reticulum Stress in Pancreatic B-Cells. *Diabetes*, Vol. 54, No.2, (Feb 1), pp.(452-461), 0012-1797

Chabot, J.M. (2002). A Report from the World Health Organization. *Rev Prat.*, Vol. 52, No.19, (Dec 1), pp.(2155-2156), 0035-2640

Chong, M.M.W., Chen, Y., Darwiche, R., Dudek, N.L., Irawaty, W., Santamaria, P., Allison, J., Kay, T.W.H. & Thomas, H.E. (2004). Suppressor of Cytokine Signaling-1 Overexpression Protects Pancreatic B Cells from Cd8+ T Cell-Mediated

Autoimmune Destruction. *The Journal of Immunology*, Vol. 172, No.9, (May 1), pp.(5714-5721), 0022-1767

Contreras, J.L., Bilbao, G., Smyth, C.A., Jiang, X.L., Eckhoff, D.E., Jenkins, S.M., Thomas, F.T., Curiel, D.T. & Thomas, J.M. (2001). Cytoprotection of Pancreatic Islets before and Soon after Transplantation by Gene Transfer of the Anti-Apoptotic Bcl-2 Gene 1. *Transplantation*, Vol. 71, No.8, (Apr 27), 0041-1337

Contreras, J.L., Smyth, C.A., Bilbao, G., Eckstein, C., Young, C.J., Thompson, J.A., Curiel, D.T. & Eckhoff, D.E. (2003). Coupling Endoplasmic Reticulum Stress to Cell Death Program in Isolated Human Pancreatic Islets: Effects of Gene Transfer of Bcl-2. *Transplant International*, Vol. 16, No.7, (Jul), pp.(537-542-542-537-542-542), 0934-0874

Cottet, S., Dupraz, P., Hamburger, F., Dolci, W., Jaquet, M. & Thorens, B. (2002). Cflip Protein Prevents Tumor Necrosis Factor-A–Mediated Induction of Caspase-8–Dependent Apoptosis in Insulin-Secreting Btc-Tet Cells. *Diabetes*, Vol. 51, No.6, (Jun), pp.(1805-1814), 0012-1797

Delaney, C.A., Pavlovic, D., Hoorens, A., Pipeleers, D.G. & Eizirik, D.L. (1997). Cytokines Induce Deoxyribonucleic Acid Strand Breaks and Apoptosis in Human Pancreatic Islet Cells. *Endocrinology*, Vol. 138, No.6, (Jun), pp.(2610-2614), 0013-7227

Devin, A., Cook, A., Lin, Y., Rodriguez, Y., Kelliher, M. & Liu, Z.G. (2000). The Distinct Roles of Traf2 and Rip in Ikk Activation by Tnf-R1: Traf2 Recruits Ikk to Tnf-R1 While Rip Mediates Ikk Activation. *Immunity*, Vol. 12, No.4, (Apr), pp.(419-429), 1074-7613

Devin, A., Lin, Y. & Liu, Z.-g. (2003). The Role of the Death-Domain Kinase Rip in Tumour-Necrosis-Factor-Induced Activation of Mitogen-Activated Protein Kinases. *EMBO reports*, Vol. 4, No.6, (Jun), pp.(623-627), 1469-221X

Dinarello, C.A. (1997). Interleukin-1. *Cytokine & Growth Factor Reviews*, Vol. 8, No.4, (Dec), pp.(253-265), 1359-6101

Dode, L., De Greef, C., Mountian, I., Attard, M., Town, M.M., Casteels, R. & Wuytack, F. (1998). Structure of the Human Sarco/Endoplasmic Reticulum Ca2+-Atpase 3 Gene. Promoter Analysis and Alternative Splicing of the Serca3 Pre-Mrna. *J Biol Chem*, Vol. 273, No.22, (May 29), pp.(13982-13994), 0021-9258

Eizirik, D.L. & Darville, M.I. (2001). Beta-Cell Apoptosis and Defense Mechanisms: Lessons from Type 1 Diabetes. *Diabetes*, Vol. 50, No.suppl 1, (Feb), pp.(S64-S64), 0012-1797

Eizirik, D.L. & Mandrup-Poulsen, T. (2001). A Choice of Death - the Signal-Transduction of Immune-Mediated Beta-Cell Apoptosis. *Diabetologia*, Vol. 44, No.12, (Dec), pp.(2115-2133), 0012-186X (Print), 0012-186X (Linking)

Eldor, R., Yeffet, A., Baum, K., Doviner, V., Amar, D., Ben-Neriah, Y., Christofori, G., Peled, A., Carel, J.C., Boitard, C., Klein, T., Serup, P., Eizirik, D.L. & Melloul, D. (2006). Conditional and Specific Nf-Kb Blockade Protects Pancreatic Beta Cells from Diabetogenic Agents. *Proceedings of the National Academy of Sciences of the United States of America*, Vol. 103, No.13, (Mar 28), pp.(5072-5077), 0027-8424

Elias, D., Marcus, H., Reshef, T., Ablamunits, V. & Cohen, I.R. (1995). Induction of Diabetes in Standard Mice by Immunization with the P277 Peptide of a 60-Kda Heat Shock Protein. *European Journal of Immunology*, Vol. 25, No.10, (Oct), pp.(2851-2857), 0014-2980

Emanuelli, B., Glondu, M., Filloux, C., Peraldi, P. & Van Obberghen, E. (2004). The Potential Role of Socs-3 in the Interleukin-1β-Induced Desensitization of Insulin Signaling in Pancreatic Beta-Cells. *Diabetes,* Vol. 53, No.suppl 3, (Dec 1), pp.(S97-S103), 0012-1797

Emanuelli, B., Peraldi, P., Filloux, C., Sawka-Verhelle, D., Hilton, D. & Van Obberghen, E. (2000). Socs-3 Is an Insulin-Induced Negative Regulator of Insulin Signaling. *Journal of Biological Chemistry,* Vol. 275, No.21, (May 26), pp.(15985-15991), 0021-9258

Feng, D., Wei, J., Gupta, S., McGrath, B.C. & Cavener, D.R. (2009). Acute Ablation of Perk Results in Er Dysfunctions Followed by Reduced Insulin Secretion and Cell Proliferation. *BMC Cell Biol,* Vol. 10, (Sep 4), pp.(61), 1471-2121

Flodström-Tullberg, M., Yadav, D., Hägerkvist, R., Tsai, D., Secrest, P., Stotland, A. & Sarvetnick, N. (2003). Target Cell Expression of Suppressor of Cytokine Signaling-1 Prevents Diabetes in the Nod Mouse. *Diabetes,* Vol. 52, No.11, (Nov 1), pp.(2696-2700), 0012-1797

Flodström, M., Welsh, N. & Eizirik, D.L. (1996). Cytokines Activate the Nuclear Factor [Kappa]B (Nf-[Kappa]B) and Induce Nitric Oxide Production in Human Pancreatic Islets. *FEBS Letters,* Vol. 385, No.1-2, (Apr 29), pp.(4-6), 0014-5793

Frigerio, S., Junt, T., Lu, B., Gerard, C., Zumsteg, U., Hollander, G.A. & Piali, L. (2002). [Beta] Cells Are Responsible for Cxcr3-Mediated T-Cell Infiltration in Insulitis. *Nat Med,* Vol. 8, No.12, (Dec), pp.(1414-1420), 1078-8956

Giannoukakis, N., Rudert, W.A., Trucco, M. & Robbins, P.D. (2000). Protection of Human Islets from the Effects of Interleukin-1β by Adenoviral Gene Transfer of an Iκb Repressor. *Journal of Biological Chemistry,* Vol. 275, No.47, (Nov 24), pp.(36509-36513), 0021-9258

Gowda, A., Roda, J., Hussain, S.R., Ramanunni, A., Joshi, T., Schmidt, S., Zhang, X., Lehman, A., Jarjoura, D., Carson, W.E., Kindsvogel, W., Cheney, C., Caligiuri, M.A., Tridandapani, S., Muthusamy, N. & Byrd, J.C. (2008). Il-21 Mediates Apoptosis through up-Regulation of the Bh3 Family Member Bim and Enhances Both Direct and Antibody-Dependent Cellular Cytotoxicity in Primary Chronic Lymphocytic Leukemia Cells in Vitro. *Blood,* Vol. 111, No.9, (May 1), pp.(4723-4730), 1528-0020 (Electronic), 0006-4971 (Linking)

Grunnet, L.G., Aikin, R., Tonnesen, M.F., Paraskevas, S., Blaabjerg, L., Storling, J., Rosenberg, L., Billestrup, N., Maysinger, D. & Mandrup-Poulsen, T. (2009). Proinflammatory Cytokines Activate the Intrinsic Apoptotic Pathway in Beta-Cells. *Diabetes,* Vol. 58, No.8, (Aug), pp.(1807-1815), 1939-327X (Electronic), 0012-1797 (Linking)

Gurzov, E.N., Germano, C.M., Cunha, D.A., Ortis, F., Vanderwinden, J.M., Marchetti, P., Zhang, L. & Eizirik, D.L. (2010). P53 up-Regulated Modulator of Apoptosis (Puma) Activation Contributes to Pancreatic Beta-Cell Apoptosis Induced by Proinflammatory Cytokines and Endoplasmic Reticulum Stress. *J Biol Chem,* Vol. 285, No.26, (Jun 25), pp.(19910-19920), 1083-351X (Electronic), 0021-9258 (Linking)

Gurzov, E.N., Ortis, F., Cunha, D.A., Gosset, G., Li, M., Cardozo, A.K. & Eizirik, D.L. (2009). Signaling by Il-1beta+Ifn-Gamma and Er Stress Converge on Dp5/Hrk Activation:

A Novel Mechanism for Pancreatic Beta-Cell Apoptosis. *Cell Death Differ,* Vol. 16, No.11, (Nov), pp.(1539-1550), 1476-5403 (Electronic), 1350-9047 (Linking)

Gysemans, C., Callewaert, H., Overbergh, L. & Mathieu, C. (2008). Cytokine Signalling in the B-Cell: A Dual Role for Ifnγ. *Biochemical Society Transactions,* Vol. 36, No.3, (Jun), pp.(328-333), 0300-5127

Gysemans, C.A., Ladrière, L., Callewaert, H., Rasschaert, J., Flamez, D., Levy, D.E., Matthys, P., Eizirik, D.L. & Mathieu, C. (2005). Disruption of the Γ-Interferon Signaling Pathway at the Level of Signal Transducer and Activator of Transcription-1 Prevents Immune Destruction of B-Cells. *Diabetes,* Vol. 54, No.8, (Aug 1), pp.(2396-2403), 0012-1797

Harding, H.P., Zeng, H., Zhang, Y., Jungries, R., Chung, P., Plesken, H., Sabatini, D.D. & Ron, D. (2001). Diabetes Mellitus and Exocrine Pancreatic Dysfunction in Perk-/-Mice Reveals a Role for Translational Control in Secretory Cell Survival. *Mol Cell,* Vol. 7, No.6, (Jun), pp.(1153-1163), 1097-2765

Heimberg, H., Heremans, Y., Jobin, C., Leemans, R., Cardozo, A.K., Darville, M. & Eizirik, D.L. (2001). Inhibition of Cytokine-Induced Nf-Kapab Activation by Adenovirus-Mediated Expression of a Nf-Kappab Super-Repressor Prevents Beta-Cell Apoptosis. *Diabetes,* Vol. 50, No.10, (Oct), pp.(2219-2224), 0012-1797

Hess, D.T., Matsumoto, A., Kim, S.-O., Marshall, H.E. & Stamler, J.S. (2005). Protein S-Nitrosylation: Purview and Parameters. *Nat Rev Mol Cell Biol,* Vol. 6, No.2, (Feb), pp.(150-166), 1471-0072

Hohmeier, H.E., Thigpen, A., Tran, V.V., Davis, R. & Newgard, C.B. (1998). Stable Expression of Manganese Superoxide Dismutase (Mnsod) in Insulinoma Cells Prevents Il-1beta- Induced Cytotoxicity and Reduces Nitric Oxide Production. *The Journal of Clinical Investigation,* Vol. 101, No.9, (May 1), pp.(1811-1820), 0021-9738

Holohan, C., Szegezdi, E., Ritter, T., O'Brien, T. & Samali, A. (2008). Cytokine-Induced B-Cell Apoptosis Is No-Dependent, Mitochondria-Mediated and Inhibited by Bcl-Xl. *Journal of Cellular and Molecular Medicine,* Vol. 12, No.2, (Apr), pp.(591-606), 1582-1838

Hoorens, A., Stange, G., Pavlovic, D. & Pipeleers, D. (2001). Distinction between Interleukin-1-Induced Necrosis and Apoptosis of Islet Cells. *Diabetes,* Vol. 50, No.3, (Mar), pp.(551-557), 0012-1797

Hsu, H., Huang, J., Shu, H.-B., Baichwal, V. & Goeddel, D.V. (1996a). Tnf-Dependent Recruitment of the Protein Kinase Rip to the Tnf Receptor-1 Signaling Complex. *Immunity,* Vol. 4, No.4, (Apr), pp.(387-396), 1074-7613

Hsu, H., Shu, H.-B., Pan, M.-G. & Goeddel, D.V. (1996b). Tradd Traf2 and Tradd Fadd Interactions Define Two Distinct Tnf Receptor 1 Signal Transduction Pathways. *Cell,* Vol. 84, No.2, (Jan 26), pp.(299-308), 0092-8674

Hsu, H., Xiong, J. & Goeddel, D.V. (1995). The Tnf Receptor 1-Associated Protein Tradd Signals Cell Death and Nf-°B Activation. *Cell,* Vol. 81, No.4, (May 19), pp.(495-504), 0092-8674

Igarashi, K., Garotta, G., Ozmen, L., Ziemiecki, A., Wilks, A.F., Harpur, A.G., Larner, A.C. & Finbloom, D.S. (1994). Interferon-Gamma Induces Tyrosine Phosphorylation of Interferon-Gamma Receptor and Regulated Association of Protein Tyrosine

Kinases, Jak1 and Jak2, with Its Receptor. *Journal of Biological Chemistry,* Vol. 269, No.20, (May 20), pp.(14333-14336), 0021-9258

Islam, M.S., Leibiger, I., Leibiger, B., Rossi, D., Sorrentino, V., Ekstrom, T.J., Westerblad, H., Andrade, F.H. & Berggren, P.O. (1998). In Situ Activation of the Type 2 Ryanodine Receptor in Pancreatic Beta Cells Requires Camp-Dependent Phosphorylation. *Proc Natl Acad Sci U S A,* Vol. 95, No.11, (May 26), pp.(6145-6150), 0027-8424

Iwahashi, H., Hanafusa, T., Eguchi, Y., Nakajima, H., Miyagawa, J., Itoh, N., Tomita, K., Namba, M., Kuwajima, M., Noguchi, T., Tsujimoto, Y. & Matsuzawa, Y. (1996). Cytokine-Induced Apoptotic Cell Death in a Mouse Pancreatic Beta-Cell Line: Inhibition by Bcl-2. *Diabetologia,* Vol. 39, No.5, (May), pp.(530-536), 0012-186X

Jun, H.-S. & Yoon, J.-W. (2003). A New Look at Viruses in Type 1 Diabetes. *Diabetes/Metabolism Research and Reviews,* Vol. 19, No.1, (Jan), pp.(8-31), 1520-7560

Kägi, D., Ho, A., Odermatt, B., Zakarian, A., Ohashi, P.S. & Mak, T.W. (1999). Tnf Receptor 1-Dependent ß Cell Toxicity as an Effector Pathway in Autoimmune Diabetes. *The Journal of Immunology,* Vol. 162, No.8, (Apr 15), pp.(4598-4605), 0022-1767

Kägi, D., Odermatt, B., Seiler, P., Zinkernagel, R.M., Mak, T.W. & Hengartner, H. (1997). Reduced Incidence and Delayed Onset of Diabetes in Perforin-Deficient Nonobese Diabetic Mice. *The Journal of Experimental Medicine,* Vol. 186, No.7, (Oct 6), pp.(989-997), 0022-1007

Karlsen, A.E., Rønn, S.G., Lindberg, K., Johannesen, J., Galsgaard, E.D., Pociot, F., Nielsen, J.H., Mandrup-Poulsen, T., Nerup, J. & Billestrup, N. (2001). Suppressor of Cytokine Signaling 3 (Socs-3) Protects B-Cells against Interleukin-1β- and Interferon-Γ-Mediated Toxicity. *Proceedings of the National Academy of Sciences of the United States of America,* Vol. 98, No.21, (Oct 9), pp.(12191-12196), 0027-8424

Kim, H.-E., Choi, S.-E., Lee, S.-J., Lee, J.-H., Lee, Y.-J., Kang, S.S., Chun, J. & Kang, Y. (2008). Tumour Necrosis Factor-{Alpha}-Induced Glucose-Stimulated Insulin Secretion Inhibition in Ins-1 Cells Is Ascribed to a Reduction of the Glucose-Stimulated Ca2+ Influx. *J Endocrinol,* Vol. 198, No.3, (Sep 1), pp.(549-560), 1479-6805 (Electronic), 0022-0795 (Linking)

Kim, H.S., Han, M.S., Chung, K.W., Kim, S., Kim, E., Kim, M.J., Jang, E., Lee, H.A., Youn, J., Akira, S. & Lee, M.-S. (2007). Toll-Like Receptor 2 Senses [Beta]-Cell Death and Contributes to the Initiation of Autoimmune Diabetes. *Immunity,* Vol. 27, No.2, (Aug), pp.(321-333), 1074-7613

Kim, H.S., Kim, S. & Lee, M.S. (2005). Ifn-Gamma Sensitizes Min6n8 Insulinoma Cells to Tnf-Alpha-Induced Apoptosis by Inhibiting Nf-Kappab-Mediated Xiap Upregulation. *Biochem Biophys Res Commun,* Vol. 336, No.3, (Oct 28), pp.(847-853), 0006-291X

Kim, S., Kim, H.S., Chung, K.W., Oh, S.H., Yun, J.W., Im, S.-H., Lee, M.-K., Kim, K.-W. & Lee, M.-S. (2007). Essential Role for Signal Transducer and Activator of Transcription-1 in Pancreatic B-Cell Death and Autoimmune Type 1 Diabetes of Nonobese Diabetic Mice. *Diabetes,* Vol. 56, No.10, (Oct), pp.(2561-2568), 1939-327X (Electronic), 0012-1797 (Linking)

Kort, H.d., Koning, E.J.d., Rabelink, T.J., Bruijn, J.A. & Bajema, I.M. (2011). Islet Transplantation in Type 1 Diabetes. *British Medical Journal*, Vol. 342, (Jan 21), pp.(d217-d217), 1468-5833 (Electronic), 0959-535X (Linking)

Kotenko, S.V., Izotova, L.S., Pollack, B.P., Mariano, T.M., Donnelly, R.J., Muthukumaran, G., Cook, J.R., Garotta, G., Silvennoinen, O., Ihle, J.N. & Pestka, S. (1995). Interaction between the Components of the Interferon Receptor Complex. *Journal of Biological Chemistry*, Vol. 270, No.36, (Sep 8), pp.(20915-20921), 0021-9258

Kutlu, B., Cardozo, A.K., Darville, M.I., Kruhøffer, M., Magnusson, N., Ørntoft, T. & Eizirik, D.L. (2003). Discovery of Gene Networks Regulating Cytokine-Induced Dysfunction and Apoptosis in Insulin-Producing Ins-1 Cells. *Diabetes*, Vol. 52, No.11, (Nov 1), pp.(2701-2719), 0012-1797

Kwon, G., Corbett, J., Rodi, C., Sullivan, P. & McDaniel, M. (1995). Interleukin-1 Beta-Induced Nitric Oxide Synthase Expression by Rat Pancreatic Beta-Cells: Evidence for the Involvement of Nuclear Factor Kappa B in the Signaling Mechanism. *Endocrinology*, Vol. 136, No.11, (Nov 1), pp.(4790-4795), 0013-7227

Lenzen, S., Drinkgern, J. & Tiedge, M. (1996). Low Antioxidant Enzyme Gene Expression in Pancreatic Islets Compared with Various Other Mouse Tissues. *Free Radical Biology and Medicine*, Vol. 20, No.3, pp.(463-466), 0891-5849

Lieberman, S.M., Evans, A.M., Han, B., Takaki, T., Vinnitskaya, Y., Caldwell, J.A., Serreze, D.V., Shabanowitz, J., Hunt, D.F., Nathenson, S.G., Santamaria, P. & DiLorenzo, T.P. (2003). Identification of the B Cell Antigen Targeted by a Prevalent Population of Pathogenic Cd8+ T Cells in Autoimmune Diabetes. *Proceedings of the National Academy of Sciences of the United States of America*, Vol. 100, No.14, (Jul 8), pp.(8384-8388), 0027-8424

Liu, D., Pavlovic, D., Chen, M.C., Flodström, M., Sandler, S. & Eizirik, D.L. (2000). Cytokines Induce Apoptosis in Beta-Cells Isolated from Mice Lacking the Inducible Isoform of Nitric Oxide Synthase (Inos-/-). *Diabetes*, Vol. 49, No.7, (Jul), pp.(1116-1122), 0012-1797

Liu, Y., Rabinovitch, A., Suarez-Pinzon, W., Muhkerjee, B., Brownlee, M., Edelstein, D. & Federoff, H.J. (1996). Expression of the Bcl-2 Gene from a Defective Hsv-1 Amplicon Vector Protects Pancreatic B-Cells from Apoptosis. *Human Gene Therapy*, Vol. 7, No.14, (Sep 10), pp.(1719-1726), 1043-0342

Lortz, S. & Tiedge, M. (2003). Sequential Inactivation of Reactive Oxygen Species by Combined Overexpression of Sod Isoforms and Catalase in Insulin-Producing Cells. *Free Radical Biology and Medicine*, Vol. 34, No.6, (May 15), pp.(683-688), 0891-5849

Lortz, S., Tiedge, M., Nachtwey, T., Karlsen, A.E., Nerup, J. & Lenzen, S. (2000). Protection of Insulin-Producing Rinm5f Cells against Cytokine-Mediated Toxicity through Overexpression of Antioxidant Enzymes. *Diabetes*, Vol. 49, No.7, (Jul), pp.(1123-1130), 0012-1797

Mandrup-Poulsen, T. (1996). The Role of Interleukin-1 in the Pathogenesis of Iddm. *Diabetologia*, Vol. 39, No.9, (Sep), pp.(1005-1029), 0012-186X

Mandrup-Poulsen, T., Pickersgill, L. & Donath, M.Y. (2010). Blockade of Interleukin 1 in Type 1 Diabetes Mellitus. *Nat Rev Endocrinol,* Vol. 6, No.3, (Mar), pp.(158-166), 1759-5037 (Electronic), 1759-5029 (Linking)

Mathis, D. & Benoist, C. (2004). Back to Central Tolerance. *Immunity,* Vol. 20, No.5, (May), pp.(509-516), 1074-7613

McCabe, C., Samali, A. & O'Brien, T. (2006). Cytoprotection of Beta Cells: Rational Gene Transfer Strategies. *Diabetes-Metab. Res. Rev.,* Vol. 22, No.3, (May), pp.(241-252), 1520-7552

Mehmeti, I., Lenzen, S. & Lortz, S. (2011). Modulation of Bcl-2-Related Protein Expression in Pancreatic Beta Cells by Pro-Inflammatory Cytokines and Its Dependence on the Antioxidative Defense Status. *Mol Cell Endocrinol,* Vol. 332, No.1-2, (Jan 30), pp.(88-96), 1872-8057 (Electronic), 0303-7207 (Linking)

Moore, F., Naamane, N., Colli, M.L., Bouckenooghe, T., Ortis, F., Gurzov, E.N., Igoillo-Esteve, M., Mathieu, C., Bontempi, G., Thykjaer, T., Ørntoft, T.F. & Eizirik, D.L. (2011). Stat1 Is a Master Regulator of Pancreatic B-Cell Apoptosis and Islet Inflammation. *Journal of Biological Chemistry,* Vol. 286, No.2, (Jan 14), pp.(929-941), 1083-351X (Electronic), 0021-9258 (Linking)

Muzio, M., Ni, J., Feng, P. & Dixit, V.M. (1997). Irak (Pelle) Family Member Irak-2 and Myd88 as Proximal Mediators of Il-1 Signaling. *Science,* Vol. 278, No.5343, (Nov 28), pp.(1612-1615), 0036-8075

Nakayama, M., Abiru, N., Moriyama, H., Babaya, N., Liu, E., Miao, D., Yu, L., Wegmann, D.R., Hutton, J.C., Elliott, J.F. & Eisenbarth, G.S. (2005). Prime Role for an Insulin Epitope in the Development of Type[Thinsp]1 Diabetes in Nod Mice. *Nature,* Vol. 435, No.7039, (May 12), pp.(220-223), 1476-4687 (Electronic), 0028-0836 (Linking)

Nikulina, M.A., Sandhu, N., Shamim, Z., Andersen, N.A., Oberson, A., Dupraz, P., Thorens, B., Karlsen, A.E., Bonny, C. & Mandrup-Poulsen, T. (2003). The Jnk Binding Domain of Islet-Brain 1 Inhibits Il-1 Induced Jnk Activity and Apoptosis but Not the Transcription of Key Proapoptotic or Protective Genes in Insulin-Secreting Cell Lines. *Cytokine,* Vol. 24, No.1-2, (Oct), pp.(13-24), 1043-4666

Noguchi, H., Nakai, Y., Matsumoto, S., Kawaguchi, M., Ueda, M., Okitsu, T., Iwanaga, Y., Yonekawa, Y., Nagata, H., Minami, K., Masui, Y., Futaki, S. & Tanaka, K. (2005). Cell Permeable Peptide of Jnk Inhibitor Prevents Islet Apoptosis Immediately after Isolation and Improves Islet Graft Function. *American Journal of Transplantation,* Vol. 5, No.8, (Aug), pp.(1848-1855), 1600-6143

Norlin, S., Ahlgren, U. & Edlund, H. (2005). Nuclear Factor-Kb Activity in B-Cells Is Required for Glucose-Stimulated Insulin Secretion. *Diabetes,* Vol. 54, No.1, (Jan 1), pp.(125-132), 0012-1797

Ortis, F., Cardozo, A.K., Crispim, D., Storling, J., Mandrup-Poulsen, T. & Eizirik, D.L. (2006). Cytokine-Induced Proapoptotic Gene Expression in Insulin-Producing Cells Is Related to Rapid, Sustained, and Nonoscillatory Nuclear Factor-{Kappa}B Activation. *Mol Endocrinol,* Vol. 20, No.8, (Aug 1), pp.(1867-1879), 0888-8809

Ortis, F., Pirot, P., Naamane, N., Kreins, A., Rasschaert, J., Moore, F., Théâtre, E., Verhaeghe, C., Magnusson, N., Chariot, A., Ørntoft, T. & Eizirik, D. (2008). Induction of Nuclear Factor-Kb and Its Downstream Genes by Tnf-A and Il-1β Has a Pro-

Apoptotic Role in Pancreatic Beta Cells. *Diabetologia,* Vol. 51, No.7, (Jul), pp.(1213-1225), 0012-186X

Oyadomari, S., Takeda, K., Takiguchi, M., Gotoh, T., Matsumoto, M., Wada, I., Akira, S., Araki, E. & Mori, M. (2001). Nitric Oxide-Induced Apoptosis in Pancreatic B Cells Is Mediated by the Endoplasmic Reticulum Stress Pathway. *Proceedings of the National Academy of Sciences of the United States of America,* Vol. 98, No.19, (Sep 11), pp.(10845-10850), 0027-8424

Pacher, P., Beckman, J.S. & Liaudet, L. (2007). Nitric Oxide and Peroxynitrite in Health and Disease. *Physiol Rev,* Vol. 87, No.1, (Jan), pp.(315-424), 0031-9333

Pahl, H.L. (1999). Activators and Target Genes of Rel/Nf-Kappab Transcription Factors. *Oncogene,* Vol. 18, No.49, (Nov 22), pp.(6853-6866), 0950-9232

Paige, J.S., Xu, G., Stancevic, B. & Jaffrey, S.R. (2008). Nitrosothiol Reactivity Profiling Identifies S-Nitrosylated Proteins with Unexpected Stability. *Chemistry & Biology,* Vol. 15, No.12, (Dec 22), pp.(1307-1316), 1074-5521

Pavlovic, D., Andersen, N.A., Mandrup-Poulsen, T. & Eizirik, D.L. (2000). Activation of Extracellular Signal-Regulated Kinase (Erk)1/2 Contributes to Cytokine-Induced Apoptosis in Purified Rat Pancreatic Beta-Cells. *European Cytokine Network,* Vol. 11, No.2, (Jun), pp.(267-274), 1148-5493

Perez-Arana, G., Blandino-Rosano, M., Prada-Oliveira, A., Aguilar-Diosdado, M. & Segundo, C. (2010). Decrease in {Beta}-Cell Proliferation Precedes Apoptosis During Diabetes Development in Bio-Breeding/Worcester Rat: Beneficial Role of Exendin-4. *Endocrinology,* Vol. 151, No.6, (Jun 1), pp.(2538-2546), 1945-7170 (Electronic), 0013-7227 (Linking)

Peter, M.E. & Krammer, P.H. (2003). The Cd95(Apo-1/Fas) Disc and Beyond. *Cell Death Differ,* Vol. 10, No.1, (Jan), pp.(26-35), 1350-9047

Petrovsky, N., Silva, D., Socha, L., Slattery, R. & Charlton, B. (2002). The Role of Fas Ligand in Beta Cell Destruction in Autoimmune Diabetes of Nod Mice. *Annals of the New York Academy of Sciences,* Vol. 958, No.1, (Apr), pp.(204-208), 0077-8923

Pileggi, A., Molano, R.D., Berney, T., Cattan, P., Vizzardelli, C., Oliver, R., Fraker, C., Ricordi, C., Pastori, R.L., Bach, F.H. & Inverardi, L. (2001). Heme Oxygenase-1 Induction in Islet Cells Results in Protection from Apoptosis and Improved in Vivo Function after Transplantation. *Diabetes,* Vol. 50, No.9, (Sept), pp.(1983-1991), 0012-1797

Piro, S., Lupi, R., Dotta, F., Patan, G., Rabuazzo, M.A., Marselli, L., Santangelo, C., Realacci, M., Del Guerra, S., Purrello, F. & Marchetti, P. (2001). Bovine Islets Are Less Susceptible Than Human Islets to Damage by Human Cytokines1. *Transplantation,* Vol. 71, No.1, (Jan 15), 0041-1337

Pirot, P., Ortis, F., Cnop, M., Ma, Y., Hendershot, L.M., Eizirik, D.L. & Cardozo, A.K. (2007). Transcriptional Regulation of the Endoplasmic Reticulum Stress Gene Chop in Pancreatic Insulin-Producing Cells. *Diabetes,* Vol. 56, No.4, (Apr), pp.(1069-1077), 0012-1797

Rabinovitch, A., Suarez-Pinzon, W., Shi, Y., Morgan, A. & Bleackley, R. (1994). DNA Fragmentation Is an Early Event in Cytokine-Induced Islet Beta-Cell Destruction. *Diabetologia,* Vol. 37, No.8, (Aug), pp.(733-738), 0012-186X

Rabinovitch, A., Suarez-Pinzon, W., Strynadka, K., Ju, Q., Edelstein, D., Brownlee, M., Korbutt, G.S. & Rajotte, R.V. (1999). Transfection of Human Pancreatic Islets with an Anti-Apoptotic Gene (Bcl-2) Protects Beta-Cells from Cytokine-Induced Destruction. *Diabetes,* Vol. 48, No.6, (Jun), pp.(1223-1229), 0012-1797

Rabinovitch, A. & Suarez-Pinzon, W.L. (1998). Cytokines and Their Roles in Pancreatic Islet [Beta]-Cell Destruction and Insulin-Dependent Diabetes Mellitus. *Biochemical Pharmacology,* Vol. 55, No.8, (April 15, 1998), pp.(1139-1149), 0006-2952

Reddy, S.A.G., Huang, J.H. & Liao, W.S.-L. (1997). Phosphatidylinositol 3-Kinase in Interleukin 1 Signaling. *Journal of Biological Chemistry,* Vol. 272, No.46, (Nov 14), pp.(29167-29173), 0021-9258

Reddy, S.A.G., Lin, Y.-F., Huang, H.J., Samanta, A.K. & Liao, W.S.L. (2004). The Il-1 Receptor Accessory Protein Is Essential for Pi 3-Kinase Recruitment and Activation. *Biochemical and Biophysical Research Communications,* Vol. 316, No.4, (Apr 16), pp.(1022-1028), 0006-291X

Riedl, S.J. & Salvesen, G.S. (2007). The Apoptosome: Signalling Platform of Cell Death. *Nat Rev Mol Cell Biol,* Vol. 8, No.5, (May), pp.(405-413), 1471-0072

Saldeen, J. (2000). Cytokines Induce Both Necrosis and Apoptosis Via a Common Bcl-2-Inhibitable Pathway in Rat Insulin-Producing Cells. *Endocrinology,* Vol. 141, No.6, (Jun), pp.(2003-2010), 0013-7227

Samali, A., Gorman, A.M. & Cotter, T.G. (1996). Apoptosis -- the Story So Far. *Experientia,* Vol. 52, No.10-11, (Oct 31), pp.(933-941), 0014-4754

Samali, A., Zhivotovsky, B., Jones, D., Nagata, S. & Orrenius, S. (1999). Apoptosis: Cell Death Defined by Caspase Activation. *Cell Death Differ,* Vol. 6, No.6, (Jun), pp.(495-496), 1350-9047

Satoh, T., Abiru, N., Kobayashi, M., Zhou, H., Nakamura, K., Kuriya, G., Nakamura, H., Nagayama, Y., Kawasaki, E., Yamasaki, H., Yu, L., Eisenbarth, G., Araki, E., Mori, M., Oyadomari, S. & Eguchi, K. (2011). Chop Deletion Does Not Impact the Development of Diabetes but Suppresses the Early Production of Insulin Autoantibody in the Nod Mouse. *Apoptosis,* Vol. (Apr), pp.(1-11), 1573-675X (Electronic), 1360-8185 (Linking)

Seewaldt, S., Thomas, H.E., Ejrnaes, M., Christen, U., Wolfe, T., Rodrigo, E., Coon, B., Michelsen, B., Kay, T.W. & von Herrath, M.G. (2000). Virus-Induced Autoimmune Diabetes: Most Beta-Cells Die through Inflammatory Cytokines and Not Perforin from Autoreactive (Anti-Viral) Cytotoxic T-Lymphocytes. *Diabetes,* Vol. 49, No.11, (Nov 1), pp.(1801-1809), 0012-1797

Sies, H. (1997). Oxidative Stress: Oxidants and Antioxidants. *Experimental Physiology,* Vol. 82, No.2, (Mar 1), pp.(291-295), 0958-0670

Stassi, G., De Maria, R., Trucco, G., Rudert, W., Testi, R., Galluzzo, A., Giordano, C. & Trucco, M. (1997). Nitric Oxide Primes Pancreatic Beta Cells for Fas-Mediated Destruction in Insulin-Dependent Diabetes Mellitus. *J Exp Med,* Vol. 186, No.8, (Oct 20), pp.(1193-1200), 0022-1007

Steer, S.A., Scarim, A.L., Chambers, K.T. & Corbett, J.A. (2006). Interleukin-1 Stimulates Beta-Cell Necrosis and Release of the Immunological Adjuvant Hmgb1. *PLoS Med,* Vol. 3, No.2, (Feb), pp.(e17), 1549-1676 (Electronic), 1549-1277 (Linking)

Stephanou, A., Brar, B.K., Knight, R.A. & Latchman, D.S. (2000). Opposing Actions of Stat-1 and Stat-3 on the Bcl-2 and Bcl-X Promoters. *Cell Death Differ*, Vol. 7, No.3, (Mar), pp.(329-330), 1350-9047

Stephanou, A., Brar, B.K., Scarabelli, T.M., Jonassen, A.K., Yellon, D.M., Marber, M.S., Knight, R.A. & Latchman, D.S. (2000). Ischemia-Induced Stat-1 Expression and Activation Play a Critical Role in Cardiomyocyte Apoptosis. *Journal of Biological Chemistry*, Vol. 275, No.14, (Apr 7), pp.(10002-10008), 0021-9258

Storling, J., Binzer, J., Andersson, A.K., Zullig, R.A., Tonnesen, M., Lehmann, R., Spinas, G.A., Sandler, S., Billestrup, N. & Mandrup-Poulsen, T. (2005). Nitric Oxide Contributes to Cytokine-Induced Apoptosis in Pancreatic Beta Cells Via Potentiation of Jnk Activity and Inhibition of Akt. *Diabetologia*, Vol. 48, No.10, (Oct), pp.(2039-2050), 0012-186X

Suk, K., Kim, S., Kim, Y.-H., Kim, K.-A., Chang, I., Yagita, H., Shong, M. & Lee, M.-S. (2001). Ifn-Γ/Tnf-A Synergism as the Final Effector in Autoimmune Diabetes: A Key Role for Stat1/Ifn Regulatory Factor-1 Pathway in Pancreatic B Cell Death. *The Journal of Immunology*, Vol. 166, No.7, (Apr 1), pp.(4481-4489), 0022-1767

Szegezdi, E., Logue, S.E., Gorman, A.M. & Samali, A. (2006). Mediators of Endoplasmic Reticulum Stress-Induced Apoptosis. *EMBO Rep*, Vol. 7, No.9, (Sep), pp.(880-885), 1469-221X (Print), 1469-221X (Linking)

Takeda, K. & Akira, S. (2000). Stat Family of Transcription Factors in Cytokine-Mediated Biological Responses. *Cytokine & Growth Factor Reviews*, Vol. 11, No.3, (Sep 2000), pp.(199-207), 1359-6101

Thiel, D.J., le Du, M.H., Walter, R.L., D'Arcy, A., Chène, C., Fountoulakis, M., Garotta, G., Winkler, F.K. & Ealick, S.E. (2000). Observation of an Unexpected Third Receptor Molecule in the Crystal Structure of Human Interferon-[Gamma] Receptor Complex. *Structure*, Vol. 8, No.9, (Sep 15), pp.(927-936), 0969-2126

Thomas, H.E., Darwiche, R., Corbett, J.A. & Kay, T.W. (2002). Interleukin-1 Plus Gamma-Interferon-Induced Pancreatic Beta-Cell Dysfunction Is Mediated by Beta-Cell Nitric Oxide Production. *Diabetes*, Vol. 51, No.2, (Feb), pp.(311-316), 0012-1797

Tiedge, M., Lortz, S., Munday, R. & Lenzen, S. (1998). Complementary Action of Antioxidant Enzymes in the Protection of Bioengineered Insulin-Producing Rinm5f Cells against the Toxicity of Reactive Oxygen Species. *Diabetes*, Vol. 47, No.10, (Oct), pp.(1578-1585), 0012-1797

Turley, S., Poirot, L., Hattori, M., Benoist, C. & Mathis, D. (2003). Physiological Beta Cell Death Triggers Priming of Self-Reactive T Cells by Dendritic Cells in a Type-1 Diabetes Model. *J Exp Med*, Vol. 198, No.10, (Nov 17), pp.(1527-1537), 0022-1007

Vandenabeele, P., Galluzzi, L., Vanden Berghe, T. & Kroemer, G. (2010). Molecular Mechanisms of Necroptosis: An Ordered Cellular Explosion. *Nat Rev Mol Cell Biol*, Vol. 11, No.10, (Oct), pp.(700-714), 1471-0080 (Electronic), 1471-0072 (Linking)

Varadi, A., Molnar, E., Ostenson, C.G. & Ashcroft, S.J. (1996). Isoforms of Endoplasmic Reticulum Ca(2+)-Atpase Are Differentially Expressed in Normal and Diabetic Islets of Langerhans. *Biochem J*, Vol. 319 (Pt 2), (Oct 15), pp.(521-527), 0264-6021

Viner, R.I., Ferrington, D.A., Williams, T.D., Bigelow, D.J. & Schoneich, C. (1999). Protein Modification During Biological Aging: Selective Tyrosine Nitration of the Serca2a

Isoform of the Sarcoplasmic Reticulum Ca2+-Atpase in Skeletal Muscle. *Biochem J,* Vol. 340 (Pt 3), (Jun 15), pp.(657-669), 0264-6021

Wang, B., Andre, I., Gonzalez, A., Katz, J.D., Aguet, M., Benoist, C. & Mathis, D. (1997). Interferon-Gamma Impacts at Multiple Points During the Progression of Autoimmune Diabetes. *Proc Natl Acad Sci U S A,* Vol. 94, No.25, (Dec 9), pp.(13844-13849), 0027-8424

Wang, L., Bhattacharjee, A., Zuo, Z., Hu, F., Honkanen, R.E., Berggren, P.O. & Li, M. (1999). A Low Voltage-Activated Ca2+ Current Mediates Cytokine-Induced Pancreatic Beta-Cell Death. *Endocrinology,* Vol. 140, No.3, (Mar), pp.(1200-1204), 0013-7227

Wang, P., Qiu, W., Dudgeon, C., Liu, H., Huang, C., Zambetti, G.P., Yu, J. & Zhang, L. (2009). Puma Is Directly Activated by Nf-Kappab and Contributes to Tnf-Alpha-Induced Apoptosis. *Cell Death Differ,* Vol. 16, No.9, (Sep), pp.(1192-1202), 1476-5403 (Electronic), 1350-9047 (Linking)

Welsh, N., Eizirik, D.L. & Sandler, S. (1994). Nitric Oxide and Pancreatic Beta-Cell Destruction in Insulin Dependent Diabetes Mellitus: Don't Take No for an Answer. *Autoimmunity,* Vol. 18, No.4, pp.(285-290), 0891-6934

Wesche, H., Henzel, W.J., Shillinglaw, W., Li, S. & Cao, Z. (1997). Myd88: An Adapter That Recruits Irak to the Il-1 Receptor Complex. *Immunity,* Vol. 7, No.6, (Dec), pp.(837-847), 1074-7613

White, N.H., Sun, W., Cleary, P.A., Danis, R.P., Davis, M.D., Hainsworth, D.P., Hubbard, L.D., Lachin, J.M. & Nathan, D.M. (2008). Prolonged Effect of Intensive Therapy on the Risk of Retinopathy Complications in Patients with Type 1 Diabetes Mellitus: 10 Years after the Diabetes Control and Complications Trial. *Archives of Ophthalmology,* Vol. 126, No.12, (Dec), pp.(1707-1715), 1538-3601 (Electronic), 0003-9950 (Linking)

Xu, L., Eu, J.P., Meissner, G. & Stamler, J.S. (1998). Activation of the Cardiac Calcium Release Channel (Ryanodine Receptor) by Poly-S-Nitrosylation. *Science,* Vol. 279, No.5348, (Jan 9), pp.(234-237), 0036-8075

Yamin, T.-T. & Miller, D.K. (1997). The Interleukin-1 Receptor-Associated Kinase Is Degraded by Proteasomes Following Its Phosphorylation. *Journal of Biological Chemistry,* Vol. 272, No.34, (Aug 22), pp.(21540-21547), 0021-9258

Yasukawa, H., Sasaki, A. & Yoshimura, A. (2000). Negative Regulation of Cytokine Signaling Pathways. *Annu. Rev. Immunol.,* Vol. 18, No.1, (Apr), pp.(143-164), 0732-0582

Ye, J. & Laychock, S.G. (1998). A Protective Role for Heme Oxygenase Expression in Pancreatic Islets Exposed to Interleukin-1{Beta}. *Endocrinology,* Vol. 139, No.10, (Oct), pp.(4155-4163), 0013-7227

Youle, R.J. & Strasser, A. (2008). The Bcl-2 Protein Family: Opposing Activities That Mediate Cell Death. *Nat Rev Mol Cell Biol,* Vol. 9, No.1, (Jan), pp.(47-59), 1471-0080 (Electronic), 1471-0072 (Linking)

Zhang, L., Xing, D. & Chen, M. (2008). Bim(L) Displacing Bcl-X(L) Promotes Bax Translocation During Tnfalpha-Induced Apoptosis. *Apoptosis,* Vol. 13, No.7, (Jul), pp.(950-958), 1573-675X (Electronic), 1360-8185 (Linking)

Zhang, P., McGrath, B., Li, S., Frank, A., Zambito, F., Reinert, J., Gannon, M., Ma, K., McNaughton, K. & Cavener, D.R. (2002). The Perk Eukaryotic Initiation Factor 2

Alpha Kinase Is Required for the Development of the Skeletal System, Postnatal Growth, and the Function and Viability of the Pancreas. *Mol Cell Biol*, Vol. 22, No.11, (Jun), pp.(3864-3874), 0270-7306

Zhang, W., Feng, D., Li, Y., Iida, K., McGrath, B. & Cavener, D.R. (2006). Perk Eif2ak3 Control of Pancreatic Beta Cell Differentiation and Proliferation Is Required for Postnatal Glucose Homeostasis. *Cell Metab*, Vol. 4, No.6, (Dec), pp.(491-497), 1550-4131

Zinszner, H., Kuroda, M., Wang, X., Batchvarova, N., Lightfoot, R.T., Remotti, H., Stevens, J.L. & Ron, D. (1998). Chop Is Implicated in Programmed Cell Death in Response to Impaired Function of the Endoplasmic Reticulum. *Genes Dev*, Vol. 12, No.7, (Apr 1), pp.(982-995), 0890-9369

Permissions

The contributors of this book come from diverse backgrounds, making this book a truly international effort. This book will bring forth new frontiers with its revolutionizing research information and detailed analysis of the nascent developments around the world.

We would like to thank Dr. Chih-Pin Liu, for lending his expertise to make the book truly unique. He has played a crucial role in the development of this book. Without his invaluable contribution this book wouldn't have been possible. He has made vital efforts to compile up to date information on the varied aspects of this subject to make this book a valuable addition to the collection of many professionals and students.

This book was conceptualized with the vision of imparting up-to-date information and advanced data in this field. To ensure the same, a matchless editorial board was set up. Every individual on the board went through rigorous rounds of assessment to prove their worth. After which they invested a large part of their time researching and compiling the most relevant data for our readers. Conferences and sessions were held from time to time between the editorial board and the contributing authors to present the data in the most comprehensible form. The editorial team has worked tirelessly to provide valuable and valid information to help people across the globe.

Every chapter published in this book has been scrutinized by our experts. Their significance has been extensively debated. The topics covered herein carry significant findings which will fuel the growth of the discipline. They may even be implemented as practical applications or may be referred to as a beginning point for another development. Chapters in this book were first published by InTech; hereby published with permission under the Creative Commons Attribution License or equivalent.

The editorial board has been involved in producing this book since its inception. They have spent rigorous hours researching and exploring the diverse topics which have resulted in the successful publishing of this book. They have passed on their knowledge of decades through this book. To expedite this challenging task, the publisher supported the team at every step. A small team of assistant editors was also appointed to further simplify the editing procedure and attain best results for the readers.

Our editorial team has been hand-picked from every corner of the world. Their multi-ethnicity adds dynamic inputs to the discussions which result in innovative outcomes. These outcomes are then further discussed with the researchers and contributors who give their valuable feedback and opinion regarding the same. The feedback is then collaborated with the researches and they are edited in a comprehensive manner to aid the understanding of the subject.

Apart from the editorial board, the designing team has also invested a significant amount of their time in understanding the subject and creating the most relevant covers. They scrutinized every image to scout for the most suitable representation of the subject and create an appropriate cover for the book.

The publishing team has been involved in this book since its early stages. They were actively engaged in every process, be it collecting the data, connecting with the contributors or procuring relevant information. The team has been an ardent support to the editorial, designing and production team. Their endless efforts to recruit the best for this project, has resulted in the accomplishment of this book. They are a veteran in the field of academics and their pool of knowledge is as vast as their experience in printing. Their expertise and guidance has proved useful at every step. Their uncompromising quality standards have made this book an exceptional effort. Their encouragement from time to time has been an inspiration for everyone.

The publisher and the editorial board hope that this book will prove to be a valuable piece of knowledge for researchers, students, practitioners and scholars across the globe.

List of Contributors

Vladimir Jakus and Dagmar Michalkova
Institute of Medical Chemistry, Biochemistry and Clinical Biochemistry, Faculty of Medicine, Comenius University, Bratislava, Slovakia

Jana Kostolanska
Children Diabetological Center of the Slovak Republic, 1st Department of Pediatrics, Comenius University and University Hospital for Children, Bratislava, Slovakia

Michal Sapak
Institute of Medical Immunology, Faculty of Medicine, Comenius University, Bratislava, Slovakia

Bruno Vergès
Service Endocrinologie, Diabétologie et Maladies Métaboliques, Dijon University Hospital, France

S. S. Soedamah-Muthu and S. Abbring
Division of Human Nutrition, Wageningen University, Wageningen, Netherlands

M. Toeller
Department of Endocrinology, Diabetology and Rheumatology, Heinrich-Heine-University Duesseldorf, Germany

Mykola Khalangot, Volodymir Kovtun, Nadia Okhrimenko, Viktor Kravchenko and Mykola Tronko
Komisarenko Institute of Endocrinology and Metabolism Academy of Medical Sciences, Kiev, Ukraine

Vitaliy Gurianov
National Medical University, Donetsk, Ukraine

Laura Nabors
School of Human Services, College of Education, Criminal Justice, and Human Services, University of Cincinnati, USA

Phillip Neal Ritchey
Department of Sociology, College of Arts and Sciences, University of Cincinnati, USA

Bevin Van Wassenhove and Jennifer Bartz
Department of Psychology, College of Arts and Sciences, University of Cincinnati, Cincinnati, Ohio, USA

M. Graça Pereira and Liliana Rocha
University of Minho, School of Psychology, Portugal

A. Cristina Almeida and Engrácia Leandro
University of Minho, Social Sciences Institute, Portugal

Ricardo V. García-Mayor and Alejandra Larrañaga
Eating Disorders Section, Endocrinology, Diabetes, Nutrition and Metabolism Department, University Hospital of Vigo, Spain

Joseph P. H. McNamara, Sarah E. Righi and Gary R. Geffken
University of Florida, Department of Psychiatry, USA

Adam M. Reid
University of Florida, Department of Clinical and Health Psychology, USA

Alana R. Freedland
University of Florida, Department of Counselor Education, USA

Fernando Valente and Sérgio Atala Dib
São Paulo Federal University, São Paulo, Brazil

Marília Brito Gomes
State University of Rio de Janeiro, Rio de Janeiro, Brazil

Stephanie N. Lewis, Elaine O. Nsoesie, Charles Weeks, Dan Qiao and Liqing Zhang
Virginia Tech, Blacksburg, VA, USA

Toshiro Arai, Nobuko Mori and Haruo Hashimoto
Nippon Veterinary and Life Science University, Japan

Lisa Vincenz, Eva Szegezdi, Richard Jäger, Caitriona Holohan and Afshin Samali
Apoptosis Research Centre, Ireland

Timothy O'Brien
Regenerative Medicine Institute, National University of Ireland Galway, Ireland

Printed in the USA
CPSIA information can be obtained
at www.ICGtesting.com
JSHW011433221024
72173JS00004B/782